Plundered Kitchens, Empty Wombs

PLUNDERED KITCHENS, EMPTY WOMBS

Threatened Reproduction and Identity in the Cameroon Grassfields

Δ Δ Δ

Pamela Feldman-Savelsberg

Ann Arbor

THE UNIVERSITY OF MICHIGAN PRESS

A CIP catalog record for this book is available from the British Library.

Library of Congress Cataloging-in-Publication Data

Feldman-Savelsberg, Pamela, 1958–
    Plundered kitchens, empty wombs : threatened reproduction and
identity in the Cameroon grassfields / Pamela Feldman-Savelsberg.
        p.   cm.
    Includes bibliographical references and index.
    ISBN 0-472-10989-8 (cloth : alk. paper)
    1. Women, Ngangte—Ethnic identity.   2. Women,
Ngangte—Psychology.   3. Women, Ngangte—Health and hygiene.
4. Fertility, Human—Cameroon—Maham.   5. Human
reproduction—Cameroon—Maham.   6. Maham (Cameroon)—Population.
7. Maham (Cameroon)—Social life and customs.   I. Title.
DT571.N43   F45   1999
304.6'32'096711—dc21   98-51223
                                                                    CIP

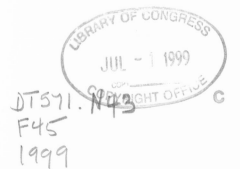

for Joachim, Anna, and Rebecca
and in memory of baby Clara

Contents

List of Illustrations   ix

Preface   xi

Acknowledgments   xvii

Pronunciation Guide   xix

Cast of Characters   xxi

Introduction: Fertility and the Politics of Identity
   in Cameroon   1

Chapter 1. The Short-lived Marriage of a King's Wife:
   Paulette's "Plugged Fertility" and Blocked Mobility   15

Chapter 2. Being Bangangté: Social Organization
   and Identity   41

Chapter 3. Cooking Inside: The Symbolic
   Construction of Gender, Marriage, and Fertility   71

Chapter 4. The Kitchen Plundered: Fear of Infertility   99

Chapter 5. Seeking Remedies: Medical Pluralism
   and the Distribution of Fear   135

Chapter 6. "Then We Were Many": The Search for
   Vitality in a Changing Context   175

Appendix: Kings of Bangangté   201

Notes   203

Glossary   219

References   225

Index   249

Illustrations

1. Elderly cowives of Paulette visiting in the first queen's quarter of the royal compound of Bangangté   16

2. Marguerite addressing her neighborhood *tontine* (rotating credit association) in Batela', near the royal compound of Bangangté   40

3. Map of Cameroon   44

4. Map of Bamiléké kingdoms   44

5. Descent and ancestor worship, patrilineal   52

6. Descent and ancestor worship, matrilineal   53

7. Ta nkap marriage system   55

8. Pam nto' (uterine solidarity) relations   56

9. Map of the royal compound of Bangangté   64

10. Jeanne preparing manioc in front of her earthen brick kitchen, royal compound, Bangangté   72

11. In a rite of reconciliation to cure infertility, disputing kin wash themselves in raffia wine surveilled by the bandansi (ritual specialists of the palace)   100

12. Bangangté typology of causes of misfortune   104

13. Mfen Meshinke', elderly healer and subchief of Bantoum village, cutting herbs for medicines   136

14. Che'elou, ca. 85 years old, watching the burial of one of her cowives at the royal compound of Bangangté, October 1986   176

Table 1. Inventory of health care specialists and institutions   152

Preface

This book about women's fear of infertility in an area renowned for its fecundity was inspired by the overwhelming concerns of the people I worked with during fifteen months of anthropological fieldwork in 1983, 1986, and 1997 in Bangangté, a Bamiléké kingdom of about 60,000 residents in the highland Grassfields of Cameroon. Despite a high birthrate in the area (the average woman bore more than six children during her reproductive years), Bangangté women were preoccupied with threats to their reproductive health. The threats that worried them so included biological infertility as well as social and supernatural impediments to good marriage, bringing a pregnancy to term, and socializing offspring to further reproduce a Bangangté life-style. Individuals were worried about the conception, birth, and survival of their own children and were anxious about the decreasing population and number of births in the royal family. What is more, women used these complaints in their everyday negotiations with kin and with neighbors about what it means to be a woman, what it means to be Bangangté, and how Bangangté people can survive and get ahead in the economic and political upheavals that have rocked Africa over the past fifteen years.

Birth and fertility are not solely "natural" or "biological" events, but are also social processes with culturally and historically specific meanings. The rural African women at the center of my research revealed for me a core of shared images of procreation and social reproduction, centered on cooking. They also demonstrated to me that not all Bangangté worry about reproduction in the same way or to the same extent. Their concerns are shaped by the multiple and changing hierarchies within Bangangté society, including both the formal rankings centered around palace life and the educational and economic mobility within the modern Cameroonian state. These dimensions of social differentiation affect the beliefs about health and society, the potential consequences of infertility, and the experience of physical and social vulnerability. The complex meanings of infertility for the lives of Bangangté women can only be understood through a combination of symbolic, historic, and political-economic analysis. Realizing these interconnections for the case at hand has convinced me that medical anthropology needs to be firmly grounded in a holistic, multidimensional sociocultural anthropology.

My interest in rural Bangangté beliefs regarding health, illness, and reproduction was stimulated both by key ideas from anthropological literature and by previous research experience. Studies of gender awakened my curiosity in the varying relevance of gender categories for organizing social life in diverse cultures and in how women's experience of recent social change differs from men's. Medical anthropological literature on therapeutic management, combined with my Peace Corps experience in 1980–81 as a female health worker in southern Cameroon, led me to inquire how change in women's status has affected their perception and experiences of illness and health care. Data collected in 1983 during preliminary fieldwork centered in Maham, an outlying village of Bangangté chiefdom, indicated that different groups of Bangangté villagers disagreed about the causes of medical misfortunes and appropriate strategies to deal with these afflictions. These beliefs appeared to have changed through time, in association with specific social, political, and economic contexts. In accounts of recent Bangangté witchcraft afflictions, women were most often cited as both causes and victims of witchcraft. The disturbance of human reproduction was a prominent theme both in these witchcraft stories and in everyday conversation. Archival research in 1984, 1985, and 1987 indicated that depressed fertility was represented as a problem throughout the past century by diverse groups of Europeans and Africans competing for Grassfields labor and allegiance.

Representations of reproductive illness thus emerged as a theme of central interest to present-day Bangangté women as well as to diverse actors with divergent interests over time. My research reflects this intense involvement in both present and past. For the entire twelve months of my 1986 fieldwork I lived in the royal compound of Bangangté, using this as a base for participant observation at the palace, in the surrounding quarter and two additional villages, in Bangangté town and at numerous health-care institutions, indigenous and biomedical, in Ndé Division. Almost as soon as I had asked *mfen* (paramount chief or king of Bangangté) Njiké Pokam for permission to live near the royal compound, he and his wives assigned me the fictive kinship status of younger sister to one of the mfen's many wives, in this case his white wife, the daughter of French missionaries born and raised in Cameroon. I was invited to reside within the two wives' quarters of the palace grounds as the mfen's visiting sister-in-law.

For the first four months I shared the two-room mud kitchen-house of Louise, the second queen. For the next eight months I lived in my own 4 × 4 meter hut in, the first queen's quarter. Since I did not have my own kitchen, I ate with my "sister" and her cowife Jeanne in their shared kitchen, informal meeting place of the entire palace population. As my friendship with the elderly Che'elou developed until she became recognized as my "grandmother," I occasionally ate with her. Living in the two women's quarters and eating at the royal wives' hearths was a unique chance to observe firsthand health beliefs and practices in everyday life, and patterns of alliance and accusation among cowives in disputes regarding fertility. I also chose the royal compound as the main research site because there the interweaving of religious and secular activities and of traditional king-centered and modern nation-state authority were most apparent.

Bangangté reactions to me and my presence, while always generous and tolerant, were as varied as the individuals involved and changed through time as we got to know different things about one another and to present ourselves accordingly. The royal wives at first described formal hierarchy in the royal compound as if it were the most important aspect of their daily interactions with their cowives. Only later were patterns of rivalry and alliance revealed, often crosscutting these formal hierarchies. Both royal wives and village women gave me schoolbook descriptions of conception, pregnancy, and childbirth for months before I discovered the extent of the belief and fear that other women, especially cowives, could steal one's fetus. As time passed, informants' trust and willingness to confide in me increased. More importantly, the sorts of things they told me changed as their perceptions of my role and personality, and thus the kind of impression they wanted to make on me, developed. For example, after my husband's first visit to Bangangté, some avenues of communication were closed, and more were opened. As the royal wives' impressions of me changed from "runaway childless wife" to "good wife waiting for her husband," they confided more to me about childbirth, sexuality in marital relations, and their cowives' alleged extramarital consorts, and less to me about their own consorts.

The effect of differences in informants' perceptions of my role as fieldworker upon the data gathered became very clear when I began doing structured interviews with women in two different field sites. I conducted 42 interviews lasting between 40 and 75 minutes with 16 women living in two hamlets near the royal compound and with 26 women in the distant village of Bantoum. I had lived among the women of Ntanleme and Batela' (two communities near the palace) for 10 months, engaging them in conversation but not conducting formal interviews or ostentatiously taking notes. They largely resisted my attempts to interview them, to change the relation from one of neighbors to one of interrogator/interrogated, over which they had less control. Both informants and myself as fieldworker experienced a conflict about my two roles of participant and observer. In Bantoum, by contrast, I had accompanied a female community development agent to the village several times over a period of eight months before I came to stay for two weeks to interview women. These women always perceived me as "stranger" and "worker" conducting a community study to help women. They were eager to be interviewed and to present their particular views of village and family relations.

My research with Bangangté women continued throughout the 12 months of fieldwork. I used French and Bangangté languages, the latter often with a younger neighbor of the interviewee as interpreter although I also managed by myself. I conducted research on health-care practitioners in segments, parallel to my work with Bangangté women.

My observations and interviews in biomedical institutions were concentrated in the first third of the fieldwork stay. As with village women, my relation to biomedical staff of all levels in the two hospitals and four clinics studied changed through time. For example, doctors who at first called popular healers "worthless" on later encounters told me about referring patients to indigenous practitioners. As their impressions of me changed from someone wanting to "weed out charlatanism" to a relative "sympathizer with traditional medicine," they gave me more differentiated information on their relations with popular healers. I returned to these biomedical institutions toward the end of the fieldwork to collect 53 written questionnaires from personnel in each division and of each status from each institution. The 20-item questionnaires asked informants to identify and rank major local health problems, discuss their familiarity with fertility and sterility cases, and discuss their attitudes toward indigenous medicine.

During the second third of my fieldwork I concentrated on the study of indigenous healing, interviewing seven indigenous practitioners (five herbal and spiritual healers, one spirit medium, and one diviner) and observing their treatments and interaction with clients. I also studied one healers' association and interviewed civil servants on their attitudes toward popular healing.

Toward the end of my fieldwork I aimed to collect the direct words of the next generation of Bangangté parents. Two hundred thirty schoolchildren, from primary school through the last year of high school, wrote essays on any one of the following four topics: family planning and the importance of children; monogamy and polygyny; therapeutic choice for women suffering from sterility; and advantages and disadvantages of indigenous medicine and biomedicine. The schoolchildren received their essay assignments through the cooperation of their regular teachers, some of whom I knew personally and some of whom were introduced to me by my "sister" from the royal compound, a lycée teacher herself.

The data presented in this book are as unchanged from their original sources as possible. In my translations of French and Bangangté quotations I have tried to be true to original nuance. To protect individuals' anonymity, I have changed the names of all informants except kings, who are public figures, and the king's French wife, who has become a celebrity after being the subject of a television documentary. I have used French first-name pseudonyms for all informants who are habitually addressed with their given French names. For the mostly older informants who are commonly addressed with their *ndap* (praise names indicating a parent's village of origin), I have retained the original ndap.

I returned to Bangangté in 1997, visiting with the widows, orphans, and successor to mfen Njiké Pokam. The issues revealed during my 1986 fieldwork were apparent in even sharper contour in 1997. A decade of economic crisis left women, and men, feeling physically and socially vulnerable. Exchange networks among kin between urban and rural areas were even more important, but there was less wealth to distribute, and patterns of flow were often disrupted. Being Bangangté was a resource for survival in economically troubled times, but could also be a liability in the national political arena. The meanings of ethnicity, gender, and fertility remained prominent topics of local debate.

A final note on language and terminology: Bangangté people call their language *Medumba.* For simplicity, I refer to Medumba in the text as *Bangangté* or *Bangangté language.* I have simplified the spelling of Bangangté words in the text, but in the glossary I have included the orthography currently used by CEPOM, a local Bangangté organization that gives summer sessions in reading and writing Medumba to Bangangté children and adults.

I have struggled with the most appropriate terminology for types of health care in a pluralistic setting. The health planning literature describes two types of health care with the words *traditional* and *modern.* When using these terms, I refer to the statements and attitudes of health planners. When discussing popular forms of healing indigenous to Bangangté and the Grassfields, I follow the most common Bangangté practice by referring to "indigenous" healing. In so doing, I hope not to offend some Cameroonian intellectuals who associate this word with the French term *indigène* and its connotations of colonial oppression. When referring to the kind of healing practiced in hospitals and clinics, I prefer the term *biomedical* to Bangangté common usage of *modern.* With this eclectic approach I hope to avoid the implication that, in contrast to biomedicine, indigenous healing in contemporary Bangangté is "unmodern" or anachronistic.

Acknowledgments

Of the many persons and institutions to whom I am indebted, I can formally thank only some by name.

I thank the following institutions that provided funds for field and archival research: the Sigma Xi Foundation for Scientific Research and the Department of Anthropology, Johns Hopkins University, for preliminary fieldwork in 1983, the National Science Foundation (Graduate Fellowship) for archival research in summer 1984, the U.S. Department of Education Fulbright Dissertation Research Program in 1986 fieldwork in Cameroon, and the Wenner Gren Foundation for Anthropological Research for archival work in 1985 and 1987. I am grateful for several Faculty Development Endowment grants and for funds from the Dean's Discretionary Account of Carleton College to facilitate writing, preparation of the final manuscript, and my 1997 return to the field.

In Cameroon, I thank the Ministry of Higher Education and Scientific Research (MESRES) and the local authorities of Bangangté for institutional support and research permission. In this context I am especially grateful to Dr. Jean Nya Ngatchou, Dr. Paul N. Nkwi, Jean-Calvin Boog of Bangangté, the late mfen Njiké Pokam François, and the current mfen Nji Monluh Seidou Pokam. For collaboration and encouragement in professional aspects of the work, I thank Prof. Jean Mfoulou, Prof. Augustin Akoudou, Dr. Alain Froment, Mme Marie-Guy Froment, Dr. Flavien Tiokou Ndonko, and Annette and Dr. Wim Thijs. Many other Cameroonians and expatriates, including the staff of USIS-Yaoundé, helped at various stages of the work. I am grateful to the director and staff of the Institut de Formation et de Recherche Demographique and of OCISCA for their generous aid and discussions during my 1997 trip, as well as to the Ndonko family for sustaining food and intellectual exchange.

None of this work could have been accomplished without the patient and generous hospitality of the people of Bangangté. My heartfelt gratitude goes to Mlle Adrienne Keyete (Bangangté), Mme Emilienne Tondji (Bantoum), Dr. Jean-Claude Kwechi and his wife (Bantoum), and especially the wives of the late mfen Njiké Pokam. My adopted grandmother

Che'elou, mothers Nda'gou and Nyombab, and sister Nteshun among them deserve special recognition.

In Europe, the personnel of numerous archives allowed me access to crucial records on the history of Bangangté society and its health-care institutions. I especially value the help of Hartmut Müller and Herr Junker of the Staatsarchiv Bremen; Herr Steinberg of the Handelskammer, Bremen; Mme Jourdan of the Archives Techniques du Service de Santé de la France Outre-Mer, Marseille; J. F. Maurel of the Archives Nationales; Marie-Christine Held of the Département évangélique français d'action apostolique (DEFAP), Paris; and Claude Tardits for the gift of his personal archives on Bangangté.

Writing the thesis on which this book is based was improved by exchanges with numerous colleagues. I am particularly grateful to committee members Gillian Feeley-Harnik, David Cohen, and Emily Martin for valuable comments on the thesis as a whole. Eugenia Shanklin and Doris Blank gave valuable comments on specific chapters. The invaluable intellectual and personal encouragement of Gillian Feeley-Harnik throughout fieldwork and write-up deserves my deepest thanks.

Chapter 3 is revised from an article originally published in *American Ethnologist* 22, no. 3 (1995): 483–501, and is reprinted by permission of the American Anthropological Association. Chapter 4 is revised from an article originally published in *Social Science and Medicine* 39, no. 4 (1994): 463–74, and is reprinted by permission of Elsevier Science. Other portions of the book have been presented at various colloquiums and conferences. In each case, and in the process of transforming a thesis into a book, I benefited from participants' or anonymous reviewers' comments, as well as from the valuable suggestions of Don Brenneis, Michael Herzfeld, Alma Gottlieb, Marcia Inhorn, Ivan Karp, Corrinne Kratz, Jessica Kuper, Joachim Savelsberg, and my knowledgeable and incredibly good-humored editor at the University of Michigan Press, Susan Whitlock.

My American and German families continued their undaunting encouragement throughout this endeavor, and some made special contributions to the illustrations. Joachim Savelsberg took many of the photos and did measurements for the map of the royal compound. Heinrich Savelsberg prepared this detailed map. Susanne Savelsberg drew the remaining maps and diagrams.

As Tangun and member of the society of nobles of Bangangté, my husband Joachim Savelsberg secured my position as royal sister-in-law Nteshun at the palace in Bangangté generally. With his patience, wit, and insight, he enlivened my life and work on three continents. Our daughters Anna and Rebecca jumped for joy when I finished the last chapter. To all three, I am eternally grateful.

Pronunciation Guide

The Bangangté language (Medumba) is a tonal language; rising and falling tones make a difference in the meaning of words. Accent marks on Bangangté words indicate tones.

The glottal stop (what English speakers would have to do to pronounce "a ark"), a common consonant in Bangangté, is indicated with an apostrophe. Nasals (e.g., "ng" or "mb") are part of the consonant blends, not separate syllables.

ng	as in *ngaka*	is pronounced as in looki*ng*
nt	as in *Nteshun*	is pronounced as in a*nd*
mf	as in *mfi*	is usually pronounced *mf,* but is pronounced *mv* in *mfen* (sounds like *mvuhn*)

The Bangangté language has many vowels that do not appear in spoken English. These are written with phonetic characters, according to the CEPOM orthography, in the glossary, and with simplified Latin letters in the body of the text.

ɑ	written *a* in the text	is pronounced between "ah" and "aw" similar to "*aw*l"
ə	written *e* in the text	is pronounced "uh" as in "th*e*"
ɛ	written *e* in the text	is pronounced "eh" as in "h*ea*d"
ɔ	written *o* in the text	is an "open o" similar to "N*oah*" (but one syllable)
ʉ	written *u* in the text	is similar to "u" in the French "t*u*"

In addition to these vowels, the consonant *c* in the CEPOM orthography is pronounced "ch" as in "*ch*erry."

Cast of Characters

The following people appear frequently in the story of this book. A complete list of kings of the Bangangté dynasty appears as an appendix.

The Kings
    Mfen François Njiké Pokam (reigned 1974–87)
    Mfen Nji Monluh Seidou Pokam (reigned 1987–present)
Wives of Mfen Njiké Pokam
    In the first queen's quarter
        Josette (the *mabengoup,* or first queen)
        Paulette (an unfortunate newlywed who fled the palace in 1986)
        Claude (daughter of French missionaries)
        Che'elou (eldest woman in the royal compound in 1986; had been the mfen's nursemaid)
        Marguerite (seamstress, secretary of the village *tontine* or rotating credit association)
        Jeanne (friend of Claude)
        Sanke (mother of Nji Monluh Seidou Pokam)
    In the second queen's quarter
        Louise (the *nzwikam,* or second queen)
        Rebecca (often Marguerite's rival)
        Corinne (married mfen Njiké Pokam around the same time as Paulette)
The Healers
    Felix
    Nana
    Mfen Meshinke' (elderly subchief of Bantoum)

Introduction

Fertility and the Politics of Identity in Cameroon

Fertility and reproductive health are intimate, physical matters. They are also deeply gendered, social matters, involving men and women and eliciting intense interest from the surrounding kin, community, and state. This book is an anthropological study of procreation imagery and of women's concerns with reproduction in Africa. It is about the symbolic language of food and fertility that expresses women's fears of infertility in a specific locale. It is also, more generally, about gender, modernity, and struggles over cultural identity.

These broad connections lead us away from single-hypothesis explanations in medical anthropology, while underscoring the relevance of medical anthropology to other anthropological specializations. Such insights regarding the mutually constituted nature of social life and idioms of affliction, however, remain empty polemic when separated from rich ethnography. The message of this book is therefore grounded in a particular setting, the Bamiléké kingdom of Bangangté in the west-central African country of Cameroon.

Bangangté is one of the five most prominent of some hundred Bamiléké kingdoms in the lush, densely populated highland Grassfields region spanning the West and Northwest Provinces of Cameroon. Over nine decades it has provided both food and personnel (laborers, merchants, taxi drivers, and scholars) for the development of Cameroon's cities and agribusinesses. But back home, "au village" or "in the village" (as Bamiléké refer to the kingdoms, towns, and hamlets of the Western Province), this agricultural and demographic wealth is lost in a cloud of existential worries and a rhetoric of complaint.

The people of Bangangté, especially Bangangté women, seem preoccupied with threats to their reproductive health. I first arrived in Bangangté planning to do research on medical pluralism, to explore how Bangangté patients and health professionals managed[1] the enormous variety of indigenous and cosmopolitan health-care alternatives. During the

1980s, the people I lived with and visited instead told me hair-raising stories of babies stolen from their mothers' wombs, of plugged fallopian tubes, and of infant deaths. They lamented that the royal household had too few children. Their concerns about their own ability to have descendants, and the future of their kingdom in the face of population decline, seemed paradoxical. Standard demographic indicators suggested that the Bamiléké people are among those with the highest birthrate in Cameroon.[2] What was it about the meaning rural Bangangté women gave to their experiences that led them to be so anxious about infertility? As I investigated women's expressions about infertility and threats to procreation I discovered indigenous conceptions of fertility and vitality linked to a strong king (*mfen* in the local language; referred to as *fon* throughout the English-speaking Western Grassfields),[3] of illness, vulnerability and decline exacerbated by the loss of political autonomy, and of the close relation among cooking, feeding, and procreation in Bangangté cosmology.

Using the same idioms of food, cooking, and provisioning to talk about both phenomena, Bangangté cosmology links women's human reproduction and royal social reproduction. But royal social reproduction does not occur smoothly; the position of Grassfields kingdoms in relation to the Cameroonian state is currently in flux. The particularities of Bangangté highlight the ways that women's complaints about the apparently physical matters of fertility are conditioned by and also comment upon political, social, and economic change. This message emerges from a specific setting but applies broadly to societies as diverse as the Gambia (Bledsoe 1997), Egypt (Inhorn 1994a, 1996), Madagascar (Feeley-Harnik 1995), Benin (Sargent 1982, 1989), Congo (formerly Zaire) (Devisch 1993), China (Greenhalgh 1994; L. Handwerker 1995), Italy (Kertzer 1993), the United States (Becker 1994; Sandelowski 1993), or England (Strathern 1992).

Fertility and Infertility Studies: Demography and Phenomenology

This focus on complex connections is gaining ever greater attention in work on fertility in anthropological demography, and on infertility in medical anthropology. Building upon insights from social theory regarding agency and structure (Giddens 1976), and from feminist anthropology regarding the politics of reproduction (Handwerker 1990; Rapp and Ginsburg 1991), Susan Greenhalgh has called for a multidisciplinary "political economy of fertility" (1990, 1995). Her approach draws heavily on anthropological concepts and methodology to examine the relation among fertility, gender, and "the political-economic dimensions of social and cultural organization" (1990:95), of which gender itself is a "pervasive force" (1995:24). Demographers working in Africa are ever more mindful of social, cultural, and economic change, largely in an attempt to explain the relative (and anomalous) stability of high fertility in sub-Saharan Africa. The Caldwells suggest that, in many sub-Saharan African societies, belief in the efficacy of ancestors to dispense fortune and misfortune and the importance of extended kin relations support high fertility (Caldwell and Caldwell 1987). Frank and McNicoll describe high fertility as a strategy women use to ensure access to land and labor within the context of marriage, bridewealth, inheritance, and land tenure institutions (1987:11). Economic insecurity may erode these social institutions as well as eroding women's motivations to maintain a strategy of high fertility (Price 1996). In a study of contraceptive use in the Gambia, Bledsoe finds that, surprisingly, reproductive mishaps (e.g., miscarriages, stillbirths) are often followed by periods of contraceptive use (1997). This look at anomalous cases of subfertility and contraception "out of place and time" uncovered previously uncharted territories of women's knowledge regarding their bodies, reproductive capacity, and aging. What is it about the meaning and experience of these reproductive mishaps for individual women that leads to these aggregate results of higher contraceptive use? The insights of work in medical anthropology on the meaning of infertility point toward an answer, even though most of this literature is based on the experiences of women in low-fertility, high-technology societies.

Studies of infertility in medical anthropology emphasize the effects that infertility has on the lives of infertile men and women. They use infertility as a tool to reveal the dynamics of gender inequality and family life (Inhorn 1996), notions of success and failure (Becker 1994), and cultural conceptions of kinship (Modell 1989). Infertility allows anthropologists to examine how people make sense out of unexpected, unfortunate events, manage the fragmentation of experience associated with perinatal loss (Layne 1992) and prenatal diagnosis of disability (e.g., Rapp 1988, 1993), and respond culturally to the "never enough" quality of conception-assisting new reproductive technologies (Sandelowski 1991, 1993).

A Cameroonian Rhetoric of Misfortune

This book builds upon these two bodies of work by examining how a rhetoric of misfortune and a culturally specific symbolism of procreation are tied to socially structured experience. It investigates how women use infertility symbolically to comment on their lives and how they struggle, through an idiom of infertility, to find a language that gives meaning and makes comprehensible the ways their lives are affected by social change.

These women enact concepts of personhood, social status, and cultural identity through their tales of reproductive threats and through their quest for fertility. In so doing, they draw upon a symbolic repertoire of procreation imagery focused on metaphors of the kitchen and cooking. These metaphors, elements of which are common to several central and east African societies (de Boeck 1995; de Heusch 1980; Devisch 1993; Douglas 1966; Richards 1956; Weiss 1996), include visions of sex as heat; the womb as hearth or cooking pot; ova, sperm, and blood as ingredients; gestation as cooking and stirring the pot; and birth as serving a meal. The imagery of marriage refers to the kitchen, simultaneously a physical and metaphoric locale that draws the wife inside the husband's village, kin group, and compound. The term for marriage is *cooking inside,* as the wife's marital duties are to grow crops and cook food for her family while metaphorically "cooking" babies within the bounds of the nuptial kitchen.

Understanding this culinary symbolism of procreation in Bangangté is essential to solving the puzzle of the fear of infertility in an area of high fertility and to specifying the connection between social structural factors and demographic outcomes. Kinship systems and socioeconomic relationships can only support high fertility if people make demographically relevant decisions influenced by these social structural factors. Human agency is the link between social structure and demographic outcomes (e.g., fertility rates). Human agency is the product of "knowledgeable actors" (Giddens 1976), and their "knowledge" is culture (Sewell 1992). Recent theory in anthropological demography seeks to take culture seriously (e.g., Hammel 1990), but could be advanced by more attention to the content of that culture (Kertzer 1995:47). Thus, an examination of the specific imagery of procreation is an essential step in linking the anthropological demography of high-fertility societies with the concern for personal experience represented in medical anthropological studies of infertility.

During this century, anthropological explorations of the imagery of procreation have been embedded in studies on kinship (e.g., Malinowski 1929), rites of passage (e.g., Richards 1956), and more recently rites of affliction or spirit possession (e.g., Devisch 1993, Boddy 1989). Concern with the broad cultural significance of gender has motivated a reemerging interest in the symbolism of procreation. Martin's *The Woman in the Body* (1987), as well as her entertaining article on the romance of the sperm and the egg (1991), deconstruct biomedical metaphors and discourses surrounding reproductive biology. Her work reveals the influence of stereotyped gender roles on the ways American gynecologists (and many of their patients) view women's bodies and procreation. Delaney's *The Seed and the Soil* (1991) relates the imagery of coming-into-being (procreation) to gender definitions, cosmology, and everyday life in a Turkish village. The most comprehensive book to date on the symbolism of procreation, Delaney asks why human reproduction, and women's role in it, is so devalued in the Judeo-Christian-Islamic world. Delaney seeks her answer in the symbolic link between men and God as "monogenetic" life-givers and thus critiques the conflation of patriarchy and male dominance in much feminist anthropology as intellectually sloppy (1991:35), a profound if sometimes disputed challenge (see Inhorn 1996:25).

My book on the Bangangté is a contribution to this dialogue on procreation imagery and gender issues. In my attempt to explain Bangangté women's laments regarding dangers to procreation, I have tried to show the significance of both gender and procreative imagery beyond the confines of compound, kitchen, and birthing in this modern African kingdom. The metaphors of cooking ingredients and stories of plugged fallopian tubes and stolen fetuses evoke cultural typifications, simultaneously providing a framework for action and controlling it (Rasmussen 1995 makes a similar point for the symbolism involved in Tuareg spirit possession). These idioms are not "mere" idioms. The ways people think and talk about procreation can be highly significant in shaping decisions and actions regarding marriage, sex, and childbearing; they influence the therapeutic itineraries people pursue to enhance fertility, for contraception, to treat perceived infertility, and to seek obstetric care. Moreover, these decisions are often statements (or are perceived as statements) regarding the politics of cultural identity. Through the lens of ways of speaking about fertility, childbearing, and population, this book examines how rural Bangangté women, as one (often itself differentiated) voice among many, comment on political and economic change and the impact it has on their lives, health, and fears.

Personal Fate and Cultural Heritage

It becomes increasingly clear that the symbolism of procreation and women's experience of their bodies are intimately tied up in social relations. In this ethnography, these social relations include both the face-to-face interactions of the relatively small, relatively bounded community of Bangangté, *and* the larger scale interconnections and events in regional (Grassfields), national (Cameroonian), and international contexts. These grand events and processes affect notions of fertility through a series of filters or relationships; they include the changing power of Grassfields kingships with regard to the Cameroonian state and to capital markets, and the effect of these relationships on women's lives. Fear of infertility emerges as a recurrent theme in Bangangté discourse, a barometer of anxiety about personal fate, the future of the kingdom and of one's cultural heritage, and a barometer of ambivalent response to modernity and cultural imports.

Several questions with broad comparative implications guide my ethnographic description and search for explanation. The first two refer to anxiety about personal fate. First, what makes women sick? What accounts for the distribution of suffering among women? Some Bangangté women may suffer biological infertility or depressed fertility due to changes in male-female relations (e.g., separations due to seasonal and longer-term labor migration, increased incidence of sexually transmitted diseases and secondary infertility) and increased economic and psychological stress. Despite global attention to overpopulation, fertility is fragile. In the high-stress environment of rural Africa, the windows of temporal, social, and biological opportunity to produce healthy children and mothers are easily narrowed, and potential medical problems loom large in women's consciousness (Bledsoe 1997). This environment is affected by regional and global inequalities, essential elements producing patterns of health, sickness, and infertility in Africa (Cordell and Gregory 1994; Doyal 1979; Feierman and Janzen 1992). For example, historical and geographical research indicates that infertility has increased along routes of labor migration in central Africa (Retel-Laurentin 1974). Bangangté has long been a labor-reserve area, supplying workers for colonial and postcolonial economic development. Nonetheless, in Bangangté infertile women constituted only a small segment of women expressing infertility anxiety in the 1980s. But one group of women, the women of the royal court, while not infertile, seem to have experienced depressed fertility in comparison to other Bangangté women. They had neither as many children as they wanted nor as many as their nonroyal neighbors and compatriots expected. The fecundity of the king's wives is of great symbolic importance for other Bangangté citizens, and low fertility within the royal family may have contributed to a generalized fear of reproductive failure.

Second, a comparative perspective on the consequences of infertility for women shows that infertility stigmatizes women and can contribute to their impoverishment (Inhorn 1994a, 1994b, 1996). Even if most rural Bangangté women are not infertile, they *fear* reproductive threats more than men or better-situated women do because the consequences of infertility would be so grave. Infertility disrupts a rural Bangangté woman's expected life course and denies her the pride and fully adult status of motherhood. In addition, infertility puts women at greater risk of impoverishment in Bangangté, through the changes it initiates in relations between husbands and wives, among cowives, and between divorced women and their natal kin, and through the loss of potential child labor it entails. The stigma and impoverishment associated with infertility has a specific historical context in Bangangté: the economic crisis and sharpened identity politics of the 1980s and 1990s. Tales of the theft of food from women's kitchens and children from their wombs permeated Bangangté women's accounts of dangers to procreation in the 1980s; in the 1990s these accusations of theft implicated the state and commercial elite in stealing the means to health and success via harmful economic policies and new forms of witchcraft (Feldman-Savelsberg 1997; see also Geschiere with Fisiy 1994; Goheen 1996; Rowlands and Warnier 1988). This violent imagery suggests that the grave consequences of infertility find symbolic expression in a particular form of discourse.

Anxiety about personal fate is intimately linked to Bangangté concerns about the future of their kingdom and their cultural heritage. The historical and political-economic context is an essential part of local idioms for reproductive illness (and other problems; see, for example, Farmer 1988). Bangangté women use infertility as an idiom to express other difficulties, regardless of their own fertility. With the language of infertility and the imagery of thieves and witches interfering in the process of baby-making, they discuss social processes they perceive to be just as threatening as infertility itself. Writing on the "body husbandry efforts" of rural Gambian women, Bledsoe points out that high fertility and child survival are social accomplishments, requiring knowledge and skills regarding bodies, time, health, economics, kinship, and ritual life (1997). Bangangté women worry that the social changes rocking contemporary Cameroon are causing these skills to falter, and that threats to fertility may surpass their and their king's ability to manage those aspects of the physical and social worlds that contribute to reproductive health. For Bangangté women, fertility is a indicator of "things in place" and of "things falling apart" (*pace* Achebe). Their reproductive fears express local ambivalence regarding the changing place of divine kingships in modern states.

Divine Kingship

Like all of the Grassfields kingdoms, Bangangté is a divine kingship. The study of divine kingships in Africa, inspired by Frazer's *Golden Bough* (1922), has a long history, revealing ongoing attention to indigenous concepts of power, legitimacy, and prosperity (Feeley-Harnik 1985:273). In divine kingships, persons are transformed into the embodiment of kingly office through installation rituals that make the king "strange," distinct from his subjects (Fortes 1968; Hocart 1936). These rituals often involve fearful images of sacrifice, cannibalism, and incest (Arens and Karp 1989; de Heusch 1982; Kuper 1947; Richards 1939, 1969), as well as nurturing or provisioning ones (e.g., Bemba sacred hearth and kitchen ceremonies; Richards 1939:48–50). They transform the king into someone who can both participate in and transcend the complexities of social life (Beidelman 1966). These special capacities (Karp 1989) lend the divine king a unique combination of religious and secular authority. But they also make the king's subjects dependent upon the king's well-being; in divine kingships, the vulnerability of persons is closely linked to the frailty of polities (Feeley-Harnik 1985:276). Indeed, the myths of regicide in Frazer's *Golden Bough* portray aging, weakening kings killed by their follower-worshippers and replaced by more vigorous counterparts who could insure the well-being of their subjects.

The kingship retains great symbolic importance in modern Bangangté. Most rural residents are convinced that their health and wealth are dependent upon the health, wealth, and reproductive vigor of the king. Even for highly educated young people, the king and the palace remain a focus of identity, an identity often formed in opposition to a state lacking in confidence, suffering from economic and political crisis (see also Goheen 1996:xii–xiii). Through inheritance of the kingship and initiation into office, the mfen of Bangangté gains sacred, supernatural powers. He embodies royal traditions in himself (e.g., through ingesting "medicines" and specially cooked food), in his relations with kin and subjects, and through rituals.

As Grassfields kingdoms became consolidated during the German (1884–1916) and French (1916–60) colonial periods, the Bangangté monarchy gained power relative to neighboring kingdoms. Nonetheless, the mfen lost his power over the life and death of his subjects, and gradually over more and more aspects of dispute management, economics, and the politicoreligious orientation of Bangangté citizens. During the 1980s it was evident that the incorporation of the local Grassfields polities into a postcolonial state, a global economy, and an increasingly global network of cultural exchange (Hannerz 1987) changed rural women's position, provided them new opportunities (den Ouden 1980), and created new vulnerabilities and threats to their pride and to their survival.

In the mid-1980s Bangangté society was differentiated not only by levels of traditional title holding but also according to differences in formal education, cash income and wealth, occupation, rural or urban residence, and religion. Gender permeated all of these differences. With the least education, income, and mobility, and the greatest orientation toward such royal institutions as death celebrations and the commemoration of past kings, rural women experience the incorporation of the Bangangté kingdom in terms of downward personal mobility. National and international policies regarding land tenure and agricultural marketing have further contributed to the dispossession of Grassfields women in the 1980s and 1990s (Goheen 1996). In the 1990s the end of the cold war was felt in terms of political upheavals and economic crisis in African countries. These events exacerbated the vulnerability of the poor rural food cultivators who made up the majority of women of the Cameroonian Grassfields. These women interpreted their vulnerability in terms of infertility-inducing witchcraft.

Thus, rural Bangangté women use culturally specific metaphors of procreation to organize their experience of social change. This experience has been mixed at best. Rural Bangangté women view their own vulnerability to impoverishment, status decline, and illness as the complex result of changes in the political autonomy and "strength" of their king, the kingship, and their kingdom, and focus much of their attention on the royal household.

All the King's Wives: The Underbelly of Power

Rural Bangangté women are such careful "royalty watchers" because they believe that the well-being of the royal family affects their own well-being, including their reproductive health. But, at a deeper level, Bangangté women closely observe the women of the court because royal power is only possible due to the symbolic, material, political, and reproductive roles of the king's wives. Although the intense polygyny of Grassfields royal courts has been described in several studies (on the Bamiléké: Brain 1972; Hurault 1962; Tardits 1960; on the Bamoum: Tardits 1985; on the western Grassfields: Goheen 1996; Kaberry 1952, 1962; Nkwi 1987), this feminine underbelly of royal power in Africa has been surprisingly neglected in studies of divine kingship. Bangangté use the same set of symbols to describe the parallel roles of the king and his wives (and women in general) as providers and reproducers. The symbolism of food and procreation cognitively and semantically connects these two activities. They are also connected in an immediate, material sense. The women of the court cultivate, prepare, and serve the food that nourishes the king, and the feasts that help reward and maintain his followership. The newly installed king is dependent upon the reproductive capacity of his wives to move from the royal initiation hut to the palace. Throughout his reign, the king remains dependent upon his wives' reproductive capacity to bear witness to his own continued vitality.

The king's wives play an important, if often hidden, role in the political intrigue of local African kingdoms such as Bangangté. Royal succession and diplomacy between kingdoms is based on the royal wives' work as mothers of heirs and as links in often diplomatically driven marriage alliances. In addition, the women of the court emerged (at least in Bangangté of the 1980s, and it seems elsewhere in the Grassfields as well; see Diduk 1989; Goheen 1996) as active commentators in struggles over identity as these kingdoms became ever more incorporated in a modern state and in international structures. Although the women of the court lead their lives under particular conditions, this book gives detailed attention to the king's wives because of their potential to reveal links between the state (in how it shapes royal power and local identities), visions of reproductive health, and the different positions of different actors.

The royal wives are an important set of actors in this story of women's fears of infertility, but are necessarily joined by other women: their sisters, daughters, mothers, neighbors, fellow members of *tontines* (the ubiquitous and "very Bamiléké" rotating credit associations), market women, nurses, teachers, and the innumerable, hardworking cultivators in the many villages of Bangangté kingdom who make up the most avid group of "royalty watchers." Social and economic variation among Bangangté women results in differing perspectives, opportunities, and life trajectories regarding reproduction. Expressed in a shared idiom of food and fertility, the distribution of images of reproductive threats among different types of rural Bangangté women indicates that a core of shared beliefs is reshaped for individuals through their experience of social differentiation. Fear of infertility and traumatic reproductive mishaps seems closely related to economic and social displacement. Even the symbolism of reproductive illness (e.g., the theft of fetuses) reflects deep ambivalence about changing values regarding reciprocity, patterns of consumption, and markers of modernity (see Gottlieb 1992:119–42; Rowlands 1996). As rural African women become increasingly dispossessed, gender becomes the most salient social differentiation; the imagery of reproductive threat is widely shared.

The Structure of the Argument

Women in Bangangté, women in similar situations throughout the Cameroonian Grassfields, and women in many other parts of rural Africa face many sources of uncertainty and vulnerability. After laying out the general analytic issues in this introduction, this book first plunges into the complexities and contradictions of one woman's reproductive ills. In chapter 1, Paulette's difficulties in marriage and her fears of reproductive illness illustrate Bangangté women's anxieties surrounding procreation, the circumstances in which they are voiced, and the actions women may take to relieve their suffering. Paulette was a deracinated, urban Bamiléké "returnee" to Bangangté, a king's wife embroiled in the sexual politics of the royal court, and a victim of unintentional "incest" within the framework of a complex kinship system. All of these contributed to her reproductive complaints; for Paulette and for other women, these issues can only be understood in the context of history and the political-economic, social, and cultural changes that have shaped kinship and marriage, gender and power, migration and the politics of identity in Bangangté.

Chapter 2 provides that context, focusing on how Bangangté notions of cultural identity are at the center of a web of practical relations that support ideas regarding procreation and women's reproductive goals. Notions of kinship, gender, and the veneration of ancestors are central to the ways Bangangté think about offspring. They are held in common across all social ranks and tie together the sociospatial categories of household, neighborhood, village, and kingdom. Despite these commonalities (shared in minor permutations by the other Bamiléké kingdoms and nearly all western Grassfields ones), Bangangté is highly diverse, made up of peoples of different origins and varying social rank. Within this diversity, integration is based upon ideas about royalty and allegiance to the mfen. Bangangté express social integration through the same basic imagery as procreation. It is created through the balanced mixing and mingling of "ingredients": genders, ranks, titles, forms of spiritual or magical strength. In parallel to procreation as largely the physical and spiritual achievement of women, the constitution of society in Bangangté is, or should be, the political and spiritual achievement of the king. However, through a process beginning with the colonial era, the king is no longer the overwhelming reference point for Bangangté identity and life strategies. World religions, schools, the market, and national politics create new reference groups, modes of action, and definitions of self and belonging. Complaints about reproductive risk and failure can only be understood in this historical context of the shifting imagery and politics of identity.

Bangangté imagery of women's role in procreation echoes that of the king's role in social reproduction. Starting with a native exegesis of the Bangangté expression for marriage, "cooking inside" (*na nda*), chapter 3 explores the links between notions of procreation and social reproduction. The imagery of procreation both reflects and shapes the ways that gender permeates a Bangangté sense of a multilayered identity, of belonging to kin groups, domestic units, the village, the kingdom, and the nation. Procreation occurs when diverse elements from man and woman are "measured" (*mfi'*), "mixed" (*nu'u*), and transformed through the "cooking" (*na*) of sex and gestation into the whole of a new being. The gendered roles of procreative cooking and the ambiguous implications of notions of inside and outside for men and women contribute to gendered differences in the perception of threats to procreation.

Symbolic construction (the focus of chapter 3) mixes with political-economic context (the focus of chapter 2) in chapter 4's discussion of infertility as an idiom of misfortune. In addition to the gender implications of the culinary symbolism of procreation, there are gendered variations in identification with the kingship and the state, and in the opportunities and constraints of the market, that further contribute to differences in the perception of threats to procreation. These variables are linked through the symbolic and material importance of food. Food figures prominently in the symbolism of fertility and infertility, referring to folk models of both physiology and social relations (e.g., hospitality and trust). Food provisioning and reproduction are both deeply gendered processes. Women and men diverge in their anxieties regarding food insecurity and infertility.

Although men and women (between and within these gender categories) differ in their life trajectories, their reproductive histories, and in the amount and kind of reproductive risk they perceive for themselves and for their community, they nonetheless express fear of infertility through a common set of idioms, the culinary imagery of measuring and cooking. Rural Bangangté find that the diverse elements of society, and especially the occult powers of good and evil possessed by different social groups, are no longer in balance (for similar analyses of Cameroonian societies see also Fisiy and Geschiere 1991; Geschiere with Fisiy 1994; Rowlands and Warnier 1988). The lack of social balance leads to disharmony and the use of witchcraft in social relations, which in turn prevent the elements of procreation from being properly measured, mixed, and cooked. As children become a rare and precious good, competition for them creates more disharmony and encourages the use of more infertility-inducing witchcraft, creating a vicious circle. The result, explicated in chapter 4, is an indigenous theory of the demographic implications of jealousy.

Women are neither equally jealous nor equally enviable regarding their personal, material, and reproductive fates. The amount and kind of rural Bangangté women's fears of reproductive threats vary according to a number of dimensions, including their reproductive histories, their exposure to various institutionalized sets of knowledge regarding health and illness, their place in the life cycle, the developmental stage of their household, and their upward or downward mobility within the highly differentiated and differentiating Bangangté society. The distribution of Bangangté women's fears parallels the material and social resources with which women can manage crises and make use of Bangangté's plural medical system. Chapter 5 examines the history of the diverse institutions Bangangté women can consult in seeking cures for reproductive illness. Resources of cure and solace for reproductive complaints are integrally related to notions of divine kingship and the ultimate causes of reproductive misfortune. Changes in health care and in the definition and redefinition of "population" problems have paralleled transformations in the sources of social disruption over time (early colonial incursions and forced labor prior to World War I, civil war and the "Bamiléké problem" of the 1950s and 1960s, the king's illness of the 1980s, and the political and economic crises of the 1990s). In this context, the idea of the king's debility (through illness or political crisis) contributing to the social ills of the community is remarkably persistent. As others have shown, the social relations of domination and power are essential elements of the power to heal, to render fertile or infertile, and even to define fortune and misfortune (Comaroff 1985; Janzen 1982; Parkin 1968). Chapter 5 also explores variations in indigenous and biomedical treatment of infertility in Bangangté of the 1980s, and how the vagaries of access and confidence contribute to women's anxieties about threats to procreation. Theses in medical anthropological literature regarding therapeutic choice and idioms of reproductive problems are placed into broader context, showing how individual variables interact and combine, and how this interaction is conditioned by historical and political-economic factors.

Fear of infertility and of population stagnation or decline in contemporary Bangangté express ambiguity regarding the dynamic of social differentiation and the politics of identity in a multiethnic, modernizing state. The place of the dynamic states-within-a-state of the Bamiléké and western Grassfields kingdoms in Cameroon has been problematic since the formation of the entity "Cameroon" in the colonial era. Individuals confronting the ideologies and practices of village life and state schools, ceremonial life and mission churches, reciprocity and "the consumption of modernity" (Rowlands 1996), diviners and biomedical surgeons must sort out a multiplicity of identities. Cultural consensus regarding "an all-encompassing scheme of identities . . . [reinforced] by systematically organized networks of social relations, is precisely what is challenged in the modern era," in Bangangté and worldwide (Calhoun 1994:11). Ironically, in the current economic and political crisis facing Cameroon, ethnic identity and difference are becoming intensely politicized, especially for the Bamiléké and Grassfields peoples of the West and Northwest Provinces (Goheen 1996; Nkwi and Socpa 1997). Sharp boundaries are drawn around what appear to be fluid entities. The sixth and final chapter of this book explores the role of the rhetorics of infertility, therapeutic choice, and divine kingship in the politics of identity. The imagery of cooking and provisioning in procreation and royal social reproduction, and the visions of theft and eating in infertility, witchcraft, and state corruption all hinge on various forms of social differentiation and access to resources. The politics of identity is closely tied to disjunctures between expectations and realities, and to struggles over who will be the haves and who the have-nots. It is then not surprising that women's complaints about fertility and infertility, markers of fortune and misfortune, figure prominently in these struggles.

While this study was motivated by the overwhelming litany of laments about infertility that greeted me in the field, infertility is only the way women *first* express their fears. Listening further, it becomes clear that rural Bangangté women are concerned about a broad range of processes from finding the appropriate sexual partner through childbearing, child rearing, and socialization, to provisioning their families with food and children, and to reproducing a viable, recognizable Bangangté society. Drawing upon a common symbolic repertoire, they are active commentators in negotiations over population management, gender relations, and the politics of identity in a multiethnic state. Connecting these areas of social action, this book is an argument for a historically and political-economically situated symbolic anthropology of women's health.

Chapter One

The Short-lived Marriage of a King's Wife: Paulette's "Plugged Fertility" and Blocked Mobility

"I am leaving, Pamé . . ." It was a late June morning, and I was typing field notes. I blew a flake of soot off the page and looked up at Paulette, standing in the doorway of my mud hut. I was living in the palace compound of Bangangté, in one of the numerous "women's houses," a kitchen built of mud brick, four by four meters, with a three-stoned hearth and an "attic" granary. I was often visited by one or the other of the royal wives during the quiet morning hours when most others were away cultivating their fields. This time Paulette had come to say good-bye. At first I thought she was just walking into town for an errand, but no. She was leaving for good. "I can't stay any more, without children. With money or not, I am going to Douala. I won't come back." Why was Paulette, this jovial, rotund twenty-one-year-old woman, leaving her marriage to the king of Bangangté? What role did her childless state play in her decision to leave her marriage? After all, she was young and had only been married for eight months.

Examining Paulette's story further, we will discover that although she was childless, Paulette's reproductive complaints underwent several transformations over the brief course of her marriage. What started as pain was redefined as infertility induced by the sorcery of competing cowives. Finally, Paulette portrayed her unhappy, unfruitful marriage as an impediment to seeking a good life. Paulette's case may not be typical of rural Bangangté women, but the drama of the story and the commentary on it by others provides a rich departure from which to study the relation between women's reproductive complaints and political, social, and cultural change.

When Paulette left, I had been living in the royal compound of Bangangté for six months, using it as a base from which to study how Bamiléké women's concerns about fertility are shaped by the symbolism of health and illness and by the changing circumstances of rural African food

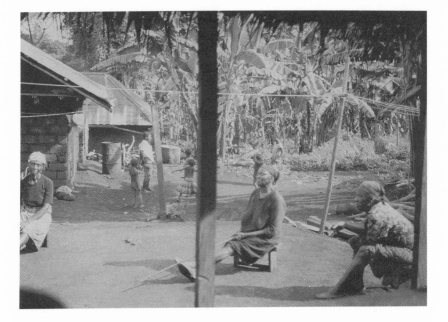

Fig. 1.   Elderly cowives of Paulette visiting in the first queen's quarter of the royal compound of Bangangté. This was a rare occasion of repose, as even elderly women are almost always engaged in agricultural or domestic labor.

cultivators. Just as the Bamiléké, Bamum, and Western Grassfields kingdoms are states within a state (Goheen 1996), the royal court of the Bamiléké kingdom of Bangangté was a village within a village. The king, or *mfen,* lived in this royal compound along with his 14 wives, their children and wards, and several royal retainers (specially initiated private servants to the king). Each wife lived in her own mud brick hut, simultaneously a kitchen and a house for a mother and her children. The mud kitchen-huts were arranged in two "quarters," each quarter presided over by wives of the king who had been invested with titles at the time of the king's coronation.

For the first four months of my fieldwork, I lived in Louise's house. Louise bore the title of *nzwikam,* the "second queen," and presided over the quarter housing Rebecca, Corinne, and several elderly women who, married to the king's grandfather, had been inherited by each subsequent king. Most elderly widows of former kings left the palace grounds to live with their grown children, but some chose to stay, married not only to the king but also to the kingship in a form of old age insurance. Louise had

been initiated as the "second queen" during the long coronation ceremonies of mfen (king) François Njiké Pokam in 1974. In 1986 she was
about 30 years old, quiet, stoic, a hard worker with three young children.

When Paulette came to say good-bye, I was already living in my own
hut, the abandoned kitchen of a deceased wife of the king's father.
Remaining my home for eight months, this hut was tucked behind the
house of Josette, the *mabengoup,* or "first" queen. The mabengoup's quarter was lively, as alliances among the cowives formed and dissolved over
shared meals, work on the farms, and child-rearing challenges. Marguerite, the seamstress, lived there, as did Jeanne, each with their two
young daughters. Both these women were daughters of rulers of other
Bamiléké kingdoms, and their marriages contributed to a dense network
of crosscutting ties among the local polities of the highland Grassfields
region. Jeanne was good friends with her cowife Claude,[1] an outspoken
woman who taught at the local *lycée* (high school). Claude, the daughter
of white French Protestant missionaries, was born in Cameroon and spent
her childhood in Bangangté. After 18 years as a teen and young adult in
France, she returned to Bangangté and eventually became one of the
king's many wives, bearing him two children. Many Bangangté admired
Claude, while a few saw the presence of a white woman in the royal family
as an indicator of the decline of truly Bangangté mores. Several elderly
wives, widows of the king's grandfather, also lived in mabengoup's quarter, including the wise Che'elou. Paulette spent most of her time in this
quarter and in the king's main house.

The king lived in a stone and cement house, built during the 1950s by
a French governor for the king's father. Here, and in a series of separate
buildings housing the customary court and the meeting places of the regulatory societies, the king received visitors—nobility coming with advice,
ritual specialists seeking to maintain the vigor of the kingdom, and subjects seeking the resolution of myriad disputes. Although a village within a
village, full of its own intrigue, the royal court remained a touchstone, a
place of both symbolic and practical relevance for the nonroyal citizens of
the kingdom. They came there to get the king's signature on birth and
death certificates, but also to participate in rituals to prevent illness and to
celebrate their common identity as Bangangté within the multiethnic state
of Cameroon. These nonroyals lived in villages and hamlets throughout
the territory of Bangangté kingdom, in places like Maham, where I had
spent two months investigating medical pluralism in 1983, and Bantoum,
where I conducted comparative research in late 1986. They also lived in the
town called Bangangté, an administrative center with a population, in the
mid-1980s, of approximately 12,000 people. Large populations of Bangangté citizens lived in the cities of Yaoundé, Douala, and Nkongsamba;

they met in "family reunions" and *tontines* (rotating credit associations, often organized along ethnic, gender, and occupational lines) and returned to Bangangté to visit relatives and perform propitiary rituals.

Most urban Bamiléké are descendants of labor migrants who began to leave the Grassfields during the early colonial period (1890s through 1910s), often through coercion, to develop the colonial infrastructure in southern Cameroon (Rudin 1938:324–27). Many Bamiléké, especially Bangangté, emigrated to seek their fortunes through wage employment in the expanding postwar cities of southern Cameroon. Some are more recent migrants, striving for a better life in an era when land shortage and a depressed market for coffee, the major cash crop, plagues their country cousins. Recent migrants include highly educated civil servants, merchants, and taxi drivers.

Population movement between the Bangangté countryside and Cameroon's urban centers flows in two directions. Kin ties and village origin remain important sources of identity for urban Bamiléké. Trips "back home" (even if one has never lived in the village) are common to celebrate births and mourn deaths. In the 1980s, many urban Bangangté built country houses, anticipating their retirement. In the 1990s, concerned by increasing ethnic tensions and occasional anti-Bamiléké violence in the major cities, urban Bangangté began to build commercial buildings. Despite changing patterns of investment over these two decades, the back and forth urban–rural movement retained a consistent spirit of urban entrepreneurship coupled with strong emotional ties to one's land of origin, family, and king.

Paulette was one of these urban Bamiléké "exiles" (as they refer to themselves). Although ethnically Bangangté and a descendant of the Bangangté royal family, Paulette had spent her entire life in Cameroon's largest port city, Douala. Royal pedigree rarely translates into wealth in the urban context, and Paulette grew up in a poor family. She attended six years of primary school, but never obtained the primary school certificate.

Shortly before the rains started in 1985, Paulette came to Bangangté for the first time. Following a common Bamiléké pattern of urban–rural movement, Paulette "returned" to the land of her ancestors, her "village" of Bangangté, to attend the death celebration of her paternal grandmother. She stayed on to help her sister, who had just given birth at Bangangté Divisional Hospital. Bamiléké women like Paulette customarily visit female kin to admire newborns and relieve the new mother of household duties during her postpartum recovery. Paulette, a full sibling, cared for her sister for two months.

As she and others told me later, during this time Paulette developed ringworm. To her great consternation, patches of her hair fell out. A young woman hoping to get ahead in the world of romance and commerce, Paulette was concerned about her appearance and sought treatment at Bangangté Hospital and from a well-known local healer named Felix. But Paulette needed to pay for her medical bills, and her double search for employment and cure would eventually keep her in Bangangté. Finding paid work was not easy in this provincial town of 12,000 inhabitants, particularly for a young woman with neither school diploma nor agricultural experience. Familiar with city houses, Paulette became the maid of an Italian businessman, a friend of the mfen of Bangangté. The king often went to the Italian's house to watch videotapes and meet girlfriends: women, usually paid, who could give the king a different kind of attention than his many wives, burdened as they were with agricultural and ritual duties. According to the rules of royal marriage, these women were not normally eligible to become wives of the king. Although a king could marry anyone he fancied, royal wives were most often daughters of royal retainers, Bangangté nobility, and neighboring kings. Paulette fell between categories; the maid of a European, a deracinated urban "returnee," a woman with little knowledge of "country fashion" (customs and practical skills of rural life), she was also a distant descendant of the royal household. She married the mfen in October 1985.

A Royal Romance?

Born in 1947, François Njiké Pokam became king of Bangangté in 1974, succeeding the 31-year reign of his father, Robert Pokam. During infancy, the wise but childless Che'elou, bride of his grandfather, had been mfen Njiké Pokam's nursemaid. He spent some of his youth in Bamenda, the booming provincial capital of the anglophone Northwest Province. There he began an auto mechanic's apprenticeship. Upon accession to the throne, Njiké Pokam inherited his father's and grandfather's widows and responsibility for their children. He married several new wives, daughters of other Bamiléké kings and nobles, establishing and solidifying patterns of alliance among the traditional elite of the region. Before he could move to the royal palace from the temporary initiation hut, la'kwa, the king had to sire a boy and a girl baby. His mother, the new queen mother, performed the ceremony of tossed beans to insure that her son would provide his people with the necessary ingredients for the regeneration of human life. After only boy babies were born the first year of Njiké Pokam's reign, the queen mother once again threw handfuls of beans from each hand (right hand for boys, left hand for girls) over the sacred fields of an abandoned palace; finally a daughter was born, and the mfen could enter his palace.

Such details of royal marriages and births were closely watched by Njiké Pokam's subjects. The king, his strength, and his fertility played a key role in how the Bangangté people thought about their futures. In 1986, after a dozen years of Njiké Pokam's rule, many Bangangté were grumbling. Their mfen, a friendly and open man to strangers, often acted against the restrictive rules of royal behavior that kept the king strange, sacred, and powerful. Perhaps seeking a kind of companionship difficult to achieve in the context of large-scale polygyny, the king casually visited foreign friends and nightclubs, drinking copiously, sharing food and seating with mere mortals. Where was his entourage on these occasions, his food specially prepared on the royal hearth by his wives alone, his throne on which no other dared to sit? Barely 40 years old, the mfen's heavy drinking was taking its toll; Njiké Pokam was very ill with cirrhosis of the liver. Rumors traveled the land regarding his inadequacies as a leader: the prefect and subprefect (prominent representatives of the Cameroonian government) could cleverly outtalk the relatively uneducated king; some found questionable his decisions regarding economic development and the construction of the new paved road; and he had failed to reopen sacred fields to cultivation by the royal wives and queen mothers, even threatening to sell the land to a developer. He occasionally broke out in rage and beat his wives. While some domestic violence was expected in royal marriages, in which "a wife should never turn her back on her husband" for fear of his immense power, the mfen may have gone too far. Twelve of the 16 wives he had married since acceding to the throne had run away, preferring self-imposed exile to palace life.

Mfen Njiké Pokam's difficulties were both personal problems *and* part of a process of loss of control and influence experienced by Grassfields kingdoms in the contemporary Cameroonian context. This process affects not only kingdom–state relations and the influence of the king over the newly wealthy or educated elite. It is also felt in the intimate relations of palace life, where royal wives throughout the Grassfields have less political power than in the past, more need for cash, and fewer means to obtain cash than women married to nonroyals. Many royal wives were given to their husbands as pawns in their fathers' attempts to curry favor with the king. As Goheen describes for the western Grassfields kingdom of Nso', "being the wife of a *fon* [mfen] today is not an enviable position," and many wives leave their marriages (1996:34).

As a naive, young urban woman, marriage to her king at first seemed a glamorous prospect to Paulette. She claimed that she was quickly married, because the king "was in a hurry." After so many of his wives had left the palace, Njiké Pokam was eager to prove marital success by acquiring two new wives in 1985, Paulette and Corinne. The king's expansion of his harem, and Paulette's royal romance, were short-lived; their marriage was plagued by a host of difficulties and lasted only eight months.

Bangangté families check genealogies to insure that a marriage will not result in incest, which they believe can cause a host of problems, including infertility. Misfortune occurs particularly easily if sensitive maternal ancestresses are angered by an improper marriage. The king's advisers did check Paulette's complex maternal kin relations for danger of incest. But in the mfen's rush to marry Paulette, no one bothered to check the usually more straightforward patriline. Paulette's great-grandfather, however, was a king of Bangangté, and Njiké Pokam was his heir. Paulette's *ndap*,[2] her praise name indicating her village of origin, was *So'nyu* or "daughter of the mfen of Bangangté." Njiké Pokam was Paulette's classificatory father. Paulette's family was angered at her marriage and had never visited her since her marriage to the king. Paulette often mentioned her family's anger and rejection sadly, explaining that her family considered her polluted through her marriage, and therefore she could not share food, drink, or utensils with her kin. Fear of pollution may have been only one reason why her family avoided Paulette. "Checking" genealogies during marriage negotiations is usually the role of parents; it is possible that Paulette's family rejected her not only because of her classificatory incest, but because she had not consulted them about her marriage. Certainly Paulette's royal marriage started off on a sad note, and she felt quite alone.

Marriage to the king of Bangangté was no fairy-tale life of a princess rescued from hardship and delivered to luxury. On the other hand, Bangangté royal marriage did not entail entering a wasp nest of jealousy, as described in the dark visions of many village nonroyals. Cowives often formed close bonds and supported each other through the trials and tribulations of agricultural and domestic labor, childbirth and illness. They also had conflicts, and there was plenty of room for intrigue as the king's wives navigated the twists and turns of both formal and informal hierarchies of court life. By late June 1986, when Paulette left the royal household, I had witnessed shifting friendships and enmities, alliances and splits among the king's fourteen wives. Paulette, groping to find her place within the complex rules of the court and the many personalities of her cowives, was often implicated in the verbal altercations that peppered court life.

Ranking and Regulation among the King's Wives

In the formal hierarchy of royal wives, only four have ranked titles, unrelated to age or marriage order. The first two, *mabengoup* and *nzwikam,* are chosen by the *nkam be'e* (the council of nine notables) and "captured" and initiated at the same time as a new mfen is "captured" for his initiation. Each of these titled queens presides over a neighborhood of royal wives, organizing work and watching over their cowives. The first queen, the mabengoup (Josette during Njiké Pokam's reign), determines the order in which her cowives "work in the palace," cook the king's meals, and sleep with him. She thus controls sexual access to the king. In the related Grassfields kingdom of Nso', the two highest ranked royal wives share this role and are thus able to choose the women who will bear the sons who could become the next *fon* (king) (Goheen 1996:34). They therefore play a central part in the physical reproduction of the royal household, the social reproduction of power, and intrigue among the king's wives. In Bangangté, strong sentiments of appropriate behavior urge the first queen to rotate wives, letting all have equal sexual access to the king and equal chances to bear his children and potential heirs. Conflicts often disrupt this order, and it is the formal responsibility of the wives with the third and fourth ranked titles to mitigate these conflicts and make the royal compound "tranquil." The king chooses these third and fourth wives, titled *makokwa* and *tsiyang,* upon concluding his nine weeks in the initiation hut. During Njiké Pokam's reign, these were Rebecca and Marguerite. They found dispute prevention and resolution challenging and often turned to their untitled cowives for help.

Although lacking formal rank, some elderly wives, often widows of the king's father or grandfather, were respected for their wisdom and skills at conciliation. Che'elou, who long ago had been the king's nursemaid, was particularly treasured as a peacemaker. Some middle-aged or even younger wives were influential through their oratorical skills or through their distribution of food and goods to cowives or their children. They gained the means to do so through hard work, gifts, or wage employment. For example, Claude, a salaried high school teacher, took on the responsibility for the school fees of several of her cowives' children. Based on her "presentability" to the modern world rather than her ability to manage a traditional royal household, the king also chose an untitled wife as his "Madame" (*zimewe*), the wife who accompanies him on official occasions. Again, Claude was often the mfen's "Madame." Agricultural productivity and childbearing contributed to each wife's respect, and also became objects of envy. The most recently born child of the king was doted on by all; its mother could enjoy occasional relief from child-rearing tasks, but also feared the jealousy of her less fortunate cowives. Some unranked wives wielded no particular influence, and the influence of all unranked wives was often quite temporary.

The young recently married wives were, and still are, assigned as "daughters" to their senior cowives. Establishing a relation of dependency, the senior cowife guides the young woman in her new wifehood and teaches her the special rules and duties of being a royal wife in exchange for services rendered by the "daughter." This places newlywed brides at the bottom of the formal and informal hierarchies of court life. Two generations ago when the mfen had many wives, some prepubescent, this arrangement also helped integrate and parent a large number of child brides.

Che'elou and Sanke as Young Wives. Two elderly wives (widows of the king's grandfather, Njiké II, who had been inherited in turn by each successor to the throne and are still considered wives of the king), Che'elou (born between 1900 and 1905), and Sanke (born 1928) were married as young girls, probably aged seven or eight years. Both recall their marriages and their years of tutelage under the guidance of a senior cowife.

> I was born in Bangwa. My father, mfen Nya, ran out of the village. They brought me when I was still a baby to Bangangté. My father, a chief, was a slave, that's to say under the authority of the king of Bangangté. It is my father who gave me to the king of Bangangté. I was not yet big, had no breasts, nothing. I stayed with the mabengoup [first queen] of the late Njiké, before I grew. It was Njiké who arranged to take care of me. I was taking care of the baby of mabengoup before I grew and became the wife of the king. I only took care of the baby. I did nothing else. (Che'elou)

> When I was a small child, I arrived at the palace. If the queen mother hadn't pointed me out, the king would not have sent his royal retainers to fetch me. My father was a noble in the king's service, and I was living with my grandmother following my mother's death. Because I arrived at the palace so young, I lived near the king, who gave me to a "nurse" [an elder cowife]. There were many of us there, and we learned to serve palm wine. Each group of girl-wives had their particular tasks, one for the laundry, one for the plates, one to bathe the king . . . It was well-organized, not like today when everyone does a little of everything. Only when I had full breasts did I become the full wife of Njiké . . . Finally, I gave birth to the children of Pokam [Njiké's son and heir]. (Sanke)

When Che'elou and Sanke were young wives, "daughterhood" was a form of fostering. The senior wife would raise the young child (her cowife), bringing her to adulthood as well as teaching her the special duties and regulations of royal wifehood (e.g., dietary restrictions for the king, schedules for cooking and sexual access to the king, restrictions on receiving guests). Each of the prepubescent royal wives was assigned one particular task and was socialized into palace life. The young wives were considered children, expected to laugh and play as well as to work and learn. Only after puberty did the young "daughter" wives obtain the wifely duties of intercourse, cooking for the mfen, and bearing his children. Che'elou and Sanke independently concur that this change of status was unmarked by ritual.

This fostering arrangement among cowives within the royal court is common in Bamiléké and Bamum palaces, and is described in Egerton for Bangangté (1938:304), Ndachi Tagne for a fictitious Bamiléké kingdom (1986), and Tardits for Bamum (1985:126). In these accounts, the young wives might live individually with their "mothers" and her children, or in a dormitory arrangement with approximately twelve girls together in one house under the tutelage of a senior cowife. Ndachi Tagne describes how such arrangements can lead to an enduring relation of mutual protection and support among two adult women. In Bangangté, the close emotional feeling "daughters" have for their cowife "mothers" may remain even after the "mothers" have died. In 1986 Josette was excited to find her "mother" among Egerton's 1937 photos of Njiké II's wives and fondly pointed her "mother" out to her cowife contemporaries.

A number of factors have contributed to the current transformation of the "mother–daughter" cowife institution. First, wives no longer are married to the king before puberty. Second, a long socialization period into royal wifehood is no longer necessary because many of the regulations of palace life either have broken down or are no longer practiced. Other changes in the royal compound may contribute to the continuation of this institution in a new form. The interests of the supporters of the institution and those socializing the young wives (the king and his senior wives) may no longer be based upon expectations of future rewards from a large group of well socialized junior cowives. Instead, they seek immediate rewards. The "mother" cowives use their adult junior "daughter" cowives as servants, exploiting them economically. Through having dependents, the "mothers" gain social as well as economic prestige. The king gains by marrying sexually mature wives in weak positions who are dependent upon their "mother" cowives and cannot easily run away. This adds to his number of wives during a time of decline, adds fertile women to the royal family, and rewards senior cowives, inducing them to stay.

Paulette and Corinne as Newlyweds in the Royal Court. After the mfen married Paulette and Corinne, the two young women were integrated into the hierarchy of *njwi* mfen, the king's wives. Paulette was "assigned" or "given" by the king to her senior cowife, Claude, the king's French wife. Corinne became the "daughter" of Louise, the *nzwikam* or second queen and my hostess for the first four months of my fieldwork in the royal compound. The foster mother cowives were to guide the two young wives in their new royal wifehood. Although Corinne and, particularly, Paulette aided their "mothers" in housekeeping and agricultural work, they slept in the palace building rather than in the houses of their "mothers." A generation before, as we have seen for Che'elou, Sanke, and Josette, "daughter" cowives were prepubescent girls and slept with their guardian mothers. Like other sexually mature wives, Paulette and Corinne slept in the palace and worked their cowives' fields. Once they became pregnant, they would acquire their own farms and their own kitchen-huts.[3] Although this was consistent with past practices, it also meant that Paulette and Corinne, adult newlyweds, had no independent resources to use for themselves or to redistribute to gain the favor of their other cowives.

"Daughterhood" was uncomfortable for both these women, but most difficult for Paulette. Corinne had retained both her ties to her family and, it was rumored, her professional connections from her time as a prostitute in Bafoussam, the provincial capital. Corinne was scorned by her cowives for her "prostitution" (this may have meant the exchange of sex for payment, or merely extramarital sexual encounters), but admired for her independence. She had options to her marriage to the king, which gave her a position of relative strength within the royal compound. Paulette, in contrast, had almost no ties remaining outside the royal compound. None of the royal wives ranked lower than Paulette, and during her eight months in the royal compound daughterhood for Paulette changed from a dependent and protective relation to a dependent and exploitative one.

In addition to her low formal status within the royal compound, Paulette suffered from the negative informal evaluations of her cowives. They were suspicious of her unfamiliar city background and associated her former employment as a maid with servility and prostitution. Her cowives also scorned Paulette's alleged lack of village knowledge; they thought that, had she been schooled in village customs, she would never have been married so unhappily to her "father" the mfen. Not trained in agriculture, she could not be very helpful to her cowives. None of them were very fond of Paulette, a slow and sloppy worker who in their eyes laughed too much.

These negative evaluations of Paulette affected her daily interaction with her cowives. During her last five months in the royal compound she became involved in increasingly serious quarrels with her cowives and was always the most vulnerable actor in these disputes. Many of the quarrels began as accusations of using another wife's cooking ingredients or kerosene, often goods that had been set aside to prepare the king's meals (and meal preparation is the key to sexual access). In March 1986, the king beat Paulette in a fit of drunken anger, and Paulette fled to the women's quarter, seeking refuge in the house shared by Claude and Jeanne. Tensions mounted when Paulette at first rejected her cowives' advice to return to the palace. Even after she had resumed her duties as a young wife, Paulette was accused by Josette that she "did not know how to make babies or find them at market" and had instead stolen Josette's baby from her belly. Even though Josette was secretly ridiculed by her cowives for tragically insisting (for months) that she was pregnant despite all evidence to the contrary, this was still a serious accusation. Josette was the mabengoup, the king's wife of highest formal rank, and Paulette was an untitled newlywed, unschooled in village life and palace etiquette. It was also an ironic accusation, given Paulette's childless state and search for conception.

Paulette's Belly and the Redefinitions of Her Plight

Based on the examination of medical records, lengthy accounts by Paulette and her "mother" Claude, commentary by other royal wives, and my direct observations, we can piece together a story of Paulette's affliction and quest for therapy running parallel to that of Paulette's failed marriage to the king. Given Bangangté assumptions of the sociogenic nature of most reproductive disorders, the two stories are closely related.

In December 1985, about six weeks after her marriage, Paulette complained to her "mother" that her "belly bothered" her. According to "mother" Claude, Paulette complained of menstrual cramps, and Claude recommended that Paulette seek the help of an unspecified healer, "for psychological reasons." Claude knew that, as a newlywed, Paulette was under stress. Paulette gave a different reason for seeking a healer. "Medical remedies" of the hospital can treat the pain (symptoms), but only a healer can identify the cause and treat the origin of the pain with "indigenous medicine." When she had a scalp condition a few months earlier, Paulette had consulted Felix, a *ngakà* (healer, person of medicine) in his mid-thirties who combined biomedical and indigenous elements in his practice. In late December she consulted him again regarding her "belly." Felix said Paulette's problems originated in the palace, which Paulette understood as a warning that her unfriendly cowives were mystically attacking her. Her aching belly became the symptom of a crisis in her new marital situation, which for Paulette was infused with drama and intrigue. She sought to keep her visits to the healer secret from the palace children and from all her cowives except her "mother," Claude. She certainly did not tell her husband, the mfen, fearing his disapproval.

Felix gave Paulette a health booklet, an individual medical record of the type used in public hospitals, in which he recorded her complaint, his diagnosis and his treatment plan. Paulette's booklet contains the entry: "28.12.85, Maladie: Ventre. Trompes bouchés. Débouchement Fegondité [*sic*]"[4] with the stamp and signature of the healer. Thus, Felix defined the physical problem leading to Paulette's complaint of menstrual cramps as "plugged tubes," and the resulting problem to be solved by treatment as "stopped up fertility." He prescribed a series of eight remedies.

Paulette received her treatment in a number of visits to the healer. At the first visit Paulette received a medicinal powder. At the second visit the healer placed an egg in Paulette's vagina and, while a cord was tied around her waist, turned the egg around, removed it, and broke it into a plate. Hair and a black substance appeared in the plate along with the broken egg. Felix said that this was something that someone had put in Paulette's uterus to keep her from getting pregnant (a common explanation of failure to conceive). At the third visit, in February 1986, Felix gave Paulette some powdered medicine with the instructions to mix it with raffia wine and take it as an enema. She did this a number of days after her third visit, and it made her feel ill. On this occasion she described her health problem, suspicions about its cause, and visits to the ngakà to me. About one week later, on February 25, Claude, Paulette, and I drove to Felix's compound on the edge of Bangangté-town. We found the healer absent, but encountered him on the road during our drive back to the royal compound. He arranged to prepare Paulette's next medicine for her to pick up the following day. After a number of irregular and unsuccessful attempts to find Felix at his compound, Paulette eventually gave up this series of treatments.

Paulette's problems in the palace and concern about threats to her reproductive capacities did not end with the termination of her treatment regimen. Many interpretations of Felix's "the problem originates in the palace," including that of royal incest, would have been possible. Paulette believed her problems, and the hair and black substance blocking her reproductive organs, were caused by the malevolent activities of her cowives. Paulette was receptive to her healer's diagnosis because of her increasingly difficult situation in the royal compound. We have seen that Paulette was particularly vulnerable to other royal wives' anger and banter. She had no house or fields of her own. Rejected by her kin and with almost no formal education, she also had no culturally legitimate escape from the royal compound. Paulette's cowives were suspicious of her city origins and that she had worked as a domestic for a white man. They were disdainful of what they perceived as her ignorance about village ways. They also disapproved of her running away from the king after he beat her.

Initially, Paulette's dependency relation with her "mother" cowife was sometimes protective, mitigating her vulnerability in the face of her cowives and husband. However, during the time when Paulette most obviously sought Claude's physical protection from the king, their relation became progressively more bitter.

At first Claude was pleased that the king had assigned Paulette rather than Corinne to her. Soon after my arrival, Claude told me that while she sometimes seemed slow or stupid, Paulette was really quite intelligent. Her initial evaluation of her "daughter" did not, however, change Claude's loyalty to Jeanne, another cowife of Paulette's age, married to the mfen for seven years and mother of two. After Paulette had fled the king's rage, all three women shared the same crowded house for seven weeks. Tension increased between Paulette and these two senior cowives. When "mother" Claude became ill and irritable in late April, Paulette's situation worsened.

Paulette made efforts to please her "mother" cowife by washing and cooking, skills she had learned through her urban socialization and at her previous job as a maid for a European. Rather than improving her position, Paulette's servile behavior only increased her exploitation.

At the same time Claude's attitude toward her ward's therapy-seeking changed. When Felix attributed the illness to the evil machinations of Paulette's cowives, a socially disruptive explanation, Claude at first responded that menstrual cramps may be exacerbated by the psychological strain of fear of one's cowives. But in May and June, already disaffected with her ward, Claude indicated that Paulette's weakness of character made her susceptible to psychosomatic problems and to accepting her healer's supernatural explanations. She did not accept that malevolent forces, sent by her cowives of long standing, were working against her ward. She also denigrated Paulette's healer. She did not call him a healer, but rather a "sorcerer" (a second gloss for *ngakà*), emphasizing his magical and potentially sinister actions rather than his healing skills. With this shift in Claude's attitude, Paulette lost her only support in her quest for therapy.

By mid-June, Paulette was quite depressed at the failure of her strategy of servility to protect or improve her social situation in the palace. She explicitly described changes in her relationship with her "mother" cowife that made her feel abandoned. She claimed that Claude was formerly her solace, had cared for her well and made her feel better in her unhappy, rashly conceived marriage to the mfen. From Paulette's perspective, Claude had since become reclusive, verbally abusive, authoritarian, and impatient.

In this context Paulette redefined her initial reason for consulting healer Felix and reassessed her precocious termination of his treatment regimen. Paulette claimed she visited Felix to seek help to conceive. She said, "it is not good to stay in the palace a long time without children," but in her position it was "better not to become pregnant." Thus, in Paulette's last weeks in the palace compound she claimed it was her wish not to conceive rather than obstacles to therapy-seeking that made her give up her treatment.

Paulette finally devised ways to escape her unhappiness. In early June 1986 she briefly left the royal compound, sleeping at and moving some of her effects to her "aunt's" in Bangangté-town. Soon after this she either invented or elaborated a story of her mother's delivery of a child, and in late June another story of the baby's death and her mother's subsequent illness. This story created a need for Paulette to leave for Douala. Paulette tried to manage her leave-taking to protect her reputation by informing the appropriate people of her intention to help her mother in Douala. No one cared about her story, and her reputation was not saved. She ran away in the morning of June 26, 1986, into self-imposed exile in Douala. Because she had fled marriage with a powerful king, Paulette could not hope to remarry. Nonetheless, she received no sympathy from the cowives she had left behind. Eleven years later, Claude, Louise, and Josette all claimed they had heard no word about or from Paulette.

Concern with Procreation and Personal Mobility: Implications of Paulette's Experience

Why did Paulette leave her marriage? What worried her so much that she chose to live in self-imposed exile rather than stay at the palace of Bangangté? Her case lends itself to two readings that, taken together, are instructive for the themes of this book.

The first reading is from the point of view of medical anthropology, focusing on the social context of the meaning of Paulette's affliction, and of the therapeutic itinerary she pursued. Her case illustrates the negotiation of definition and redefinition, explanation, and treatment in the complex interactions typical of African therapeutics (see, e.g., Feierman 1981, 1985; Janzen 1978a, 1987). Paulette's reproductive health difficulties began with lower abdominal pain. Paulette's pain appeared when she was under strain in a new marriage and rejected by her family because of her incestuous marriage. On the advice of her guardian and senior cowife, Paulette sought the help of a tradipractitioner, a healer she had previously consulted and who she believed could discover and treat the underlying cause of her pain. This healer redefined her pain as a symptom of "stopped-up" fertility and plugged fallopian tubes. He found that the cause of the illness originated in the palace. Paulette suspected the malevolent activities of her cowives, further interpreting the healer's attribution of cause. When her guardian cowife rejected this explanation of Paulette's affliction, Paulette became increasingly isolated. Facing problems of access, she failed to complete her treatment regimen. Later, Paulette redefined her withdrawal from therapy as a change in her goals; she was no longer seeking conception but rather searching for an escape from an untenable situation.

This story of problem definition, quest for therapy, and termination of treatment could be retold in a different light. A young naive woman expected a fairy-tale romance of royal marriage, a strategy seemingly certain to enhance her social status and quality of life. Instead she found herself at the bottom of the status hierarchy in the complex, confusing, and unfamiliar world of court life. After eight months, she wanted out.

Paulette did not appear to be trying hard to get pregnant. In everyday conversations with me and with her cowives, she spoke more frequently and elaborately about making money and the indignities of being a junior cowife in *la grand polygamie* (large-scale polygamy) than about children, parenthood, or childlessness. When she did mention childlessness or children, it was in terms of how parenthood would improve her miserable status within the hierarchy of the royal compound. Nonetheless, Paulette's two stories of reproductive illness and an ill-fated strategy for personal mobility are linked. Paulette somaticized her psychological and social difficulties as pain in the belly and interpreted them in the rubric of threats to her procreative capacity. *Why did Paulette couch her woes about a crisis in her marriage and her relationship to her cowives in the language of reproductive illness?*

Paulette's perception of reproductive threats emerged from her difficulties as a newlywed in the royal compound, that household made up of the mfen, his wives, children, foster children, and a limited number of royal retainers. The challenges she faced (adapting to a new environment and marriage, proving her domestic skills and her fertility) confront all other Bangangté newlywed women as well, but are drawn into sharp relief by the particularities of Paulette's biography and of court life. Achieving motherhood was a ubiquitous goal for Bangangté women, essential for identity as a Bangangté woman, and an important element in attaining success in life. At a time when the means for success seemed out of reach to so many, Bangangté women feared for their ability to achieve motherhood as well. As for other Bangangté women, Paulette interpreted her struggles with identity and status in a framework of procreation and the metaphors of cooking, commensality, kitchens, and thieving, interfering witches that permeate Bangangté notions of procreation and social life.

Social Status and the Interpretation of Misfortune

In the context of a pervasive fear of infertility in Bangangté, Paulette used the idiom of procreative failure to organize and explain her experience of her marital difficulties and her declining social status. Paulette's concern with her unenviable social status and her wish for upward mobility helped create her crisis and shaped its outcome.

Bangangté are intensely aware of status, which they conceive of in terms of ranks of prestige and privilege.[5] The statuses engendered by a promotion system of titles centered in court life were an important source of personal identity in the past. But now the royal compound and its surrounding entourage of nobles and retainers is no longer the sole reference point for marking status. Like other Grassfields groups, Bangangté now have a number of status systems offering new opportunity structures and creating new dependency relations (den Ouden 1987). The worlds of commerce, church, education, and national politics also challenge a singularly Bangangté scheme of identities, combining it with a multiplex, ambiguous palette of identities typical of modernity (Calhoun 1994). Bangangté citizens like Paulette must negotiate among these new status and identity systems to maximize their health, wealth, and well-being.

Despite these shifting centers of reference, the community of the royal compound was sufficiently well-defined and relatively closed that the status system and social interactions within it became an overwhelming context during the history of Paulette's illness. The royal compound was all the more important as a reference point for Paulette due to her tiny social network in Bangangté and her lack of mobility both within and beyond Bangangté-town. Within the royal compound, Paulette was at the bottom rung of the formal status hierarchy among the king's wives. Within the informal status system, the evaluations of her cowives as played out in daily interaction within the royal compound and at the royal farms were also unfavorable. The older wives in particular were suspicious of Paulette's urban origin, since for them city life embodied threatening changes in images of tradition, Bangangté-ness, and gender. Paulette suffered from the often conflicting relations among her cowives and between the mfen and his wives. She became increasingly isolated and vulnerable in the verbal altercations that expressed and negotiated the informal status system of court life.

For Paulette, the formal and informal status systems among the king's wives meant a spiral of dissolving rewards. She did not meet her mostly rural cowives' expectations of a good wife and woman. Her marriage to the king did not meet her own expectations of upward personal mobility. In addition, Paulette's involvement in the quarrels so integral to large-scale polygyny, a "lack of tranquillity," made Paulette vulnerable in local belief. Many Bangangté believe that disruptions of authority relations—between husband and wife, among senior and junior cowives, between parents and children, and between the mfen and his subjects—contribute to envy and an uncontrolled practice of witchcraft. Paulette shared these images of social order and disorder playing themselves out in the realm of procreation. They became central to her perception of affliction.

Perception of Affliction

Both the importance of motherhood and assumptions about the dangers of court life contributed to the interpretation of Paulette's physical and psychosocial pain as an attack on her reproductive capacity. For untitled royal wives the only means to gain an enduring rise in status is through one's children, especially if one's son becomes the next mfen. Any of the king's sons could become the next king. Chosen officially by the king himself and announced by the council of nine highest nobles only after the king's death, no wife knows whose son is the heir apparent. This leads to competition among cowives for having children, and suspicions that a cowife might harm one's procreative ability.

Widely held assumptions about the sociogenic etiology of misfortune, and reproductive illness in particular, further contributed to Paulette's perception of her affliction. Most Bangangté women with little schooling, as Paulette, first think of "custom" (*ndonn,* including witchcraft, taboos, and ancestral wrath) when they search for causal explanations of their problems, especially those concerning reproductive health. While Bangangté women also believe in naturalistic causes of illness, such explanations are rarely invoked in cases of infertility. Against the background of widely shared beliefs regarding marriage, fidelity, envy, and witchcraft, Paulette redefined the problem of her aching belly. She assumed that malevolent acts initiated by her cowives would attack her reproductive rather than other bodily functions.

The emotional climate of the royal compound, the criticisms of the elderly wives, Paulette's dissatisfaction with her marriage, and the squabbles she became involved in all made Paulette receptive to her healer's diagnosis that her menstrual cramps were nothing so simple as a symptom of a normal physiological event. In her eyes, they must be a sign of the evil machinations of her cowives, the pain of her bad position in a bad marriage. Healer Felix's diagnosis, in turn, confirmed and perhaps increased Paulette's suspicion of the ill wishes of her cowives until she could stand it no longer and fled.

Paulette easily accepted her healer's attribution of cause due to particular features of her position in the royal compound. First, she was well aware of her low status within the palace and thus felt vulnerable to her cowives' malevolent activities. Second, she suspected that her cowives might be jealous that she was the powerful Claude's "daughter" and therefore might have access to more resources. Third, as a recently arrived young wife, she feared that her cowives might view her as a usurper of their sexual access to the mfen.

Paulette's position in the royal compound does not, however, explain why she did not regard her breaking of kinship and marriage regulations or ancestral wrath as the source of her illness. By ignoring this likely explanation, Paulette was reiterating images of contentious and dangerous relations among royal cowives. In this nest of jealous and competing women, as it was seen by many, Paulette was weak and vulnerable—and knew it. She was also putting the blame for her misfortunes on others, and neither on her own negligent behavior nor on that of the mfen, a powerful public figure who would be invulnerable to her feeble attacks.[6]

Paulette was faced with the dilemma of defining childlessness as a problem, on the one hand, and seeing motherhood as an impediment to gaining independence, on the other. But this was most likely only a temporary dilemma. Although becoming a parent is only one way Bangangté men and women seek to advance themselves under current conditions in Cameroon, the question even the most educated, urban woman faces is motherhood now or later. Paulette redefined her difficulties according to the strategies she chose. Paulette identified childlessness as a problem in her current social context, saying it is not good to be childless at the palace. In her attempts to gain independence within that context, Paulette viewed her most serious problem to be her low social status in the royal compound of Bangangté. When she finally fled palace life, Paulette decided to attempt personal advancement as an independent urban woman.[7] Thus, her case concerns not only a problem of reproductive illness, but also one of social mobility within the changing, differentiating context of contemporary Bangangté life.

As with much of Bangangté social interaction, the situations in which Paulette talked about her affliction centered around food. These situations arose during walks to market to buy cooking ingredients, chats around the hearth while preparing meals, and eating with cowives, guests, or, occasionally, kin. The prominence of cooking and eating metaphors in the imagery of procreation used by Bangangté women will become more evident in chapters 3 and 4. With regard to Paulette's case, healer Felix's diagnosis of plugged-up tubes fit with the fears of many rural Bangangté women of childbearing age that someone or something would interfere in the potential mixing of the procreative ingredients of semen and blood.

Paulette's abandonment and declining status was underlined by the refusal of Paulette's kin to eat with her. For Paulette, the image and reality of a warm and welcoming hearth disappeared.

Seeking Remedies

Compared to other Bangangté cases of seeking cures and solace for repro-ductive illness, Paulette's quest for therapy was uniquely narrow. Her small social network and her unfamiliarity with Bangangté limited her knowledge of health-care facilities, both indigenous and hospital-based. Paulette's relations with the various members of the royal household also affected the therapeutic advice she could seek from them. Paulette pre-sented her story differently, at turns confiding, utilitarian, secretive, or nonthreatening, to her various audiences within the royal court. Paulette's social isolation led her to attempt to create allies, relating her stories to some in confiding terms, keeping secrets from others. She needed to be dis-creet because she was weaker than her cowives. Paulette feared their wrath, and the malevolent activities it could lead them to, if they thought she were gossiping about them. Paulette also needed to prove, with her own case, that she could keep confidences in order to receive gossip about others. Being unfamiliar with Bangangté, gossip was Paulette's main avenue of information about her surroundings. Gossip about her neigh-bors' illnesses was also the major way to learn about health-care facilities and her contemporaries' evaluations of them. Paulette's social isolation thus decreased the flow of information to her.

Paulette made a clear distinction between "modern" and "indigenous" health-care institutions, as do most rural Bangangté women.[8] Consistent with her fears of witchcraft, Paulette sought a traditional healer's therapy. Felix, the healer she chose, gained legitimation and reputation via the sta-tus of his clients, some of whom were part of Bangangté's civil service elite. He was well-known and had been consulted by Paulette earlier for her ring-worm. Thus far Paulette's therapeutic itinerary appears typical.

While Bangangté women often complain of difficulties having chil-dren to lower level health workers when they go to hospitals or clinics for other health problems, they rarely consult caregivers from the hospital-based sector for infertility problems. Most assume a nonbiological cause out of the doctor's or nurse's realm of competence. On the level of practice in searching for alleviation from suffering, patients do not at all limit themselves to seeking a healer of the same category with which they label their illness, although that is generally where they start their therapeutic itineraries. They and their escorts will try many if not all available thera-pies, depending upon how long and through how many attempts at therapy the affliction persists before meeting success. Their search may or may not be accompanied by a redefinition of the illness to justify seeking help at another institution. This is an area where patients do not appear to be bothered by the very different premises of alternative forms of health care. Rather, they develop strategies of integration.

Paulette had no need to integrate multiple forms of health care because she consulted only one healer for this health problem. Here, her case is atypical for seeking a cure for reproductive afflictions. Paulette lacked not only knowledge, but also the social and material resources she needed when misfortune befell her. Not trained in village ways or agriculture, she could not be very helpful to her cowives, and they in turn showed little interest in investing resources for her care. They felt little sympathy for her. They observed no life-threatening symptoms and their sense of moral responsibility was not awakened. Only Paulette's "mother" and the mfen had jural responsibility for her well-being. Of these two, only Claude participated in Paulette's quest for therapy, and herself soon lost interest. Having grown up in Douala, Paulette had no acquaintances in Bangangté to whom she could turn for help. She also could not solicit aid from her kin, who had broken off relations with Paulette since her disapproved marriage to the king.

Because Paulette was a new wife with no fields, she had no income with which to pay for treatment, medicine, or transportation. She also had no skills that would allow her legitimate employment, and no capital to start a trading business to earn needed money. Not only did her social isolation prevent her from getting needed material resources from others, her position as a new wife prevented her from gaining these resources herself.

Paulette's surprisingly narrow quest for therapy, while reflecting her lack of knowledge, social, and material resources, may also have been a function of what she was trying to accomplish by visiting a healer. Paulette may have been using her affliction to gain recognition and support. Initially, this strategy worked for Paulette. She was able to solicit advice and help from her cowife "mother" and awakened the curiosity of the resident ethnographer. In the end, however, Paulette lost her "mother's" interest and failed to gain support from other cowives and kin. Once she left the palace, her cowives derided her and seemed to imply that her affliction was an attention-getting fake.

Paulette appeared to be using her affliction and search for cure as a means to social ends. She was concerned with more than relieving physical symptoms. Building upon Parson's notion of the sick role (Parsons 1951) numerous studies have investigated the at least ephemeral power of affliction, especially within African possession cults. They posit that affliction focuses attention on the dispossessed and affords the muted the license to express their concerns (and sometimes resistance) to the more powerful members of society (Boddy 1989; Lewis 1966; Rasmussen 1995; V. W. Turner 1968). For example, Karp examines rites of possession among the Iteso of Kenya in terms of indigenous concepts of power, asserting that for Iteso women, "possession can be resistance, a form of female assertion against males or competition with co-wives, play, or even relative deprivation" (1989:93). Among the Iteso, undergoing the possession and curing rituals brings about a change in the relationship of women to power, through changing definitions of "the person, her rights, duties, and the attitudes displayed towards her" (1989:105), and this transformation allows women, at least temporarily, to act against the male sources of jural power.

Karp's analysis is both compelling and instructive, but cases like Paulette's expression of social difficulties through reproductive affliction are more diffuse and individualistic than instances in which such problems can be channeled into known, recognized possession cults. Paulette's search for remedies represented the attempt of an individual to seek solace for her declining ability, and it only marginally challenged male jural authority, if at all. Shaw's study of Temne women's consultations with diviners in Sierra Leone (1985) provides comparative material that more closely fits Paulette's case. Public divination searching for the cause of affliction tends to reiterate a view of Temne society in which maleness is considered a symbol of order and femaleness a potential menace. Temne women, however, consult private diviners, seeking supportive diagnoses that they nonetheless keep secret "because of the antagonism with which their husband's families would probably react" (1985:296). A woman's private diagnosis, kept secret, does not allow her subjective experience to be publicly objectified, but reaffirms her own experience of reality. Shaw contrasts more common analyses of the "politics of definitions" in divination with a "politics of experienced reality" (1985:300). Paulette at first sought the power that attention to her plight might bring her, as implied in Karp's analysis. When she failed, her visits to healer Felix became a search for solace and affirmation that her misfortunes were something done to her. This solace was largely private, shared with a few and kept secret from her husband and more and more of her cowives. In the end, solace alone was inadequate, and Paulette withdrew from her difficult situation by running away.

The Wider Context: Personal Mobility and Images of Royal Decline

Paulette's case illustrates one woman's images of threats to her reproductive capacities and the action she took to alleviate her problems. Other

Bangangté observing Paulette's case referred to it as an example of the decline of palace life and the strength of the kingship. They often described this decline in the concrete terms of this and similar cases, using Paulette's alleged sterility and flight as metaphors of a kingdom that has become sterile and cannot hold on to its population. Three aspects of Paulette's case refer to prominent images of decline in Bangangté: depressed fertility among the royal wives, and by extension of the kingdom's population and agricultural land as a whole; contentious relations among royal wives and other Bangangté citizens, indicating the breakdown of rules of respect and mechanisms of dispute management; and Paulette's flight from the royal compound, the last of thirteen young wives who allegedly ran away from mfen Njiké Pokam.

The king's wives, including those more favorably positioned than Paulette, are preoccupied with threats to their reproductive capacities. They experience recent change in Bangangté traditional organizations as a dissolving reward system and thus as diminishing social status. For example, with the disappearance of *masou* (an association of the mfen's wives, sisters, and queen mothers), their political power has been pushed entirely behind the scenes. The royal wives also view changes in the institution of kingship as decline, as the prestige and material rewards of kingship are closely linked to their own status. Since the mfen is no longer omnipotent, but must share power with the state, it is no longer very prestigious to be a king's wife. The mfen can no longer demand tribute and is poorer than past kings. He is also not the richest in the land since his subjects may be better able to take advantage of new economic opportunities. As a result the king has fewer riches to share with his wives than some of his subjects, should he choose to be generous with the women who feed him. Due to the breakdown of norms governing relations between husbands and wives, the current king is less willing to share his albeit minimal wealth with his wives than oral and written accounts suggest for past mfens. Because the royal wives' participation in outside economic activities is restricted, they often suffer more material hardship than their village neighbor women. They receive no help from these neighbors in agricultural labor, but must produce a surplus to support the feasts hosted by the king. Royal wives' hopes of reaching the top of the social hierarchy for women are disappointed by these harsh realities.

Other changes further complicate the royal wives' position. Differences in formal education, alternative forms of income earning to traditional food crop agriculture, and the need to interact with such modern institutions as hospitals, schools, and the registry office make differentiations among royal wives that did not exist previously. In addition, many young women have new expectations from marriage, including romantic love and economic support, that cannot be met in the context of royal marriage. This difficult situation has led Paulette and a dozen of her cowives to run away.[9]

The changes in palace life that contributed to Paulette's unhappiness are viewed as unfavorable change only by certain social segments, those who perceive benefits from the maintenance of strongly traditional social structures in Bangangté. Those who do not suffer, and even advance through the changing reward and prestige systems in Bangangté, view these changes as progress. While many say palace life and the power of the king are declining, the images they use to describe social change are those found in the state-run media to rally the population into a unified and prosperous modern state: development, democratization, autonomy, and progress. By contrast, recent changes in Bangangté offer the least attractive new opportunities and diminish the honor and rewards of the women with whom I worked. These women also describe social change and their downward social mobility with images of violence, trickery, and reproductive failure. Divergent views of both social change and reproductive illness emerge from Bangangté citizens' experiences with the structure and process of social differentiation, and thus from their varying interests and points of view. The differing ways these two groups of Bangangté view social change and health indicate the importance of status changes in the distribution of beliefs about health and society.

The kind of status change one experiences (i.e., downward or upward mobility) is often a function of gender. Men are in the majority in the group profiting from recent changes, even if they must often migrate to do so. Although rural Grassfields women (and rural African women in general) have been described as dispossessed (Goheen 1996; Moore 1994), the experience of rural Bangangté women confronted with profound changes varies as well. We can predict some of this variation by examining different women's position in terms of prestige and reward within households, and of the household within a developmental cycle of domestic groups. Further differences emerge if we include the new, educated, salaried or commercial elite. Women who are part of this group mostly migrate to towns and cities for employment and/or marriage, and are not the focus of this book. Paulette's situation offered some similarities to that of many young newlyweds in a rural polygynous household, although royal wifehood is a special case and her degree of social isolation was extreme. Distinguishing among categories of women and men helps us to understand the interaction of the structure and dynamics of social differentiation with variation in health beliefs in a changing context. The process through which new distinctions among social groups are made, and old distinctions gain new meaning, engenders new idioms about reproductive illness and alters the distribution of health beliefs among different social segments.

Paulette's case has illustrated the complexities and contradictions of one woman's reproductive ills. Her story is unique, but emblematic of the multiple contradictions of life in Bangangté and in similar communities throughout Africa. Paulette was caught among several tugs-of-war in negotiating status and identity: between the city and the country, modern life and tradition, natal family and marriage, economic productivity and the search for status. Women's roles emerge through this case study as multifaceted, even when limited to a special subset of rural women, the royal wives. On the one hand, the court women serve as pawns and labor in the maneuverings of male politics and marriage alliances. On the other hand, these women participate in these games of gender and power through their roles in regulating sex and reproduction, contributing or withholding food from royal feasts, safeguarding or disrupting the details of royal protocol, and in socializing the next generation of royalty. These women nonetheless face many sources of vulnerability and uncertainty. For Paulette, the contrast between her role expectations and her social status is brought out in sharp relief. This contrast, however, is present for all Bangangté women as they struggle with what it means to be Bangangté and how to manage the practical relations that tie together kinship, household, village, and kingdom. In the following chapters we shall see how the imagery of social integration reiterates the imagery of procreation, linking the two closely in Bangangté consciousness.

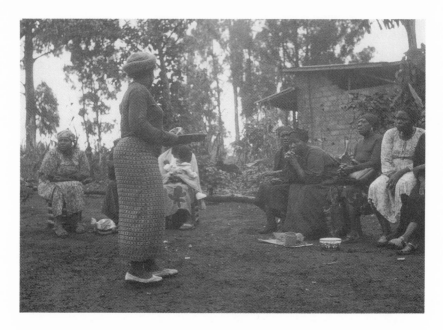

Fig. 2. Marguerite addressing her neighborhood *tontine* (rotating credit association) in Batela', near the royal compound of Bangangté. Cameroonians recognize that the Bamiléké, more than any other ethnic group, have developed the tontine into a powerful form of social cohesion.

Chapter Two

Being Bangangté:
Social Organization and Identity

Vignette 1:   Learning to Be Cameroonian or
Learning to Be Bangangté

*André, a 10-year-old boy living at the royal compound, was chatting
with my husband about where various acquaintances were from. They
were talking about the familial, village, and national identity of both
André's friends and Joachim's relatives. Without any prodding, André
announced, "I am Cameroonian." Surprised, Joachim then pursued the
issue, reminding André that he is a son of the king. André insisted that
he is Cameroonian first, Bangangté second.*

*André grew up speaking only Bangangté, just like his preschool half
siblings and neighbors in Batela' village. He witnessed and participated
in funerals, royal convocations, and tagged along with his mother to
tontine (rotating credit association) meetings. He thus took part in
some of the daily traffic holding adult Bangangté life together. In his
imaginary play, André reenacted contemporary Bangangté household
life, building a play house and practicing gender roles with his brothers
and sisters. But starting at age three or four, André learned poems and
songs in French while attending* école maternelle *(nursery school). In
primary school he sang the national anthem, indicating that the earth
cradling his ancestors' skulls and tying him to his homeland was not just
the earth of Bangangté, but of the nation: "O Cameroun berceau de nos
ancêtres . . ."*

Elderly Bangangté say things have changed more since independence than
during the colonial era. They refer to the prestige and power of the mfen,
economic relations, missions, schools, and to their grandchildren who, like
André, seem to be weakening their identification with the kingdom.
Indeed, a significant challenge for Bangangté men and women of all ages
is managing the sometimes contradictory demands of Bangangté royal

41

authority and the centralized Cameroonian state. Within this context, Bangangté are concerned with getting ahead, and sometimes just getting by. Their well-being is closely tied to being Bangangté, both in terms of the effect they believe the spiritual and political strength of the kingship has on their health and fortune and in terms of the use to which they can put ethnic ties when seeking their fortune in Cameroon, and even abroad. Many Bangangté fear that their small kingdom is losing population and power in the midst of Cameroon's economic and political hardship and increasingly global involvement.

Bangangté worry nowadays about social reproduction, about what it means and will mean to be Bangangté and where they fit in. In particular, rural Bangangté women worry about their ability to contribute to social reproduction through procreation and the socialization of their children. They have a particular vision of what kind of Bangangté individuals and society they would like to reproduce. Their vision of being Bangangté is one among many in contemporary Bangangté, a society with multiple and shifting centers of orientation. To best understand why Paulette was worried about her womb, and why her cowives and neighbors were worried about Paulette, we need to examine rural women's vision of being Bangangté and to situate their way of being Bangangté in the context of other experiences of Bangangté life.

From rural women's point of view, kinship, marriage, neighborliness, and actively participating in royal festivals are all part of being Bangangté. Children and food are essential to maintaining each of these forms of affiliation. Raising children and sharing food draw families together and are the purpose of family life among the living. Children (having descendants) and food (making offerings) please the ancestors and establish ties between generations living and dead. Children and food also draw the kingdom together, in a homologous polity-family relationship. The king, through his initiation and coronation ceremonies, becomes procreator- and provider-in-chief. In the context of shifting and multiple centers, in which identity systems are unclear and complex, the relative weakness of the divine kingship has been experienced in terms of an existential threat to provisioning the family with food and children. Thus, this structured set of relations that makes people Bangangté also promotes a particular understanding of procreation and frames women's high fertility goals.

This chapter is about these multilayered aspects of experience that make people feel "Bangangté" and how these individuals—in all their variety—who identify themselves with Bangangté are organized to constitute Bangangté society.[1]

Bangangté's Context: Cameroon and the Bamiléké

The contemporary sense (or senses) of being and feeling Bangangté is embedded in a web of practical relations among kin, neighbors, villages, and the hierarchy of the system of royal titles and promotions. These relations only make sense in a wider setting, placing Bangangté of the 1980s and 1990s within the context of the historical, political-economic, social, and cultural changes confronting the Bamiléké peoples and Cameroon.

The Republic of Cameroon is an ethnically and geographically diverse country on the "hinge" between west and central Africa (see fig. 3). Numerous peoples have passed through and sometimes settled in its territory over the past two thousand years of African history and population movement. One of the most historically dynamic regions of the territory is the Bamiléké highlands of the eastern Grassfields, a high plateau region wedged between dry savanna and sahel to the now predominantly Muslim north and rain forest to the now predominantly Christian south. It is currently one of the most densely populated areas of Cameroon, whose 167 inhabitants per square kilometer in parts of the Western Province in 1966 (Koenig 1977:58) contrast with Cameroon's average population density of 16/km^2 at the time of the 1976 census (Dongmo 1981:21). Together the circa one hundred Bamiléké kingdoms comprise about 25 percent of Cameroon's population. Bangangté is one of the most prominent of the Bamiléké kingdoms, and one of the five Bamiléké administrative centers in the Western Province (see fig. 4).

The earliest Bamiléké kingdoms were formed during the sixteenth century, a result of a complex dynamic of conquest, ruse, and shifting allegiance when population movements in Adamoua pushed the "pre-Tikar" Ndobo into the Bamiléké plateau (Notué and Perrois 1984:10–14). This epoch is portrayed in the "hunter-king" legends of the founders of many of today's rulers, including Bangangté.[2]

Succession disputes, the search for new hunting grounds, and demographic pressure led to the emergence of new kingdoms from the first core polities. The number, size, and shape of Bamiléké kingdoms continued to change until European colonization, when interkingdom warfare was curtailed and the limits of territories were frozen at borders partly determined by the colonizers (Dongmo 1981:45; Tardits 1960:17; interviews). This history of shifting borders, alliances, and the influx of refugees from neighboring kingdoms makes each kingdom a political composite of diverse peoples owing allegiance to the king (*mfen* in Bangangté, *fo* or *fon* in other kingdoms) and established royal institutions (Notué and Perrois 1984:10).

Relations among kingdoms included economic exchange and cooper-

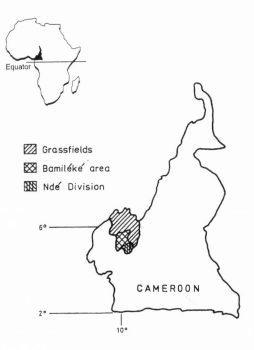

Fig. 3.   Map of Cameroon

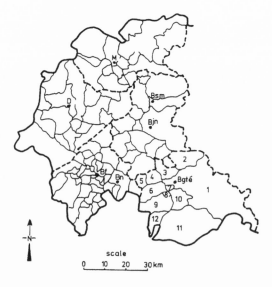

Fig. 4.   Map of Bamiléké kingdoms, showing the kingdoms of Ndé Division, of which Bangangté is the administrative capital (adapted from Dongmo 1981:46)

ation as well as territorial belligerence. In the seventeenth, eighteenth, and nineteenth centuries, regional trading networks linked the Grassfields polities, including Bangangté and other Bamiléké kingdoms, to parts of what would become Cameroon and Nigeria (Warnier 1985). Ivory, palm oil, wood, iron implements, and slaves flowed through these networks and on to Europe (Koenig 1977:77; Warnier 1985). The slave trade in the Grassfields was surrounded by mystification, "medicine," and deception, as heads of households, occasionally overwhelmed by obligations, allegedly sold their young relatives in secret (Warnier 1985). The cultural legacy of insecurity is evident in fears of population decline and of secret wealth and power gained, through sorcery, at the expense of one's own kind. In fact, this trope of forces draining the wealth, health, and population of the kingdom organizes Bangangté and other Grassfields peoples' collective memories of colonial rule, civil war, independence, and multi-party strife.

European contact with what is now Cameroon began with the arrival of Portuguese traders in 1472. The colonial period began on July 12, 1884, when the Duala kings made a treaty with the German Empire. Between 1914 and 1916 the German colony of Kamerun was conquered by French and British forces. It was divided between the two nations by League of Nations mandate, and continued as a UN Trusteeship after World War II. The division between French and British Cameroon ran through the Grassfields; Bangangté and most other Bamiléké kingdoms were on the French side.

The early colonizers found a rich and cultivated territory, maintaining multiple commercial relations as evidenced by paths and markers, as two German colonial officials, Strumpell and Müller, reported from their 1902 and 1904 expeditions into Bamiléké territory (cited in Tardits 1960:66). Then, as now, women were the primary producers of food crops (maize, beans, and peanuts). Men's cash crop cultivation of coffee and cocoa, shop-keeping, and taxi and truck driving have replaced precolonial involvement in animal husbandry and war. Oral and archival evidence shows Bangangté, among the Bamiléké kingdoms, to be a relative latecomer to the production of coffee.[3] Mfen Njiké II, who reigned from the end of the German colonial period until 1943, discouraged the production of coffee; he feared cash crop production would loosen his control on the fortunes of his subjects and distract labor from politically and symbolically important food production. French agricultural policy from 1920 through 1950 also favored production of food crops (Tardits 1960:77), but with different intent than that of Njiké II. Aiming to feed the growing cities and commercial plantations, French agricultural policy encouraged the small-scale commercialization of women's food crops, starting in the 1930s.

The confluence of colonial and indigenous policies contributed to changes in gender relations and household economies that had begun at the turn of the twentieth century. Both German and French colonizers used forced labor for public works, officially ending only in 1946. The Grassfields was a major labor recruitment area for road, railroad, and plantation work (DeLancey 1978; Rudin 1938:324–27; Tardits 1960). Responding to an expanding need for cash, and seeking to escape restrictions imposed by the kings, young Bamiléké men increasingly migrated to southern commercial centers during the French colonial period. The Bamiléké area continues to be a largely agricultural region from which large numbers of youth emigrate in search of work, sometimes temporarily, sometimes permanently (Dongmo 1981:44). This long history of labor migration has demographic consequences and also poses a challenge to a Bamiléké cultural identity based on ties to the land and to one's king. In the late 1980s, the overall population of the Bamiléké was approximately two million, only one million of whom resided on the Bamiléké plateau. Since the 1950s, Bangangté kingdom has remained one of the most consistent sources of labor migration from the Bamiléké region to other parts of Cameroon.

The comparative absence of young men facilitates the polygynous marriages of older men (about half of rural Bangangté marriages are polygynous) and means that wives are often considerably younger than their husbands. As we shall see in chapters 3 and 4, male labor migration leaves many rural women as de facto heads of households, at least temporarily. It increases the repertoire of tasks women must do and may give them more independence, but also renders them more vulnerable. The impact of colonial and postcolonial regimes in Cameroon on rural women's lives endures.

Political steps toward independence, especially the outlawing of the trade union–based Union des Populations Camerounaise (UPC), led to civil war in the years surrounding independence (gained in 1960), concentrated first in the Bassa and then in the Bamiléké area (Joseph 1977). Personal and political scars from these "troubles" are still visible in the Western Province today. Ndé Division, of which Bangangté is the capital, remained at least through 1986 officially in a state of emergency. But more importantly for our subject of fear of infertility, many believe that the civil war of 1958 through 1972 gave potential witches "the taste for blood." The memory of the vindictiveness of the times, combined with the recent political turmoil since 1990, contributes to mistrust of the state and a sense of vulnerability to mystical attack. Women in particular fear attacks on their reproductive capacity.

Cameroon's colonial history left a legacy of official bilingualism and dual legal and educational systems. This complexity combines with further heterogeneity in religion, ecology, demography, and ethnic affiliation. Approximately 250 ethnic groups reside within its borders. Its variety of ethnic groups, forms of local political organization, and heterogeneous colonial heritage faced the politicians of newly independent Cameroon with the challenge of forging national unity out of diversity. A solution was found via Cameroon's one-party government with power centered in the president. Ahmadou Ahidjo, president from independence in 1960 to 1982, pursued a policy of regional balance. Paul Biya, his successor, developed a philosophy of "communal liberalism" and national integration during the first five years of his rule (Biya 1987). During this time he introduced some democratic innovations. Recently coronated mfen Nji Monluh Seidou Pokam benefited when his faction won in the first multiple-slate municipal elections, held in 1987. A constitutional change in December 1990 permitted the formation of new political parties, which grew in number from one in 1990 to 123 in 1995 (Nkwi and Socpa 1997:138). In January 1996, a new constitution codified the resulting ethnicization of politics (Nkwi and Nyamnjoh 1997:9).

Biya's constitutional innovations did not change authoritarian practice and were not enough to prevent major unrest when economic recession and the fall of eastern bloc dictatorships coincided in the early 1990s. The "Ghost Town" or "Villes Mortes" movement, a long-lasting general strike, forced the convocation of the first multiparty elections for the National Assembly in March 1992. In Bangangté, the immediate economic results of the strike, however, have interrupted the mfen's plans for economic and cultural rejuvenation. And despite denials by the king (Nji Monluh, personal communication, June 1997), most Bamiléké associate their kings with Biya's party, the Cameroon People's Democratic Movement. In the analysis of Cameroonian social scientists:

> The state manipulates traditional authority so as to convert chiefs into clients capable, in turn, of legitimating state action and contradictions; their financial needs have turned them into political beggars and once honoured [they] can now be treated shabbily by the political elite and by their own disaffected subjects. Traditional rulers are no longer sacrosanct in their powers, as they are subject to the same deficits of legitimacy suffered by those who manipulate them for support. (Nkwi and Nyamnjoh 1997:11)

Political as well as economic constraints limit the king's effectiveness. Rural Bangangté women perceive this weakening of the divinity of the king and the ambivalent respect he is afforded as a threat to their well-being and fertility.

Bangangté town has slightly over 12,000 inhabitants (Boog 1986), most of whom are ethnically Bangangté or from the surrounding and closely allied "villages" or chiefdoms owing allegiance to the king of Bangangté.[4] As the capital of Ndé Division and of Bangangté Subdivision it contains offices of the prefect, subprefect, mayor, representatives of the ministries of labor and agriculture, a party building, a divisional hospital, and a preventive medicine center. The rural area of Bangangté Subdivision, 923 km[2,] has a population estimated in 1984 as 45,519 (Boog 1986).[5]

Rural Bangangté residents frequently talk about the "push factors" (lack of agricultural, educational, and employment opportunities) that encourage them sometimes to leave their kingdom to seek their fortune elsewhere. They most often mention the lure of wage labor and urban life as part of numerous drains on the demographic, political, social, and spiritual strength of their kingdom. In the context of the push and pull between the rural kingdom and the cities, Bangangté worry about cultural authenticity and cultural survival. Rural Bangangté women voice these concerns in terms of the procreation and socialization of children. They understand all too well that being and becoming Bangangté is a matter both of being born and of becoming enmeshed in the webs of affiliation (Simmel 1964) that tie kin, neighbors, the king, and the ancestors together.

These sets of relationships formed among the living are crucial to understanding how pairs come together to reproduce, and how this process is regulated by social and cultural practices. Since women worry not only about having biological offspring, but also about having properly socialized offspring who will honor them in old age and ancestorhood, these sets of relationships that make people Bangangté are of central importance. Relations among the living and the dead illuminate the intergenerational dimension of reproduction as well as the spiritual source of protection and threat to reproductive health. Two aspects of governing Bangangté subjects relate directly to reproductive issues. First, ideas about the strength of the mfen, including his reproductive vigor, figure into women's concern about their own fertility. Second, the Cameroonian state helps to shape health-care alternatives for women with reproductive problems through its relations with the kingdom and its traditional healers, and by creating hospitals and clinics.

Arenas of Social Connection and Identity

Bangangté value being "with" others. The highest expression of this is *nchu' ntu',* being of one heart. Bangangté describe nchu' ntu' as a spiritual quality fostered by sharing a meal. Commensality connotes a plethora of meanings for Bangangté, including quieting the pangs of hunger and calumny that reside in the belly and implying trust that one is feeding and being fed rather than poisoning another. Bangangté also achieve togetherness by exchanging gifts and visits, working and trading together. Paulette's inability to achieve or maintain such togetherness contributed to her misery and early departure from her marriage to the king.

Bangangté recognize that their connection to others is the essence of their identity as persons. They explain the multiplicity of names each person has in reference to various forms of social connection. A person's *ndap* (praise name) indicates one's parents' village identity; one's given Bangangté name commemorates a relative, chief, or friend of one's father; and the father's name, now used as a second surname, identifies patrisiblings. Pronouncing lists of names indicating knowledge of a conversation partner's real or fictive kinship relations and village membership is the best way to honor a person; forgetting them is an insult. Learning names and ndap proved to be an awesome task during the early months of my fieldwork, and a proud accomplishment toward the end. A person who cannot state his or her own social connections is suspect of being untrustworthy at best, a witch at worst. Coming from outside the Bamiléké world, I was given fictive kin and village connections. I was instructed in how to identify myself to other Bangangté, "so they won't be afraid." I used the ndap Nteshun that I shared with my "older sister" Claude, the king's French wife.

Bangangté speak readily about the importance of four interrelated arenas essential to Bangangté social life and identity: kin and ancestors, house and compound, neighborhood and village, and the kingdom. I discuss each of these social arenas in turn.

Kinship Ties among the Living and the Dead

Vignette 2:   Melon Vines

I have two daughters, aged eight and ten. They attend the école primaire *at Batela'. Their ndap is So'nyu, that is, they are daughters of Bangangté. Their father is mfen of Bangangté, so all the kings of Bangangté are their* ma' ngut nze' *["melon vines"], their ancestors. They are daughters of Bangangté, the kings are their fathers.*

I am happy that I have two daughters. I can tell you why. My own mother has only one daughter, and that is me. Of all my mother's children, only I am a girl. Only I can be her heiress. My brother is part of my pam nto' *[uterine group] and also part of my mother's lineage. But only my children can continue the pam nto', and since they are girls, their children continue it too. Yes, my mother and her line, her ancestors, are also ma' ngut nze' to my daughters. Everyone has two lines.*

Pam nto' is different from lines; it's not ancestors, but being from the same womb. That's why I am happy to have my two daughters.

(Marguerite)

When telling me about her daughters, Marguerite showed me once again how readily Bangangté can identify and put into practice rules of descent, alliance, and uterine relation. These rules are part of "law" (*kan*), and Bangangté refer to them constantly to explain who they visit, who they marry, who they name their children after, and who they call upon in times of trouble.

Descent. Marguerite referred to the two "lines" with which her daughters were affiliated, their two sets of ancestors. These two sets of ancestors constitute Bangangté's system of dual descent. At the center of descent groups are lineages (referred to as *ntun nda,* the "foundation" of the house) of heirs and heiresses who inherit the property, titles, and skull custodianship of their ascendants. Each lineage head chooses a single heir or heiress, who "becomes" that person in terms of titles in customary associations, and rights and duties toward all dependents (his or her noninheriting siblings and, in male inheritance, the father's widows). For example, Jeanne, the young king's wife and mother of two who shared Claude's house, explained that she followed her brother's marriage advice because, as her father's heir, he was simultaneously her full sibling *and* her father.

Bangangté individuals invoke their two lineage affiliations in different social settings. Patrilineal descent determines village membership and the inheritance of titles, land, compound, and wives. In recent times, it also determines one of a person's many names. Matrilineal descent determines inheritance of titles, movable property, and moral and legal obligation to lineage members.

Because only men head polygynous compounds and have house sites that can be inherited, patrilineal descent is more visible than matrilineal descent. Patrilineal descent groups tend to be localized. Young men often try to set up their compound near that of their father or his heir. Marriage is virilocal, giving men more control over their choice of residence than women. By contrast, members of a matrilineage may owe allegiance to different villages or even different kingdoms. The dispersal of matrilineal ties and the ideal localization of patrilineal ties casts doubt upon the long-standing descent–residence dichotomy guiding African kinship studies. This now questioned framework may have contributed to anthropologists' misunderstanding of Bamiléké kinship and the ways it affects reproductive goals and ideas about misfortune. Perhaps because of their greater visibility and importance in inheritance, most anthropologists have focused on agnatic relationships in Bamiléké kinship.[6] Bangangté themselves concentrate on agnatic links when discussing inheritance, but emphasize matrilineal links when discussing supernatural sanctions, and uterine links when discussing solidarity, personality, and witchcraft potential.

Ancestors. Like Marguerite, Bangangté call ancestors *ma' ngut nze'*, literally, "melon vines," graphically linking the living and the dead and the influence they have upon each other. Bangangté believe that both their matrilineal and patrilineal ancestors act upon the fortunes of their descendants. It is the ancestral skull (*tu*) that can "seize" a descendant with illness, and it is to the ancestral skull that descendants perform their propitiary rites (talking to, feeding, and sheltering the skull from the elements). Ancestors influence the lives only of those descendants who are morally obliged to sacrifice to their skulls (Hurault 1962; Tardits 1960). Likewise, the living only sacrifice to the skulls of those ancestors who can influence their lives (see figs. 5 and 6). For nonheirs, the obligation to sacrifice to patrilineal skulls ceases after two generations. In theory, the obligation to sacrifice to matrilineal skulls does not diminish with structural distance (that is, with generational distance from a direct heiress). In practice, facing misfortune often motivates people to renew their obligations to matrilineal ancestresses.

Ancestors are omniscient; Bangangté say they "know" or "see" all that their descendants do, how children act toward their parents, whether one steals, defames a sacred grove of trees, or breaks marriage and inheritance rules. Ancestors are quite sensitive about how they are treated by their descendants, and jealous if they feel shortchanged in relation to another ancestor. They do not like to suffer in the hot sun or feel chilled in the damp of the rainy season. They like to eat special foods. Thus heirs and heiresses exhume the skulls of their ancestors within a few years of burial, protect them in clay pots or specially built tombs, and "feed" them offerings of specially prepared food. Bangangté say ancestresses are particularly "complicated," a trait that combines contrariness and sensitivity with spiritual power (kings, witches, medico-ritual specialists, and sacred land are all likewise "complicated").

Ancestors angered by their treatment or by the behavior of their descendants may bring misfortune to the perpetrator of the bad act, or more likely to the perpetrator's close kin, "so he can see the effects of what he has done." These misfortunes include illness, accident, a business loss, failed bid for promotion or failed school exam, and infertility. The ancestors send these troubles either as simple punishment, or as warnings of

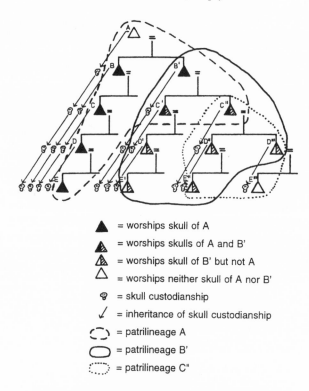

▲ = worships skull of A

⬗ = worships skulls of A and B'

⬔ = worships skull of B' but not A

△ = worships neither skull of A nor B'

☻ = skull custodianship

↙ = inheritance of skull custodianship

⊂⊃ = patrilineage A

◯ = patrilineage B'

⸝⸍⸍⸝ = patrilineage C"

Fig. 5. Descent and ancestor worship, patrilineal

more to come if a pattern of behavior continues. Offenses against marriage rules almost always result in misfortune affecting the couple's offspring (sterility, stillbirth, stunted growth of children).

Bangangté use their belief in the effects of ancestral wrath as one of several interpretations of unhappy events. Like Zande witchcraft, the action of the angered Bangangté dead upon their errant descendants is one of the most important elements in "a natural philosophy by which the relations between men and unfortunate events are explained and [that provides] a ready and stereotyped means of reacting to such events" (Evans-Pritchard 1937:18).[7]

Marriage. Knowing about one's ancestors, and thus principles of descent, is crucial in determining potential spouses. When parents arrange a marriage, or more recently when a couple decides to marry, lineage elders are asked to review the genealogies of the couple, often in consulta-

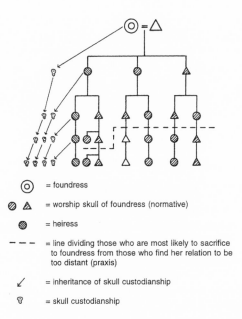

(○) = foundress

⊘ ▲ = worship skull of foundress (normative)

◉ = heiress

– – – = line dividing those who are most likely to sacrifice
to foundress from those who find her relation to be
too distant (praxis)

↙ = inheritance of skull custodianship

☻ = skull custodianship

Fig. 6. Descent and ancestor worship, matrilineal

tions with a diviner or spirit medium. Marriage is exogamous, preventing
all matrilineal kin and any individuals with patrilineal links up to the
fourth generation (i.e., as far back as the grandfather's ritual obligations)
from marrying (Hurault 1962).

Two forms of exchange govern relations between wife-givers and wife-
receivers. In bridewealth marriage, the groom gains reproductive, sexual,
and domestic rights by giving gifts of palm oil, goats, and money to the
bride's father, giving blankets and clothes to the bride and her mother, and
performing services such as gathering firewood for the mother. Bridewealth
payments may continue years after the couple has lived and even borne
children together. The wife gains a legitimate father for her children, a
house, and the right to cultivate a particular plot or plots of land.

In ta nkap marriage, no exchange of bridewealth occurs between
father and groom (Brain 1972; Hurault 1962; Tardits 1960). In this form of
marriage, which Bangangté describe as "when my father did not pay *nkap*

[bridewealth; literally, "money"] for my mother," the husband only gains rights to the woman's domestic duties (*in uxorem*). The bride's father retains rights (*in genetricem*) over the marriage and patrilineal identity of his daughter's daughters, thus becoming their *ta nkap* ("father by money"). The rights of a ta nkap can be accumulated through inheritance, or through transfer to whoever pays bridewealth for a woman married in this system (see fig. 7). The French regarded this way of capitalizing on matrimonial rights as leading toward economic abuse and uncontrolled concentration of power, and outlawed it in 1927 and 1928 (Tardits 1960:22). Nonetheless, it continues in Bangangté,[8] although no one seems to be able to identify the powerful marriage lords who hold rights over a large number of women as described in past accounts (Brain 1972; Hurault 1962; Rolland 1951; Tardits 1960).

Bangangté follow the rules regulating marriage closely because they fear the supernatural consequences of breaking them (infertility, stunted growth of children, illness). Solutions to reproductive illness are often sought by completing bridewealth payments, or paying bridewealth to a troublesome ta nkap. Many cite stories of greedy fathers who have asked for a daughter's bridewealth even though he had not paid bridewealth for her mother; such fathers bring misfortune upon their daughters, who often are ignorant of the circumstances of their mother's marriage. We have already witnessed the havoc wrought upon Paulette's marriage by her unintended incest.

Uterine Solidarity.   Expressing her joy over her two daughters, Marguerite mentioned that only her girls could continue the diffuse uterine group of those from the same womb, the pam nto'. This group encompasses one's own matrisiblings, one's mother, mother's mother, and mother's matrisiblings (see fig. 8).[9] The pam nto' group differs from the matrilineage because it does not involve the inheritance of property, custodianship of skulls, or succession to office. Instead, it involves sentiment and the idea of genetic linkage through shared blood and shared origin in one belly or uterus. Uterine kin help each other in the face of adversity and are the most reliable members of support and therapy management networks when someone falls ill. For example, when one of Marguerite's daughters fell out of a tree and cracked her skull, Marguerite called on her brother for help because she and her daughters were part of his pam nto'. Pam nto' members can also take each other's place in ordeals to prove guilt or innocence in witchcraft accusations.[10] Full siblings ("children of one mother") show support and affection for each other vis-à-vis their half siblings ("children of one father"). This solidarity is extended to the

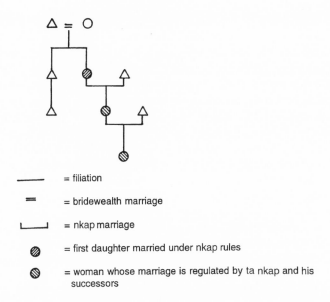

———	= filiation
⚌	= bridewealth marriage
⌞___⌟	= nkap marriage
⊘	= first daughter married under nkap rules
⊗	= woman whose marriage is regulated by ta nkap and his successors

Fig. 7.   Ta nkap marriage system (adapted from Tardits 1960:20)

mother's matrisiblings, just as affection and moral obligations to one's mother are extended to the mother's mother.

The experience of growing up together around the same "hearth" provides much of the basis for uterine solidarity. Sharing a hearth means sharing stories, companionship, and especially food. As we shall see in the next chapter, the hearth is a key symbol within the cluster of cooking metaphors through which Bangangté explain procreation. When talking about ties that bind, Bangangté use the hearth as a symbol to evoke both the nurturing warmth of matrifocal ties and the solidarity of pam nto' groups. Uterine solidarity is also promoted by the moral obligation one has toward one's mother. Bangangté often talk about "the mother who has borne me" and express the wish to honor her with grandchildren or goods.[11]

The Bangangté system of kinship and marriage affects the ways people think about offspring. Women have children to please ancestors, to be able to become ancestors themselves, and to continue the multiple links between the living and the dead constituted by a system of dual descent and uterine solidarity groups. Women gain pleasure from their sons as well as their daughters. Sons can become the patrilineal heir of their fathers.

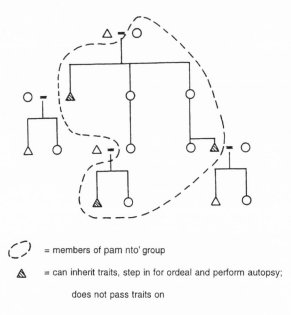

(͡) = members of pam nto' group

⚐ = can inherit traits, step in for ordeal and perform autopsy;

does not pass traits on

Fig. 8.   Pam nto' (uterine solidarity) relations

Daughters insure matrilineal continuity and bring bridewealth to the family. Bangangté relations with their ancestors shape the ways they think about marriage and sex, the usual prerequisites to procreation, and the ways they conceive of misfortune, including reproductive illness.

Bangangté notions of kinship are held in common across all social ranks. Regardless of their status within the promotional system of the royal court, as commoners, or as descendents of slaves, all Bangangté belong to patrilineages, matrilineages, and uterine solidarity groups. They all make distinctions between lineage heads and noninheriting dependents. They all venerate their ancestral skulls. With the exception of kings who pay no bridewealth, they all practice both bridewealth and ta nkap marriage, and include both monogamists and polygynists in their midst. Ideas about the rights and obligations of kinship tie together the sociospatial categories of household, neighborhood, village, and kingdom that are essential to a multilayered Bangangté identity. The emotions of solidarity and competition bound up in Bangangté kin relations extend, through notions of the shared hearth, to relations of people sharing residence, people of the same house and compound.

House and Compound

Bangangté experience the household at two distinct levels, the polygynous or monogamous compound (*la'*, same term as used for village), and the matrifocal household (*nda*, house). The segments of a compound at these two levels operate semiautonomously in some fields of activity, but coalesce in others. There is thus no such thing as a "household" as an undifferentiated, solidary decision-making unit in Bangangté (Guyer 1981:100).

Nda means house; it refers both to the structure and to the people within it. In polygynous compounds, a house is a domestic unit, the kitchen-hut of a mother surrounded by her children. Its members share day-to-day subsistence activities, affective ties, and the socialization of children. The mother organizes daily subsistence activities, assigning tasks to her children with an eye both to getting things done and to training them in household roles and skills. Household members rise at or before dawn, heat up yesterday's food or buy baguettes for breakfast, fetch water, sweep the yard, and feed any livestock before moving on to fields or school. On school holidays, children help in the fields and gather firewood. Older children watch after their younger siblings, and older girls may sometimes cook the evening meal in the mother's place.

Children are very mobile within the compound (between different matrifocal households) and in and out of it. Bamiléké consider child fosterage an appropriate strategy to deal with scarce resources and to help teach the child to interact with a variety of personalities. When a child is between six and ten years old, he or she may be sent or may ask to live in another household where more resources are available, a school is near, an old person needs help and company, or a favorite playmate lives.[12] Foster children are never as close to other household members as those sharing uterine group ties, but their treatment may range from the doting affection of a grandmother to the exploitation of a nonrelated shopkeeper (den Ouden 1987:16–17). Because fosterage is so common, resources for child rearing rarely figure into women's overall reproductive decision making.

The compound (*la'*), or the composite household (den Ouden 1980:43), is a jural, political, and spatial unit. Relationships within the compound are held together by jural ties of descent (between the male compound head and his children) and alliance (between the compound head and his wife or wives). The larger the compound, the greater is the compound head's prestige and political power. Having a sizable, polygynous compound is a requirement for some titles of nobility.[13] In the largest compounds, politics complement kinship in deciding residence, as the compound head may gather clients about him, giving shelter and gaining the labor of the clients or their children.

The spatial characteristics of the compound contribute to the shape of daily interactions and thus to the experience of being Bangangté from different social "locations." Seen from the point of view of the male compound head, his house is in the center, facing the road. Behind or next to the man's house is his wife's kitchen. In monogamous compounds, the wife and children sleep in the man's house. In polygynous compounds, each wife has her own kitchen-house where she lives with her own children. These wives' houses are clustered around the man's house, and in larger compounds they are divided into two rows or quarters "belonging to" the first and second wives, as we have seen for the royal compound. In fact, many of the features of household organization and daily life in the royal compound, described in chapter 1, apply to other polygynous compounds on a smaller scale.

A set of contrasts gives the space between and around this cluster of buildings meaning for its Bangangté inhabitants. In the cleared and inhabited space surrounding the buildings, where everyday activities take place, the earth is beaten and swept, under control. It contrasts with the "complicated" wooded space behind the compound, the sacred groves and uncontrolled bush. The cleared area is generally toward the public road and higher than the bush behind the compound. Its height is associated with dryness and sterility, the lowness of the bush with moisture, coolness, and fecundity.[14] The closed space in the women's quarters (in the past fenced in) contrasts with the open space before the man's house, a place to receive guests. The often ostentatious graves of antecedents are usually in front or directly to the side of the deceased's house, in the open, public area of the compound.[15] The open, public space, as well as the man's house, is dedicated to male activities, while the closed space of the women's quarters is the venue of women's activities where even the husband rarely makes an appearance.

In polygynous compounds, male and female spheres are highly segregated in economic as well as in social and spatial terms. In addition, the household of each wife is largely economically independent from those of her cowives, despite some food-sharing. Nonetheless, implicit and explicit contracts of rights and duties link household members economically.

The husband is responsible for buying palm oil, salt, dried fish, and meat for his wives and children, as well as paying for clothing, school fees, and medical care. He earns the money to do this through coffee or cocoa cultivation, selling small livestock, wage employment, commerce, or occasionally by practicing special skills such as healing. The husband also assigns plots to his wives from the land allocated to him by the quarter king. Both women and men in Bangangté deny the competition for land described for more densely populated Bamiléké regions (den Ouden

1980:52) and do not intercrop.[16] "How can I be angry with my husband if he plants coffee on my plot and I have to start a new one," asked one Bangangté woman in 1983. "After all, he gave me the land." Nonetheless, women often must walk long distances to their fields when their husbands take over fields nearer to the compound for coffee, and they do complain about the distance. The wives may work on their husband's coffee farm,[17] but their main responsibility is to feed their husband and children with foodstuffs they have cultivated themselves. They also prepare and serve food to receive the husband's guests. Women's agricultural, cooking, and serving skills become evident on the grandest occasions on which the entire household cooperates, festivities commemorating the dead.

In practice, husbands often do not meet their economic duties. Women sell produce and sometimes sell prepared food at the weekly and biweekly markets to earn cash for oil, salt, clothing, and school fees. They show their disapproval to their impoverished or irresponsible husband, however, by preparing the husband's food without the necessary palm oil. Bangangté associate foodstuffs, cooking, and full bellies with procreative ingredients, pregnancy, and houses full of children. As we shall see in chapters 3 and 4, complaints about irresponsible husbands and empty cooking pots constitute a discourse on threats to reproductive health.

Neighborhood and Village

Food is simultaneously the basis of solidarity and an arena of conflict not only within households but also in the local community. Sharing food and drink while visiting is the epitome of neighborliness; refusing it is an open statement of mistrust. The neighborhood and village crosscut kinship to draw people together to share information, work, and food. The *quartier,* quarter or neighborhood, is both an informal designation that Bangangté use to talk about nearby people and establishments, and a territorial unit (*tan la'*) of royal governance. Quarter and village are also units of Cameroonian state administration. But most importantly, the neighborhood is the arena of daily, extrafamilial interaction. The village is the touchstone of origin, the most readily available marker of identity. These localized, territorial connections contribute centrally to the multilayered sentiment of being Bangangté.

Roads, courtyards in front of compounds or clusters of compounds, and markets are the main arteries through which Bangangté people pass, meet, and socialize. These arteries of neighborly interaction are also communication conduits through which information about community affairs flows. Critical for women of reproductive age, this information concerns who might be suspected of witchcraft against pregnant women and what

health-care options are available to prevent or cure witchcraft and reproductive maladies. Gossip about who has had what, consulted whom, and
experienced which results is the main way women learn about and evaluate the health-care alternatives available to them. This gossip, as well as
goods and money, is exchanged in small neighborhood groups, at gatherings around a respected plantain seller's stall at a central market corner,
and at meetings of voluntary associations.

As a member of a quarter or village, one is expected to participate in
at least one voluntary association. Nobles and royal retainers take part in
title societies concerned with royal administration and ritual. *Manjo,* an
age-grade association organizing male youths into work and military parties for the king, is proudly referred to in life histories by men in their late
fifties and sixties, but appears to have ceased functioning by the early
1960s. The most significant voluntary associations for women are rotating
credit associations, which function as savings, credit, and mutual aid societies. A number of people belong to dance societies, groups drawing their
members from one specific quarter and specializing in a particular dance.
Members of both dance and rotating credit associations gather together to
share work, dance, and money, and travel together to honor and enliven
the death celebrations of members' kin. "Modern" voluntary associations
include task-oriented committees, headed by social workers from a variety
of government agencies, such as the community development program of
the Ministry of Agriculture.[18]

Village membership, determined by the father, is the basis of pride and
creates a sense of kinship among strangers, similar to the institution of
namesake kin among the Ju/Hoansi of the Kalahari (Lee 1984). One of the
first things a Bamiléké asks when meeting a new acquaintance is *ndap su ba
we?* (what is your praise name?). *Ndap,* thanking[19] or praise names, indicate
the village origins of the bearer's mother and father. The ndap given a man
or woman from a particular village alternates from generation to generation, stressing village continuity in a cycle where grandparents and grandchildren are equated in wordplay.[20] This wordplay is also used by nonkin,
who refer to their ndap-sharing acquaintance as parent, child, or sibling.
Younger, urban Bangangté who may be unfamiliar with the intricacies of
praise names ask simply, "what village are you from?" Both village origins
and their expression in ndap create a sense of connection between strangers
originating from the same local community within the kingdom.

Kingdom

The fourth arena of social connection and identity in Bangangté is the
kingdom (*ngo*), a territory with set boundaries, the land where one's ances-

tors rest and where one's king rules. Bangangté subjects are unified by their allegiance to the mfen, despite their diverse origins as noble, slave, refugee, and children of mothers from other kingdoms. Bangangté are also drawn together by common allegiance when living outside the territory of their kingdom, operating rotating credit associations and collecting funds for the emergency repatriation of their members in case of illness or death (den Ouden 1987:15). The mfen frequently visits these associations to oversee the affairs of his urban subjects and sometimes to ask them for money for his projects.

The Palace. The king's residence, *nchwed,* the royal compound, is central in Bangangté consciousness. It is the locus of collective and individual rites assuring the well-being of Bangangté subjects. These rites, including funerals, coronations, and convocations of "the children of Bangangté," link living Bangangté subjects to their deceased rulers, just as private rites link the living to their immediate ancestors. Bangangté subjects are called to the royal compound to pay tribute to the mfen in labor or cash, to pay taxes, and to demand the king's services as justice of the peace, a state function.

Bangangté subjects also spend much of their conversations contemplating palace developments. They perceive that what happens in the palace affects their well-being in direct and indirect ways, from its role in settling land tenure disputes to its spiritual guardianship of the country. The royal compound is the focal point of concerns about threats to procreation within the kingdom and thus the focal point of this book. The royal wives fear their fertility to be more threatened than others'. This is due to a number of perceptions as illustrated in chapter 1, including co-wife jealousy and competition to produce an heir among the royal wives, and the "bad" and "unhealthy" ways of the mfen.[21] Bangangté who do not belong to the royal family also perceive the royal wives to be at a higher risk of depressed fertility than other Bangangté women. Some even express their impression that the overall birthrate of Bangangté is increasing while the royal compound has "too few children."[22] In traditional Bangangté cosmology, as in many symbolic systems of societies ruled by divine kings, the wealth, health, and reproductive vigor of the mfen and his household is closely tied to the well-being of his subjects and the land. Therefore, even nonroyal households satisfied with their reproductive success are worried when the reproductive vigor of the royal family is threatened. Because of its importance for reproductive issues in Bangangté, we describe the royal compound in detail.

The royal compound of Bangangté is the administrative, religious, and cultural center of the kingdom. The web of relations among its residents is simultaneously full of the mystique of things royal and considered the exemplary polygynous compound by most Bangangté subjects. For this reason, Bangangté worry when news of the many altercations among the king and his wives leaks out.

The spatial organization of the royal compound of Bangangté resembles all Bamiléké royal compounds (Hurault 1962; Notué and Perrois 1984). One can best read the complex map of the Bangangté royal compound by imagining oneself on a walking tour of the palace grounds (see fig. 9). Visitors enter through a tall gate of decoratively worked spines of raffia palm fronds resembling bamboo, topped with a seven-peaked corrugated tin roof. The gate is located at the top of a hill, which for over fifty years has carried the traffic of the old Yaoundé–Bafoussam road. A wide double avenue leads down the hill toward a second gate. Wooden palisades and thirteen square "bamboo" structures with thatched roofs flank this avenue, shielding the two quarters of the mfen's wives from public view. The second gate at the foot of the avenue separates the three districts of activity within the royal compound: the two wives' quarters above the second gate, the residence of the king beside it, and *mâfen,* the sacred forest below it. Mâfen, the "complicated" area below the second gate, contains structures housing the royal skulls, secret society meeting places, offering sites, and the king's secret water source. Rituals are performed here to resolve disputes and to protect the well-being of the king, the kingdom, and the fertility of its populace.

Royal Authority. Traditional Bangangté government is highly centralized, with authority concentrated in the institution of kingship. The mfen's official rights in the past included taking any unmarried woman for his wife, exacting tribute and labor from his subjects, receiving payments from nobles who buy titles, displaying royal insignia (leopard skins, copper bracelet, necklace), and deciding on the life and death of his subjects. In the context of the Cameroonian state, he still receives wives as gifts from his subjects and from fellow kings, but can no longer demand them. He can request funds and labor from his subjects, but they are not required by Cameroonian law to comply. He continues to have the right to display royal insignia and receive payments for titles of nobility. He still hears cases from his subjects, but his status as judge is curtailed by the state. Officially he may only hear civil cases, while in practice his subjects continue to come to him for a variety of complaints. He no longer has the right to decide over the life and death of his subjects. His duties include not only judging disputes among his subjects, but also general responsibility for the physical and spiritual well-being of the kingdom. In the modern context, he is justice of the peace, signs all birth, marriage, and death certificates of his rural subjects, and supervises the collection of tax by his deputies.

Kingship in Bangangté embodies ideas of the mutual dependence of the wealth, health, and reproductive vigor of king, kingdom, and subjects. The king (mfen) in Bangangté is divine in a limited sense. He is not considered a god (*Nsi*), but through his inheritance of the kingship and initiation into office the mfen gains sacred, supernatural powers (*kà*) and a combination of religious and secular authority shared by no other individual. This authority is transmitted from father to son through the extended initiation and enthronement ritual. The mfen's right to govern is considered a legacy of the ancestors. The idea of royal history and descent is very important to Bangangté kingship, and dynasty lists are displayed at royal enthronement ceremonies. His religious and secular authority, now specified into separate duties by the Cameroonian state, were hardly distinguishable in traditional Bangangté. Part of a divine king's divinity is his "strangeness," or his distinction from his subjects.[23] The mfen is made "strange" through his fearful possession of kà, which can be used for good or bad, and through installation rites that transform the mfen-as-individual into the representative of his enduring, legitimate office.

The King's Men.   Because the mfen is one of many brothers who share equal patrilineal links to the predecessor, not only kinship but also rules of impartible inheritance are necessary to legitimize his succession. Nonetheless, Bangangté appreciate strength and do not condemn the usurpation of power (confirmed by den Ouden for other Bamiléké groups, 1987:13). Thus the mfen has to have something to do with his royal relatives, potential challengers to his succession to the throne. As Richards describes for the Bemba (1961), some royal relatives cluster around the office of kingship to display the size and strength of the royal dynasty at events such as funerals and receive special titles of nobility that include particular duties in royal rituals. Contrary to Richards's description (1961:144), the mfen will appoint his otherwise eligible noninheriting brothers to posts as quarter chiefs of distant quarters, chancing secession of these areas. In the past, this was a risk, although the greater risk was war with neighboring kingdoms and the sultanate of Bamoum. Nowadays, kingdom boundaries determined by the state prevent secession. In addition, royal nonheirs now seek their fortunes outside the kingdom, where educational and economic opportunities are much greater.

Forming no potential threat to the mfen's succession, queen mothers (*mamfen*) are significant supporters of the mfen's rule. They receive their high office through the mfen and are therefore interested in keeping him in power. They are important advisers to the mfen and attend meetings of the *nkam be'e* (council of nine, the highest group of nobles). They are very visible leading dances and in women's social and economic groups, commu-

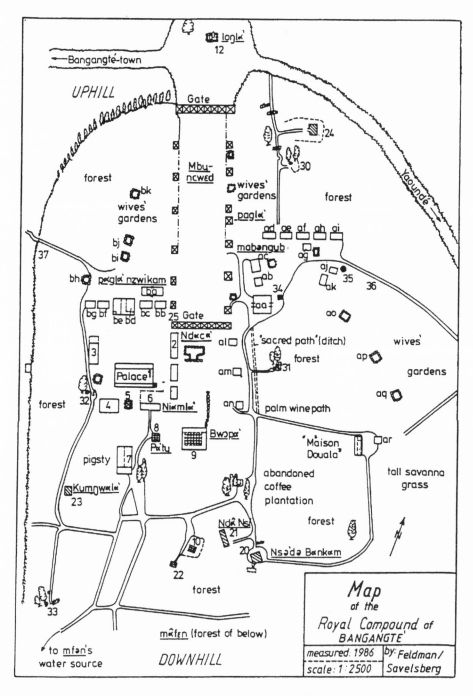

Fig. 9.   Map of the royal compound of Bangangté

1 palace
2 ndɑcɑ', courthouse
3 former garage
4 mfən's sleeping house
5 site of lɑ'kam
6 niam lɑ', mfən's kitchen
7 pigsty
8 pɑ'tu, skull house
9 bwopɑ', former palace
10 burial house of mfen Tchatchoua
11 "maison douala," house of Njiké II,
      where Egerton stayed in 1937

20 nse'de bɑnkɑm, nobles' meeting house
21 ndâ nsi, the house of god
22 unused meeting house
23 kum ngwɑlɑ', ngwɑlɑ' meeting house
24 meeting house

30 mbə, sacrifice site
31 --- " ---
32 --- " ---
33 --- " ---
34 site of mabəŋgup's burial
35 site where royal wife's skull exhumed
36 banana grove toilet area for pɑglɑ' mabəŋgup
37 toilet area for pɑglɑ' nzwikam

Houses of Royal Wives

aa	mabəŋgup	am	abandoned	ba nzwikam
ab	Marguerite's kitchen	an	abandoned, site of	bb Kikam
ac	Marguerite		burial, Fig. 1	bc abandoned
ad	Claude and Jeanne	ao	abandoned	bd Koku
ae	Sankə'	ap	abandoned	be Kikam
af	abandoned	ap	---"---	bf makokwa
ag	Cəlu'	aq	---"---	bg Tongtan, died 3/86
ah	Nyombab	ar	former house,	bh abandoned
ai	Nteshʉn		Njiké Pokam's mother	bi ---"---
aj	Jeanne's kitchen			bj ---"---
ak	construction site			bk ---"---
al	anthropologist, formerly abandoned			

KEY

□ house (mud brick)

⊠ house (traditional "bamboo")

⦂⦂⦂ house (ruin)

ø small tree

Ⓨ large tree

⇔ tree trunk

e clay bowl for sacrifices

⌇ hedge

⦙ stockade fence

▨ kum secret society (royal regulatory +
     title holder) meeting house

▦ site with ancestral skulls

nicating royal affairs and acting as mediators to interpret news and steer opinion. Although there is only one mfen, there are many mamfens. The mother of each past mfen in the dynasty has her own line of heiresses, who are referred to as *mamfen* plus the name of the original queen mother (e.g., mamfen Peto', mamfen Kemajou). One reason royal wives are so concerned that their son become mfen is that the stakes are very high; mamfen is the highest office a woman can achieve.

The royal wives do not participate directly in the governing of the mfen's subjects. They support the mfen's rule, however, in a variety of ways. They are responsible for the smooth functioning of domestic life in the royal compound, and for the protection of the mfen's powers by observing special dietary rules. They act as model subjects, displaying elaborate deference to the mfen in the presence of nonroyals. Royal wives grow the surplus and prepare the food that the mfen distributes to his subjects to cement their loyalty. Perhaps most importantly, they are responsible for producing an heir and demonstrating the mfen's potency by bearing children.

Besides royal relatives, others help the mfen rule and balance his powers. These are the nobles, sometimes royal relatives but often not, holding a variety of ranked, inherited titles (e.g., *nkam, tâ mfen, sop*), members of secret societies (e.g., *Ku'nga, ngwala', bandansi*), and royal retainers (*che' mfen,* the hats of the king). The highest ranked nobles are the *nkam be'e,* the council of nine who are the only subjects with the right to speak to the mfen as an equal. They not only act as his most important counselors, but are crucial in the initiation and enthronement procedures of royal succession.

The secret societies are associations (*kum*) with limited entry and closed meetings. Some, like Ku'nga, are masked societies, acting in the past as the mfen's police of the night by making nocturnal raids on the concessions of wrongdoers. Many more secret societies were active in the past, all meeting in structures in the sacred forest in the depths of the royal compound.[24]

Royal retainers range in function from manual laborers for the king to his trusted guards and emissaries. They are recruited at a young age, and in the past were often given a wife and some land after some years of service and residence in the royal compound. Currently, few young men wish to be royal retainers, and the corps of *che' mfen* has diminished considerably. No more retainers sleep in the palace, and most are quite elderly. Some royal retainers now live in cities far from the royal compound.

Further away from the royal compound, the mfen is aided in governing by a variety of hereditary and nonhereditary nobles. The kingdom is divided into subkingdoms, quarters, and subquarters in a highly centralized hierarchy of spatial and administrative divisions. The most important division is the quarter, which is administered by committee. The position of quarter chief (*nkam tan la'*) is originally appointed by the mfen and then inherited by the dignitary's successor. The mfen always retains the right to replace him with another, however. In practice, a committee of quarter members may choose a new quarter chief upon the death of a nkam tan la'.[25] Quarter chiefs are responsible for keeping the peace, collecting taxes, and allocating land. The land is considered land of the mfen and of the kingdom, managed by the quarter kings who allocate rights to its use to patrilineages and to nonheirs just starting out.

Two developments during the colonial era disturbed the quarter system and led to land disputes sometimes in the guise of witchcraft accusations. Hurault describes how colonial census takers reconstituted quarters as they pleased, breaking them up into smaller units that had nothing to do with the traditionally legitimate quarter system. Those made quarter heads by the actions of the census takers did not want to give up their newfound posts to kingly quarter heads. This led to hard feelings and imprecise borders, disrupting royal attempts to govern. Hurault cites Bangangté as the worst example, dislocated into 58 quarters (1962:101–2). The second development was the resettlement of hamlets along the roadside to ease security and surveillance during the civil war preceding and following independence. Because of this resettlement, the nkam tan la' were further away from the farmland they had allocated to their constituents and less able to supervise land use and prevent disputes. These disputes sometimes led to witchcraft accusations (Feldman 1984).

In the past, Bamiléké lived by their farms, dispersed in the countryside. Since the civil war of 1955–65, populations have been regrouped along roadsides. This means that cultivators, particularly women, must walk long distances to their fields. This recent pattern of settlement may also contribute to land disputes, since regulatory bodies are now far from the disputed land parcels (see Feldman 1984). The land is the property of the entire collectivity (citizens of the kingdom) and is managed by the king (mfen) and his representatives, the quarter chiefs (nkam tan la') (Tardits 1960:69). Some private ownership of land began with the introduction of coffee (Tardits 1960:70). These gradual changes in land tenure are still under way.

The mfen's ability to govern is affected not only by those who surround him, but also by the double nature of kingship. Like many divine kings, the mfen has "two bodies," an everlasting, sacred body and a temporal, mortal, human body.[26] The first sacred body is gained through a period of investiture that makes the mfen "other," powerful, and capable of changing himself into a panther. The second body is that of the mfen as a human individual, a product of his times, containing human fallibilities.

Because of this second, temporal nature, the hold of kingship and of some ancestrally sanctioned customs is weakening. Subjects find other paths to wealth and honor than traditional titles and constant allegiance to the mfen. Currently, allegiance is situational. The mfen needs new wealth acquired in modern ways, with the help of his subjects, and must relate to the Cameroonian state.

The Kingdom and State.   Managing contradictions between the traditional Bangangté kingdom and the modernizing Cameroonian state is one of the greatest challenges facing both the mfen and his subjects. Relations between the state administration (prefect, subprefect) and the mfen have not always been easy, as they demand a double allegiance from their constituents. Mfen Njiké Pokam wished to modernize, but did not have the scholastic education to make his case heard by the administration. As a result he was caught between critical Bangangté nobles, who worried he would ruin the dignity of the kingship, and the local administration backed by the force of the state. His successor, mfen Nji Monluh Seidou Pokam, during his initiation from February to May 1987 promised to improve relations on both fronts (Ndonko 1987a). Director of the parastatal coffee cooperative, and since October 1987 second deputy mayor of Bangangté, this mfen is himself highly placed in the local state apparatus. At the same time he plans to rejuvenate defunct secret societies and other palace associations to "restore tradition." His plans have been impeded by economic recession and general strikes calling for democratization in the early 1990s.

Bangangté subjects must deal with both the kingdom and the state administration, even for state-ordered bureaucratic acts. While the mfen, as justice of the peace for Bangangté Subdivision, must sign all birth, marriage, and death certificates, records for these documents, essential to attend school or to obtain wage employment, are kept in the various offices of the state bureaucracy in town.

When subjects seek legal means to settle disputes or are charged with a crime, they may have to present themselves both before the mfen's court and at the divisional courthouse. If they do not come of their own accord, they may be fetched by the mfen's emissaries or by the Cameroonian police. The mfen's legal jurisdiction is ambiguous, and he is not even president of the *tribunal coutumier* (customary court), an interim state institution hearing civil cases. The state (or parts of it in the court system) clearly intends to gradually do away with traditional dispute settlement procedures. Nonetheless, rural Bangangté in particular are mystified by and mistrustful of state legal process, which encourages the success of the mfen's dispute settlement.[27]

Bangangté experience other, perhaps less intrusive, aspects of the

Cameroonian state that do not directly contradict royal power. Children attend schools, which are run by the state, by the Protestant and Catholic missions, and as private lay enterprises at the secondary level. For rural residents, state primary schools are the main contact with educational institutions. The Ministry of Agriculture presents Bangangté cultivators with a variety of extension services and a community development program, seeking to modernize the community from above. Women's groups, teaching knitting, crocheting, and food preservation techniques, introduce new visions of women's role in modernizing Cameroon, visions not always supportive of women's traditional independence.

Finally, Bangangté villagers' health-care options are significantly shaped by the state. Not only are government hospitals and clinics widely available in Ndé Division, the government differentially supports private health-care alternatives. Mission hospitals and private clinics are officially approved. In recent attempts to organize traditional healers, attempts encouraged only by limited members of the state apparatus, herbalists have received more attention than practitioners utilizing less empirically based healing methods. The latter are denounced by most government officials as charlatans. This puts the legal status of a large body of practitioners treating women's reproductive ailments at risk.

Concluding Remarks: Social Cohesion, Exclusion, and Shifting Centers

In this chapter I have discussed various contexts in which Bangangté interact with their living compatriots, with their ancestors, and with those who govern them. I have emphasized forms of association that draw Bangangté together. But the flip side of social connectedness is exclusion; for each group of affiliates some are in and others are out. The forces that push Bangangté apart are an important aspect of everyday life.

At the level of kinship, the distinction between heirs and nonheirs creates bitterness between brothers and even cuts ritual ties. In addition, although wife-givers and wife-takers are drawn together through marriage alliance, the differences in wealth and prestige thus created are sometimes insurmountable. At the level of the compound, intense competition between cowives often leads to accusations of thievery, calumny, and witchcraft. This strife, particularly in later years, often extends to their children, pushing half siblings apart.

At the level of the quarter or village community, differences between heirs and nonheirs, peasants and salaried employees make themselves felt through differences in wealth (in capital, land, and in the labor of many wives). This yields disparities in privileges and prestige in both traditional and modern terms. Titles of nobility must be bought, and initiation involves expensive gifts to all previous members of the same rank (Hurault 1962:102). Wealth can pay for formal education, allowing one to use rather than be used by the state bureaucracy. Concrete houses, gilded with fanciful iron bars and even surrounded by a wall, serve as badges of prestige and physical reminders of difference in fortune. Highly differentiated opportunities to promote one's interests (den Ouden 1987), as well as strife between heirs and their disinherited brothers, literally push people apart by urging many to migrate.

While migrants vary widely from each other in wealth and power, they are nonetheless drawn together by common allegiance to the mfen and kingdom of Bangangté. The hold of the mfen on his subjects, however, was slipping in 1986. The mfen is now only one of a number of shifting centers of reference, especially for Bangangté migrants whose daily experience is in the urban world of wage labor. Migrants are also drawn back to kingdom territory by the pull of the ancestors. These ancestors draw shallow kinship groups together in their need to placate ancestral wrath, but having to sacrifice to one's ancestors through the solitary heir once again serves to underline the exclusiveness of descent.

The extremely hierarchical nature of traditional Bangangté government, with its system of ranked titles among men and women, clearly submits Bangangté subjects to a strict discipline of knowing one's place. This is somewhat countered by new opportunities for wealth, prestige, and power in commerce and state bureaucracy. Rather than alleviating inequality, however, these developments add a new hierarchy to the old one, where educational achievement and wealth are used as measures to render large numbers of individuals ineligible for positions of advancement.

What remains at all levels of Bangangté social life is an intense consciousness of status differences, based on prestige, privilege, and wealth in traditional and modern terms. A marked area of difference is gender. All scholars of the Bamiléké have noted the high degree of gender segregation in economic, spatial, and social fields. Den Ouden, in his exploration of notions of importance, complicatedness, and dangerousness, cites evidence indicating that "the world of women is quite puzzling for men" (1987:8). Bangangté have very specific notions of different rights and duties for men and women, as well as their different "natures." Hierarchical divisions within and between the categories of men and women are highly articulated. This is true for all of the shifting contexts within which Bangangté live their lives—in the royal compound, in their local communities, and in the commercial and bureaucratic institutions in which they work or receive services. The next chapter explores these issues of gender difference in the context of beliefs regarding procreation.

Chapter Three

Cooking Inside: The Symbolic Construction of Gender, Marriage, and Fertility

Na nda, the Bangangté expression for marriage, literally means "to cook inside." According to Tamveun, an elderly male informant:

> Na nda is marriage. An unmarried woman cooks on the road, in the open where just anyone can smell the delicious aromas from her cooking pot. A married woman cooks *inside,* cooks inside her kitchen. Only her husband tastes her food, and sniffs the aroma from her cooking pot. Her husband builds her the kitchen. Then she does not have to cook on the road. Later her kitchen is full of children.

Tamveun's expression alternated between seriousness (in my husband's absence I should understand the importance that young married women only cook inside) and that twinkle in the eye that indicated his enjoyment of the double entendre of cooking food and sex. Tamveun's exegesis of the expression *na nda* was shared by the rural women of all ages with whom I lived and worked during my fieldwork in Bangangté. These women also shared his mirth at the thought of flirtatious cooking aromas contained in the marital kitchen. While making clear that this was also serious business, Bangangté women made cooking, sex, and sharing food the basis of many jokes.

"Cooking inside" is central to the symbolic construction of gender, marriage, and fertility. It refers to both the cooking of food and the metaphoric "cooking" of sex and children inside the mud brick walls of the kitchen and the social walls of marital relations. The kitchen and cooking are key symbols that designate women's place and skill, and socialize the physical mysteries of procreation. In Bangangté kinship ideology, notions of culinary skill, procreative cooking ingredients, and vessels are integral to the complementary and sometimes conflicting demands that every person faces by belonging to both a matrilineage and a patrilineage. These

71

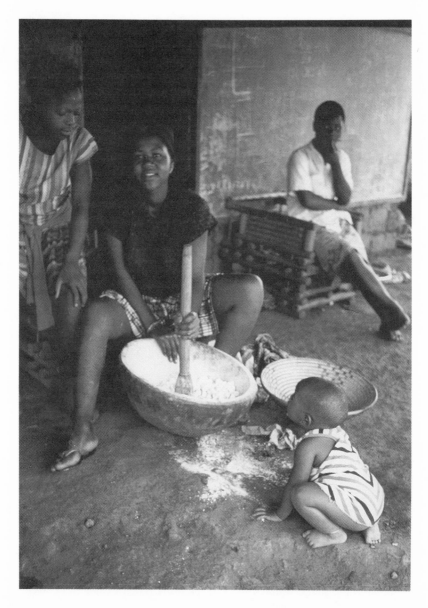

Fig. 10. Jeanne preparing manioc in front of her earthen brick kitchen, royal compound, Bangangté. She will mix the pounded manioc flour with water and cook it on the three-stoned hearth inside her kitchen. This entire process of food preparation is reiterated in the symbolism of procreation.

images of procreation figure prominently in Bangangté concerns with managing allegiance to these crosscutting kin groups, and also to village and kingdom. The same set of culinary metaphors, of recipes, cooking, and kitchens, describes procreation and the work of royalty in the constitution of Bangangté society.

Thus, notions of procreation are central to the conceptualization of both individual and group identity. Bangangté women's pleas for the revitalization of Bangangté group identity are voiced in an idiom of reproductive affliction, the difficulties of creating individuals. This process of creating individuals is deeply gendered. Its symbolism both reflects and shapes the ways that gender permeates Bangangté identity, and the spiritual and existential stake women have in the maintenance of a distinctive cultural identity. The imagery of procreation, like kinship ideology and ancestor veneration, is shared across social ranks. It draws women together with a common set of concerns, despite significant differences in women's vulnerability to misfortune. By examining women's lives and the imagery of gender, marriage, and procreation, we get closer to understanding the puzzle of Bangangté women's preoccupation with reproductive health.

Gender Distinctions: Space and
Labor in the Context of Marriage

While nearly all Bangangté citizens seem worried about issues of procreation, and while not all Bangangté mothers are married, the women who expressed their concerns to me in the most poignant detail were married women approximately between the ages of 18 and 85. In several Grassfields kingdoms, and perhaps throughout Africa, extramarital childbearing may be a strategy to avoid some of the burdens of gender inequality while maintaining pro-natalist values, an acceptable if not preferred option (Goheen 1996:179–80, 229). In contemporary Bangangté, however, marriage continues to figure prominently in notions of gender identity, the division of labor, and the blessings and travails of procreation.

In Bangangté, a wife's kitchen is the basis of marriage. Marriage brings the wife—who comes from outside the village and outside the husband's patrilineage—inside the husband's village, his compound, and the kitchen he has built. Marriage brings the potentially unruly maiden into a socially circumscribed role. It also insures that the newlyweds' children will belong to the husband's patrilineage and village.

The symbolism of the wife's kitchen and hearth looks different from the point of view of matrilineality. The center of the kitchen is the mother's hearth, which also symbolizes her womb. A mother and her hearth are the center of every uterine group (*pam nto'*), whose members are all affiliated with the same matrilineage. The solidarity of these "one womb" kingroups is based on the emotional warmth of the matrifocal household gathered round the mother's nurturing hearth and cooking pot. Ndachi Tagne expresses the power of the image of the mother's hearth in his novel *La Reine Captive* (1986), in which the kidnapped girl-queen receives solace at the hearth of the senior cowife she calls "mother."

In Bangangté gender ideology, the ideal woman is warm like her hearth. The ideal woman is a mother, a preparer of food, sweating over her cooking pot and gathering her children around her to eat and tell stories. While many fathers dote on their youngest children, Bangangté generally describe fathers and husbands as cool, distant, and authoritarian. They have nothing to do with hearths and cooking, and receive but do not serve food.

Na nda, to cook inside, expresses both the ideology and practice of a wife's incorporation, but also the gender segregation within the household, locating the "cooking" wife at her hearth. The married woman's hearth is no longer an open fire, but enclosed by her husband who acts in spatial and social realms outside the kitchen. While the term *na nda* emphasizes capturing and enclosing a wife's allegiance and her children's affiliation within the husband's patrilineage, the extension of this culinary imagery in Bangangté notions of procreation provides women an arena of expertise and the basis for alternate kin ties in the face of a largely agnatic (patrilineal) ideology.

The images of marriage and procreation reflect current Bangangté gender roles and, to some extent, their changing economic circumstances. Who shares food with whom, who feeds whose children, and who provides the parcels of land on which to grow the food all influence how people choose to affiliate with different groups of kin. In these times of economic hardship, married women are losing some of their claims upon their natal kin, particularly their patrikin, for help and land. In an ironic tug-of-war, marriage is becoming even more the key to the means of production and thus economic survival for rural women at the same time that others are avoiding marriage with unemployed or underemployed men. The symbolism of marriage does not reflect these contradictions; it emphasizes the transformation of a woman's allegiance as she is enclosed in her husband's compound. The symbolism of procreation reiterates her husband's concerns with patrifiliation, but also forefronts the warmth and feminine skills that hold together matrilines and pam nto' groups, insuring future cooperation in times of scarcity. These marital and procreative images, centering around kitchens, cooking, and food, emphasize women's space and roles.

The imagery of wives cooking inside (and men acting outside) is based on readily observable social relations in Bangangté. Many authors have noted the great extent of gender segregation among the Bamiléké (den Ouden 1980, 1987; Dieckmann and Joldersma 1982; Egerton 1938; Hurault 1962; Tardits 1960), and indeed this separation of men's and women's activities is visually striking. A visitor's first glance at Bangangté catches the sexually segregated groups of people socializing and working together. Men and women cultivate on different fields, and they cluster in separate groups on public occasions and at market. Every polygynous compound has men's and women's areas. On "country Sundays" (days commemorating past kings through the prohibition on labor with the women's hooked, iron hoe)[1] and times when women stay home to watch their and their cowives' children or to cook for their husband, they work in locations of the compound made "female" through the gendered division of labor and expressed by "cooking inside." Women prepare food, and live with their children, whom they nurture, in their kitchens (see fig. 10). When women receive their own guests, they do so most often in their kitchens, or outside in the yard between their kitchen and the main house (the husband's realm). When men receive guests, serving food prepared by the wife, they do so inside or in front of their main house. Much of the spatial segregation of men and women has its roots in the division of labor by gender.

The precolonial division of labor by gender has changed little, but the same types of labor have acquired new significance in the context of an international market economy. Between 1930 and 1950, French colonial policy made it necessary for men to earn cash to pay taxes and for increasing household needs (bridewealth payments, consumer items). They obtained this cash either through wage labor, which generally entailed emigration, or through growing cash crops. The cultivation of coffee and cocoa fit with Bangangté conceptions of male labor, which focused on the cultivation of tree crops such as raffia, plantains, avocados, and oil palms. It also fit with European notions of the division of labor, which led new, commercialized crops to be introduced to men only. Men's previous duties of fence-building, hunting, and warring have declined or disappeared. New opportunities such as commerce, taxi driving, and wage labor allow men to acquire cash.

Women's economic position in the household has become more independent (den Ouden 1980:64). Women have cultivated food crops (maize, beans, and peanuts) as long as Bangangté can remember. As we saw in chapter 2, their economic role as food crop producers was consolidated during the French colonial period before the introduction of coffee. The growth of towns led to the commercialization of women's food crops by 1930 (den Ouden 1980:49). In addition to the independent source of income they now gain through the commercialization of food crops, that is when they choose to sell their subsistence products, women, including married women, also sell prepared food on roadsides and at market, literally "cooking on the road." This allows them to buy the oil and salt their husbands often "forget" and to purchase the meat their husbands no longer hunt.

Husbands do not only "forget" about their contributions to the household economy, but are also often absent in search of wage labor. This leaves women behind in the villages, surviving better than men in the traditional economy, but also suffering from increased work loads and land scarcity. Dieckmann and Joldersma (1982) point out that Bamiléké women, like men, have increasing needs for cash to meet their two main responsibilities—providing food and raising children. School education has increased women's work, both by creating a need for cash to pay school fees and by diminishing a mother's help from her children. Women's duty to produce food leaves them little time or energy for more lucrative income-earning activities (1982:76). Difficulties meeting household needs lead to less material exchange between households with a woman's extended group of kin. This in turn leads to the growing individualization of the matrifocal household, which through diminishing support networks puts women at risk in case of illness or other misfortune (Dieckmann and Joldersma 1982:157; see also Feierman 1981).

Both men and women seek cash for everyday needs and for the special events they hope will contribute to their personal mobility by participating in rotating credit associations. Rotating credit associations allow their participants to save money, and they provide emergency credit when their members face special difficulties. These groups are segregated by gender in rural Bangangté.[2] Since women's groups operate with smaller individual contributions to weekly or monthly meetings than do men's groups, gender segregation in these associations leads to different amounts of material resources. Since these associations are among the primary venues of socializing that reach beyond kinship relations, their segregation by gender means that men and women have widely divergent social networks upon which they can call for support in case misfortune strikes.

When this misfortune involves illness, gender segregation results in differential access to types and quantity of health care. As in Europe and the United States, Bangangté women visit health-care providers more frequently than men, being responsible for their own and their children's health. In the past women were not free to do this on their own, being largely confined to enclosures under the threat of kidnapping by members of other chiefdoms for wives or slavery. Now, with their increased economic independence, many women seek out healers independently. Women are more often accompanied by men when they visit hospitals and clinics than when they visit traditional healers. Village women depend upon men's greater experience dealing with modern institutions and speaking French. Thus, their independence is limited when they become patrons of nationally and internationally oriented institutions.

Unequal access to health care is only one example of the different interactions Bangangté men and women have with a variety of institutions. For example, the need to sell one's products and buy necessities brings men and women into contact with different persons and institutions outside their kin network, or brings them into contact with the same institutions but in ways of very differing quality. Women sell food crops at market. Because types of products are clustered together in the biweekly Bangangté market, female sellers of food crops and palm oil are in a different section than male sellers of small livestock and ritual and medicinal objects. Thus, by selling their crops, women come into contact with other women at market. In contrast, men come into contact with parastatal planters' cooperatives run on bureaucratic principles when they sell their coffee and cocoa. Men thus gain experience in dealing with modern, state institutions, an experience beyond most women's reach.

Women are now trying to learn new skills, with the encouragement of the central government's community development efforts. These skills relate to women's traditional domain, the household. But what skills do these village women learn, and what effect does it have upon their well-being? The women's community development group at Bantoum (a Bangangté village) in 1986 learned crochet and knitting, food preservation techniques, and soap-making, and grew a demonstration communal field. The women of Bantoum viewed the communal field as a burden, creating more work. Crochet and knitting were the most popular activities. Some women are able to use such skills to advance themselves economically; these, however, are generally women who have benefited from formal education beyond primary school. For example, the eldest daughter of a former missionaries' aide first gained a job as a teacher of sewing in a vocational school, then quit her job to open a sewing boutique.

Not all women are able to take advantage of the education they have been fortunate enough to receive. Marguerite, aged 30, claims her position as mother and royal wife keeps her from using her home economics diploma. Instead, she must seek help from maternal kin to send her own two young daughters to school. A number of frustrations stand in the way of women seeking to advance themselves through education under present conditions in rural Bangangté: low expectations of girls' education, ideas of appropriate kinds of schooling for girls, work in the home, responsibility for younger siblings, and early marriage.

Gender Images

The images Bangangté have of maleness and femaleness are inextricably related to the varieties of male and female experience of Bangangté social life. Bangangté of both genders assume that certain characteristics are typical of men or women. These ideas both arise from and help form and maintain such basic varieties of experience as the sexual division of labor, as well as a form of gender segregation that leads to competition among individuals of the same gender and much ignorance about the lives of the other gender. That ignorance, the mystery of the unknown, often leads to men's fearful evaluations of women and women's negative evaluations of men. These critical images contrast sharply with the ones men and women have of themselves.

Women comment freely about themselves as a group, identifying what it means to be a woman, their image of "the good woman," and even negative views of women they share with men. Being a woman means reaching sexual maturity and bearing children. Sanke', although a royal bride when she married mfen Njiké II at age eight, said, "I was not yet a woman." Nkanyam, an elderly, childless woman of a village near the palace, bemoaned that she has never "walked like a woman." She had missed out on an important aspect of womanhood by never bearing children.

Being a woman also means doing what women do: working in the fields, cooking, caring for children, fixing hair, shopping, and paying particular attention to maintaining social ties through visits and attending ritual activities. There is nothing at all unwomanly about doing things few women do (being a doctor, a civil servant, a deputy to the national assembly), as long as one participates in those activities that most women do. Many women claim that women learn languages faster than men.[3] Women spend a great amount of time in conversation doing women's things. "One picks up expressions in the other language bit by bit" (Marguerite, aged 30).

Na nda, the Bangangté expression for marriage, paraphrases the attributes of the good woman in Bangangté thought. The good (married) woman cooks inside within the controlled, bounded area of her husband's compound and kinship group. The "cooking" she does within this space refers both to food preparation and the forming of children by "cooking" male and female waters and bloods during gestation.

Part of being properly inside and controlled for a woman is controlling her speech, keeping information inside. Bangangté women are very careful not to repeat what they view as hearsay. To avoid relating things they have not directly experienced (usually expressed as "seeing") themselves, women will tell an overly insistent interviewer that they are *ta' mbu' tu* (one empty head, idiot). Literature on other Bamiléké groups indicates that this care controlling the flow of information is widespread among Bamiléké women. A widow, expressing her inability to sing and dance using lyrics about any situation other than her very own, asks a researcher "what could I say about the other?" (Ongoum 1985:283–84). Women also teach their children never to repeat hearsay. The source of Bangangté women's concern with keeping information inside is the fear that uncontrolled speech and gossip fuel the jealousies and conflicts among crosscutting kinship affiliations that lead to witchcraft attacks—and witchcraft harms women's procreative chances.

Contrary to women's accounts of themselves and my observations of their actions, men view women as gossips. Miaffo, in his study of Bamiléké public autopsies in the northwest corner of the Bamiléké area, cites this reason as one of the male practitioners' rationales for shutting women out of public autopsies. Women are called "les raconteurs sans avoir vu" (taletellers without having seen) by Miaffo's informants, who also claim that "you speak like a woman" is an insult to men (1977:62).

The royal wives discussed the case of their unfortunate young cowife, Paulette, in terms of what attributes women consider important in judging each other. A good woman should have a known background. She should avoid the taint of "prostitution" and promiscuity, which could endanger both her honor and her fertility. She should have "village knowledge," that is knowledge of customs with regard to kinship and ritual, as well as knowledge of how to get along in a rural environment. Finally, a woman should have skill in agriculture and trade, with skill in agriculture seen as most important for rural women.

Both Bangangté women and men share negative images of women as dangerous and emotionally volatile. Women, who find themselves in close quarters with their competing cowives, are notoriously contentious in Bangangté. European observers investigating Bangangté dispute settlement practices in the 1930s noted that "calumny was regarded as a peculiarly feminine vice" (Egerton 1938:242). Currently the royal wives are particularly famous for expressing jealousy, considered a female trait, through word and deed. Many fear entering the royal compound for this reason.

They are afraid. It is witchcraft. Yes, it's true. *It's because there are so many women. It doesn't come from strangers, but from all the women.* (Christine, aged ca. 32, Ntamleme)

Men also fear women, believing their jealousy will lead them to use supernatural means to harm them.

You the women can do things to destroy men. (Ngangome Daniel, diviner of Nenga, near Batela', after divining that a woman would destroy my husband's job chances)

It was my first wife who poisoned me. It's always women—you really must watch out for them. And this was my Bamiléké wife, the one from Bazou . . . Be careful with women, they can kill you! (a Bangangté taxi driver, upon showing a scar from abdominal surgery to a mission doctor in Mbo)

For men, these images of women's dangerousness are imbued with a sense of mystery; the world of women is unknown and feared by Bamiléké men from many chiefdoms (den Ouden 1987:8). One area of women's knowledge, the interpretation of dream symbols,[4] is frightening and mysterious to men who are not healers but is viewed as an everyday ability by women. "All women know it," said a teenage schoolgirl living at the royal compound.

Women are viewed by Bangangté of both genders as emotionally volatile, more given to uncontrolled bursts of anger, grief or joy than men. Women are not believed to be capable of "holding their hearts" as well as men. The royal wives describe one of their cowives as prone to become "crazy with anger." Miaffo's northwestern Bamiléké informants believe women to be fragile, to catch *crises* (fits, illness) with the least shock and thus to provoke scandals at public autopsies (1977:62). Women's greater emotional sensitivity is believed to continue into ancestorhood; some explain making sacrifices more frequently to ancestresses than to ancestors because ancestresses are more apt than ancestors to be angered by the transgressions of their descendants.

Tondji: Women [ancestresses] make sickness hold children.
Q: More than men?
Tondji: Yes. (Tondji, a healer of Banekane, near Batela')

Bangangté men say that women's lack of emotional discipline leads them to commit adultery. Even Bangangté women agree that only women can commit adultery, explaining it in terms of hierarchy between the sexes.

Before God even created the world, men were on top of women. Thus, a man can do what he pleases, but a woman can know only one man. (Marguerite, aged 30)

The consequences of women's extramarital sexual relationships makes them dangerous to themselves, their husbands, and their lovers. If a woman who has ever committed adultery views her sick husband, or enters the house in which he is staying, the husband will die. The same consequence occurs if the woman's lover visits the sick husband. If husband or lover looks at the woman when she is sick, she too will die. In any of these cases, the woman is ultimately blamed for the misfortune since it is she, in her emotional weakness, who committed adultery.

These images Bangangté men and women have of female characteristics neither exist in a village vacuum nor are static. In its efforts to direct economic "development" and social "progress" (phrases often heard on national radio or printed in the national paper, the *Cameroon Tribune,* in the 1980s), the Cameroonian government has been trying to shape the image and legal status of women (Geary 1986). How, though, are these ideas communicated to rural Bangangté women and men who can neither read the newspaper nor understand French-language broadcasts? One carrier[5] is the network of women's groups run by the community development section of the Ministry of Agriculture. The women's group of Bantoum held a festival, the "Journée de Mari," in May 1986 to demonstrate their good works to their husbands and to various officials from the division and province. The speeches of the numerous participants reveal the variety of images of women communicated through the contemporary Cameroonian rhetoric of development.

The local president of the women's group, an articulate woman with four years of primary school education, opened the ceremonies. Her speech, in the Bangangté language, welcomed the participants and appealed to the officials for financial support for the group's communal fields. Her speech reflected the attitude of the members of the women's group that they had done good work and deserved a reward from official quarters. Her request was evaded or ignored by the four subsequent speeches. Local officials of the political party, of the Ministry of Agriculture, and of the local administration praised women's role in maintaining Cameroon's national food self-sufficiency, women's unity, and women's efforts at making the home nice. The Bangangté president of the women's branch of the political party, a European-educated pediatric nurse, praised women's role in agriculture as the basis for Cameroon's national food self-sufficiency, party phraseology that made a good impression on her fellow officials but did not address local concerns. The speech of the Provincial Delegate for Community Development, read in absentia, also spoke of the importance of women. The statement that the community development women's group unifies women and therefore makes them strong, paraphrasing a Bamiléké proverb that one hand alone cannot tie up a package, received enthusiastic applause. The male Agricultural Delegate addressed the husbands at this "Journée de Mari." He stated the women's group serves the purpose of pleasing the husband and making the home nice. He exhorted the men to encourage their wives to join the group. The Subprefect of Bangangté Sub-Division did not address the issue of women directly. His speech stressed nationalism and praised President Biya. Traditional culture was vilified for "getting in the way of progress," but what this meant for women was never specified. Fertility and women's role in procreation, the seeming preoccupation of everyday conversation, never was raised in these official speeches.

Views of male character, while not the focus of this research, put Bangangté images of women into the context of gender complementarity. Women and men differed greatly in their images of maleness. Women concur with men that men are "on top of women," that a hierarchical relationship exists to men's public advantage. Women speak of needing to obey their husbands, and they defer to their husbands nearly all decisions that have to do with dealing with strangers. This does not mean that men can prevent women from manipulating them or from having a full, rich social life among themselves. Men, whose major reference groups lie outside the household, often disappoint their wives, failing to live up to their duties as household heads. When women talk about men, they often complain. Two women eating together teased the hostess's husband about the cheap fish, attributing their "poor" meal to the husband's stinginess, a trait women often attribute to men. Women also distrust men, fearful of being trapped in an unhappy love affair or left pregnant and alone. One unmarried woman complained, "You know, sometimes men are so nice in the beginning. They want to trap you. But then later they might not be nice anymore. They are not always honest" (Anne, aged 24, Bangangté). Like men's fears of women's mysterious powers, women's complaints about men center on what they do not know about them. Women feel cheated in their ignorance of men's pocketbooks and of men's sexual affairs.

Men, by contrast, name their own qualities as counterpoints to those of women. They see themselves as straightforward, emotionally controlled, sexually potent (only women are sterile), and gregarious and modern in outlook. Men do not need to avoid the taint of promiscuity, although they must sometimes be circumspect regarding their extramarital sexual activities. During my field stay, only the mfen was criticized for neglecting the sexual (i.e., reproductive) needs of his wives in favor of those of prostitutes in town. Men should have knowledge of kinship and ritual rules, but do not need to get along in a rural environment to be manly. A rich man would not be denigrated for not getting along in a rural environment, for men in the household should be waited upon. But any man with wives who farm would be expected to do manual work or to pay laborers to clear his wives' fields.

Two inversions, situations in which women act like men, indicate shared male and female views of what is expected of adult Bangangté men. The first inversion involves Claude, the king's white wife, who was often described, by her cowives as well as others, as "like a husband" to the other women of the court. Claude had a steady cash income as a *lycée* professor, took care of her cowives' financial needs, transported them to distant farms, often fed them, and cared for the most children in the royal compound. Although it is often the wives who support their husbands and children, this account of a cowife/ husband indicates expectations that men should meet at least women's needs for cash and transport. The second inversion concerns the image of menopausal women. The elderly male pharmacist of the Bangangté Divisional Hospital reminisced about the life of royal wives in the past. Then, only menopausal women of the palace were allowed to go to market alone, with the justification that they are "a bit like men." Likewise, menopausal women were allowed to attend public autopsies among northwestern Bamiléké groups because they shared male qualities and had lost some female qualities. Elderly women were believed to have "hard hearts" and social experience, and to have "seen a lot." With elderly women there was no risk of spontaneous, unfounded, or uncontrolled remarks (Miaffo 1977:63).

Men and women concur about a number of images of each other's gender. They also disagree sharply about other images, generally attributing more positive characteristics to themselves than to the mysterious, dangerous, or stingy other. Some of these various images of femaleness and maleness arise from gender roles (e.g., women as food producers and child nurturers), and from differences in male and female experience (e.g., adult men do not compete with members of their own household; they have more contact with modern institutions and are seen as more "progressive"; women live in situations of competition with their cowives and are seen as jealous and contentious). Where men and women disagree about gender images, they are often complaining about the other, part of a point–counterpoint of anxiety and failed expectations with regard to the other in a society where men and women share very little social space.

Bangangté women continue to regard food and children as the two most important things they "serve up" or give to their kin and their world. A married woman cooks food and lives with her children, whom she has "cooked" through gestation and now nurtures inside the marital, procreative kitchen. In the ideal household economy, the husband provides his wife with meat, oil, and salt to add to the culinary ingredients she produces herself (maize, beans, and peanuts). The woman mixes these male and female ingredients to cook a final product, the meal. The imagery of measuring the ingredients of conception and the cooking of gestation mirror the gender roles of home economics in the realm of procreation. Wives seem more aware than husbands that their food and children link people together in numerous webs of kinship affiliation.

Cooking and Sex

When Bangangté speak of sex, whether seriously describing "what needs to be known" to children and ethnographers or joking with sexual innuendos, their language is full of culinary imagery. Bangangté men and women, old and young, say that sex is hot and therefore contains enormous transformative powers and danger. Sex is also hot in the same way that good music, a good joke, or a freshly cooked meal one just cannot wait to taste is hot: "ça chauffe!" (it's hot!) interject young Bangangté, using slang from the pop music world. Bangangté men talk about sex and procreation using imagery of the cooking fire.[6] When a man impregnates a woman, he "cooks the woman" (Goldschmidt 1986:58). A woman who has conceived before marriage has not "cooked" in the proper way; she is called *chongwa,* "oversalted," and her parents are given an oversalted meal by her affines to let them know that their daughter did not guard her hearth prudently (Nzikam Djomo 1977:34).[7] Men refer to repeated sex acts during the course of their wife's pregnancy as "tending the fire."

Women also talk about sex in terms of cooking, and stress *their* perception of cooking. Cooking, and sex, are work for rural women, and are referred to as work in everyday language. As work and as flirtation, cooking and sex are closely related; when a woman cooks a meal for a man, it is an expression of love and of the desire to have sex (Njiké Bergeret 1997:14–45). Sexual intercourse is seen as one of the duties of wifehood, and the means to become pregnant with the ubiquitously desired child.[8] Women describe that during sex, the husband provides his wife with ingredients (water, blood) to mix with her own water and blood to "cook" a child. Husband and wife "measure" (*mfi'*) these ingredients to procreate (*mfi mentun,* "to measure a person").[9] Just the right amount of blood and water, and just the right amount of sex, are necessary for successful conception.[10]

The sex act mixes (*nu'u*) the ingredients as the good cook stirs the sauce thickening and taking form in her pot. Thus Bangangté believe procreation occurs when diverse elements from man and woman are "measured" (*mfi'*), "mixed" (*nu'u*), and "cooked" (*nâ*) through sex and thus transformed into a new being.

The Procreative Kitchen

Just as food production and preparation are women's tasks in Bangangté's sexual division of labor, women's role in the *process* of procreation is dominant. The pregnant woman is both the fire and the cooking pot. She provides half the ingredients and is the cook who measures, stirs, and adds ingredients until the meal, the baby, is ready to be presented through the act of childbirth. Her experience and understanding of procreation reinforce her awareness of the importance of matrifocal and matrilineal ties despite the realities and rhetoric of cooking inside the kitchen her husband built.

Conception and Ingredients

Bangangté believe that women and men contribute equally to the *substance* that makes a new human being. During the act of sexual intercourse, the "waters" (*ntse*), or sometimes the "bloods" (*lem*), of the man and the woman mix to form a fetus. Bangangté call semen "water," but also speak of the need to cleanse an infertile woman of "bad water" to regain her fertility. Likewise, blood is a medium of inheritance. Bangangté describe resemblance in terms of which parent's blood is stronger, or in terms of a child "having the blood" of one of its parents. In discussions about procreation, Bangangté say blood is "just like" palm oil, an essential element in cooking. In wedding ceremonies and royal coronations, palm oil is a symbol of fertility and the blood of childbirth. After mixing, the two bloods or waters are then "measured" into a person.

> The woman possesses something on which the man comes to depose his own and the two touch to measure [create] a person. (Tamveun, male, aged 65, Batela')

While the sex act between two persons is recognized as necessary to produce offspring, sexual relations are considered merely adjunct to the work or gift of *nsi,* god (Nzikam Djomo 1977:23). Angered ancestors may interfere with a person's fertility, but they do not actually make couples conceive. Conception is a mystery about which only god can know (Goldschmidt 1986:58).

> Isn't it God who gives the child to the woman? (Nyombab, elderly woman, Batela')

> To make children depends on blood and God. (Charlotte, aged 18, Ntamleme)

God does it. When a woman sleeps with a man, he throws his water on the woman and she becomes pregnant. (mfen Meshinke', Bantoum)

Nsi, God, is also the original creator of humankind. Rebecca, a 28-year-old wife of mfen Njiké Pokam, stated that Nsi formed the first people out of clay from the earth and then blew life (*zwiak,* breath, spirit) into them. In nearby Bandjoun, Nsi the creator is also described as "god the potter of all things" (Goldschmidt 1986:210). As a potter, Nsi not only blows breath into the people he creates but like all good potters must bake or cook his pottery.[11] Contrasting sharply with monogenetic procreation ideology in the Judeo-Christian-Muslim world (Delaney 1991), conception involves the active participation of women as well as men, and female as well as male substance. In Bangangté, divine action is not male action; in fact, the nurturing firing of clay pots closely parallels female cooking labors.

Gestation

Once the fire has been lit and the water put up to boil through sex and conception, Bangangté women view gestation as the continuing, slow process of cooking a good sauce. The continual mixing of the central procreative fluids, water/sperm and oil/blood, is essential to produce a smooth and tasty meal, and for the proper gestation of the fetus. Bangangté women describe their feelings during pregnancy as swelling or growing, as maize meal expands when the woman cooks foofoo (porridge). While waiting for a prenatal checkup at a mission-run maternal–child health clinic, a mother in her twenties described the development of her fetus.

Pamé, you can hear noises in your belly. It is like a bubbling pot, and the doctor hears it through his horn [stethoscope]. (Celeste, Bangangté)

Bangangté regard repeated sexual intercourse during the mother's pregnancy as the normative way to accomplish the continual mixing of good cuisine. Sexual intercourse during pregnancy "tends the fire" and "opens the way" to ease childbirth (Nzikam Djomo 1977:61). As an essential ingredient, the father's semen ("water") fortifies and feeds the fetus.[12] Perhaps most importantly, when the mother has sex repeatedly with the child's father, the fetus "gets to know its father." Having sex with her fetus's father is a good deed the mother performs for her child, for it introduces or "names" the father to the child. In fact, if the mother has difficulty in childbirth it is assumed that her child results from an extramarital affair and that she has "named" the father neither to the child nor to the public. If the pregnant woman has sex with someone other than the fetus' father, the "strengths" or "bloods" of the two men will fight over the fetus, endangering its health. This set of beliefs reflects Bangangté concern with verifying a child's patrifiliation. "Cooking inside" encloses the wife's sexual and childbearing activities within the bounds of marriage and keeps her children inside her husband's patrilineage.

While concern with patrifiliation is central whenever Bangangté discuss the ins and outs of marriage and procreation or "cooking inside," attitudes toward sexual relations during pregnancy are more varied among younger women. Not all interviewed women agreed that continued sexual relations are beneficial during the period of gestation. A slight majority approved of sex during pregnancy for the nourishment of the fetus, acquainting the fetus with its father, and opening the vaginal passage to ease childbirth. Others complained that sexual intercourse had a deleterious effect on the pregnant woman's energy or health, or that sex is unnecessary if one is already pregnant. Underlying this latter opinion is the general orientation among Bangangté women that the purpose of sex is to conceive. As one woman remarked regarding sex during pregnancy, "is it food?" (Bwoda', aged 31, Bantoum). Some women declined to describe norms, saying that each woman has her own way. One was particularly uncertain about the benefits of the fetus becoming acquainted with its father through the sex act, saying:

> There are times that you are pregnant and for a certain child, it kills
> . . . He does not like his father. (Sanke', aged 28, Bantoum)

This variety of opinion leaves us with an underlying symbolic framework of ideas about measuring, mixing, and cooking, of specific ingredients controlled and kept "inside," away from the contamination of other ingredients (other men's semen). But it also reveals how a symbolic framework might be hegemonic, but not "doxic" (Bourdieu 1977). Bangangté women are quite aware that their symbols are just that—symbols. They choose to invoke them in certain circumstances, but at times ignore or override a set of symbols to express other sets of ideas, in this case ideas about the work and stresses of pregnancy and sex.[13]

Childbirth

Before Bangangté women developed a preference for giving birth in hospitals and clinics, childbirth occurred at the woman's home in the husband's compound (Nzikam Djomo 1977:69). This venue underscores the containment of the wife's sexual and childbearing duties within an area "belonging" to the husband's patrilineage. The procreative kitchen, however, is woman's space within that compound. Exemplifying the conflicting loyalties and demands on every Bangangté child and wife, the birthing mother was surrounded by other women—the neighbor-midwife or an experienced older woman and, time permitting, a mother or sister, female members of her matrilineage. Men and children were not allowed to attend births, which, like cooking, are still considered women's business.

While the skills of traditional midwives are virtually unknown to the younger generation of Bangangté mothers, Goldschmidt's nearby Bandjoun informants continue the culinary analogy by referring to the actions of traditional midwives. The movements of preparing *nkwi* (a viscous sauce considered the Bamiléké meal par excellence) are equivalent to the movements of the midwife's massage; cutting the gluey threads of the sauce is like cutting the umbilical cord (1986:159).

Presently, the high density of biomedical facilities in Ndé Division contributes to the disappearance of traditional midwifery.[14] Nearly all Bangangté women now give birth in a nearby hospital or clinic, where most nurse-midwives are men. My informants considered hospital births the medically prudent choice, by no means a conscious withdrawal from their husbands' territory or control. In fact, husbands usually pay for their wives' hospitalizations. Bangangté mothers and their husbands felt that hospital convalescence, typically one week, was more restful for the mother because it removes her from household duties and potentially argumentative cowives.

Although they no longer give birth next to their cooking hearths, Bangangté women talk about the full-term fetus as cooked food, the final outcome of a long process of cooking. Once born, the baby is a "fresh person" (*men fi*), no longer referred to as metaphoric food. Following childbirth, the symbolism of food switches from a focus on the mother's cooking skills and on the developing fetus to the textures, shapes, colors, and nutritive values of foods for the recovering mother and her infant. As soon as she returns from the hospital to her kitchen, the mother is surrounded by female neighbors, cowives, and kin who nourish her with food they cook on her hearth.

After the Meal: Postpartum and Infant Care.   In Bangangté, the gooey sauce nkwi is fed to the mother of the newborn. A food prepared only by Bamiléké cooks, nkwi is considered nutritious and easy to digest. Its smooth, viscous consistency is thought to help the expulsion of the afterbirth. Nkwi is also considered "our food" by Bangangté, a quality that makes it good to give strength and encourage the mother's milk production.

Bangangté women liken the period immediately following birth to *nja,* a now nearly defunct but well-remembered pre-betrothal puberty rite involving seclusion and fattening.[15] The mother is kept in semiseclusion and fed special foods, takes special care of her bodily cleanliness, and is not supposed to work. For up to two months, her female kin arrange their visits so that someone is always there to do housework and to bathe and admire the newborn.[16] The mother is massaged with warm water to aid the parting of blood and decrease the size of the belly (Nzikam Djomo 1977:97). The placenta and umbilical cord are buried under a banana or plantain tree somewhere near the mother's kitchen within the child's patrilineal compound, even when the child is born hundreds of kilometers away in the hospital of one of the large cities. Mothers, concerned with the lure of the cities, remind their older children to "never forget where your placenta is buried." They admonish their children to remember the multiple affiliations signified by the place of burial: the compound of patrifiliation and the father's patrilineage; the kitchen of matrifocality, pam nto', and matrilineal food exchange; and the "home" of one's village and kingdom, symbolic loci of cultural authenticity identified through kinship ties.

Infant care is the mother's responsibility, aided by the surrounding women and children who visit her during her convalescence. Mother's milk is considered best, being of the "same blood."[17] The mother is given special foods to help her lactation, and she refrains from sexual intercourse until she has weaned the child in order to "prevent her milk from spoiling." Some Bangangté women (especially the more experienced royal wives) stated that, while the "official" reason for abstinence during lactation was to protect the quality of breastmilk, sexual abstinence also prevented mothers of infants from becoming caught up in fights among cowives regarding sexual access to the husband. Keeping the mother calm is considered best for her and her baby's survival chances. Farmer suggests that the bad blood–spoiled milk complex in Haitian illness concepts is a "disorder of experience" that submits the private problems of pregnant and lactating women (poverty, abuse) to public scrutiny (1988). In the Haitian case, breastmilk is spoiled through bad social relations. Bangangté try to prevent such bad social relations by forbidding sexual intercourse to lactating women.

Soon after birth, the infant is given an enema to cleanse its belly, whence all disease is supposed to originate. Although local physicians deplore the practice of herbal enemas given to infants because it induces diarrheal disease, Bangangté women do not seem deterred by physicians' reactions. Instead, they vigilantly wash the infant; water fortifies the child as the father's water fortified the fetus in the womb. For its first month, the child remains nearly continually in the procreative kitchen, within the walls that contained its mother's procreative and culinary arts. Gradually, the child's experiences expand from the "inside" of its mother's kitchen to the larger "inside" of its father's compound, and eventually to the "outside" world of neighborhood, school, and work.

"Inside": Marriage and Controlling Threats to Procreation

Marriage (*na nda*) establishes the procreative kitchen in which the cooking of food and offspring occurs. In Bangangté eyes, it is the contract that brings procreation under social control, preventing the new wife from "cooking on the road." The Bangangté concept of married women refers to the cooking of food and offspring within the bounded, legitimized marriage relationship. Marriage, from the point of view of the groom and his patrilineage, assures the groom of eating; fiancées' appeal to their future fathers-in-law is exemplified by the typical opening line, "I have no one to cook for me." It also assures him of having descendants, as children born in wedlock belong to the patrilineage of their fathers.

The symbols of cooking and measuring ingredients that permeate Bangangté imagery of procreation are evident in the marriage exchanges made over the period of betrothal and continuing after the couple is living together. The groom and his family bring gifts of palm oil, goats, firewood, blankets, clothing, and cash bridewealth payments to the bride's family. The size of these gifts is clearly affected by market forces and varies with the wealth of the groom, his family, the bride's family, and the bride's skills and education. A ceremony, during which the bride asks her family's blessing, marks the bride's new status and change of residence to her husband's compound.[18] The groom's family brings the elements necessary for a good kitchen—palm oil, meat, and firewood—to the bride's natal compound, which the bride's family *cooks* and serves as a meal to the entire assembly. Palm oil, mixed with camwood powder, is smeared on the bride's chest and feet by her father to insure her fertility. It is likened to blood, an essential ingredient of the *procreative* kitchen. The high point of the ceremony occurs when the bride serves her father palm wine, stating "this wine is poison in your stomach should I ever divorce." The daughter's horrifying patricidal oath is considered an encouragement to the longevity of the marriage.

The substances exchanged, cooked, and manipulated in the family's blessing contain multiple layers of symbols of women and fertility. The lump of earth the bride receives from the ancestral skull house is the material in which women cultivate. Water used in cooking brings fertile moisture and is essential to conception. Oil is a symbol of peace and fertility, an ingredient of meals, and makes the woman soft and sexually appealing (Nzikam Djomo 1977:49–50). The new wife carries her gifts and the artifacts of her blessings to the kitchen her husband has built in his compound. Thus, the marriage ceremony establishes the procreative kitchen as a woman's space enclosed in a man's space and imbues it with the many-layered meanings of culinary symbolism. Essential to the Bangangté conception of marriage (and sex unencumbered by potential supernatural sanction) is that the wife cooks only inside this kitchen.

Marriage, "cooking inside," literally encloses the newlywed wife within the walls of the kitchen her husband has built for her. In precolonial Bangangté, marriage also enclosed women within the palisade walls surrounding their husbands' compounds, protecting them from raids by citizens of neighboring kingdoms seeking slaves and wives. As we saw in chapter 2, in polygynous compounds, a wife's kitchen is where she both cooks and sleeps, shares food and tells stories with her children, and receives her private guests. In monogamous compounds, the wife and her children may sleep in the main house, but the woman's daily activities center around her kitchen and her fields.

Bangangté marriage brings the woman inside in a number of figurative ways as well. Before marriage, the bride belongs to the patrilineage of her father and the matrilineage of her mother, both kin groups outside the groom's patrilineage. Marriage does not cut off the bride's kin ties, but contains her sexual and childbearing services within the rights and duties of marriage. Norms governing marriage in Bangangté prescribe exogamy, forbidding marriage of both "close" and classificatory kin, and through the institution of *ndap* (praise names indicating parents' village of origin), of partners descending from people of the same village. Since postmarital residence is virilocal, the wife, formerly a stranger, has moved socially and geographically "inside" the husband's compound and village. The very term for marriage, *na nda,* refers to the transformation of the *woman* from someone who cooks outside to a *wife* whose cooking is enclosed in the marital, procreative kitchen.

The movement from outside to inside so vividly depicted by the expression *na nda* is a social process perceived from the point of view of the husband and his patrilineage. When Bangangté speak of "inside," they usually refer to an inside defined by patrilineal and virilocal principles: inside the kingdom characterized by allegiance to a patrilineal heir, inside one's village that is also the village of one's father, inside the compound where the only links among half-siblings are patrilineal, and inside the kitchen built to enclose a wife's cooking. Bangangté matrilineages do not have the same association with place, and thus cannot have an inside. Only matrifocal households have a specific locality, and that is a kitchen within a larger compound held together by affinal and patrilineal ties. Upon marriage, a wife will acknowledge that she has moved from outside to inside her husband's realm and the domain of his patrilineal relations. She has left her mother's kitchen and father's compound, but has never moved "outside" her important links to them as kin.

Themes of enclosure or containment of women as potential strangers recur in Bangangté gender images and, in the past, in times of explicit, ritual enclosure. In addition to sex, childbearing, and children's belonging, marriage attempts to enclose women's speech and knowledge, and their volatility and dangerousness.

Keeping Sex and Children's Belonging Inside

Bangangté bring the procreative powers of women, their potentially volatile heat and fire, under social control through institutions that regulate how pairs come together to make children, and under what conditions pregnancy and childbirth can occur. Bangangté are concerned with controlling sexual intercourse through norms regarding marriage and infidelity for two reasons: assuring patrifiliation and preventing affliction.

Controlling sexual intercourse by keeping it within the bounds of marriage insures that the child's patrifiliation is known and legitimate and its kinship affiliations unambiguous. To Bangangté, matrifiliation is made obvious by the act of birth. Mother–child bonds are strengthened further through the child's care and socialization within the matrifocal household. Sharing this household with mother and full siblings fosters the child's identification with its matrilineage. The child's connection to its matrilineage is nurtured in addition through visits of its mother's sisters, mother's mother, and even more distant matrikin, starting with the care matrikin give the new mother and her infant. Patrifiliation, in contrast, is only made certain by the parents' submission to rules governing marriage choice and beliefs discouraging extramarital sexual relations. Importantly, patrifiliation determines the child's membership in a patrilineage, claims to inheritance, and village belonging.

In addition to assuring patrifiliation, keeping sexual intercourse within an approved marital union also assures the proper mix of the ingredients of a new being: the water and blood of appropriately paired parents. Using the right ingredients is necessary to keep the pot and its contents from spoiling, or in more prosaic terms to prevent the misfortune of reproductive illness.

Bangangté women speak of a recent past when nearly all marriages were arranged between the parents of the betrothed. Until about twenty years ago, parents bargained spousal choice and bridewealth without telling the children until after the marriage negotiations were completed (Ngomsi 1986). Marriages arranged by parents resulted in beneficial political and economic alliances for the parents. Arranged marriage also meant that the bride's and groom's genealogies were thoroughly checked, preventing risk of incest for the new couple. Arranged marriage was a way that parents contained the choice of mate, keeping alliances within (*inside*) their control.

Presently the question of choice of mate has changed in degree; fathers (with mothers bargaining in the background) still often choose their children's prospective spouses, but are not always successful in implementing their decisions. Take, for example, the story of Jeanne's marriage.

> *Mfen Njiké Pokam of Bangangté, soon after succeeding to the throne, asked his friend the mfen of the Bamiléké chiefdom of Bapi to honor him with the gift of a wife. The first woman chosen as a bride for mfen Njiké Pokam ran away to the port city of Douala. Jeanne was then given as a gift to the mfen by her classificatory father, also her full brother, the mfen of Bapi; she became one of the mfen of Bangangté's younger wives (born 1964). Although an outside observer would classify Jeanne's marriage to mfen Njiké Pokam as an arranged, gift marriage, Jeanne considers this marriage a choice she made, at age fourteen, to save her brother's honor.*

Earlier, a daughter could not refuse her father's choice, on threat of beating, ostracization, or even death according to one young female informant. Now she may refuse, but she always risks suffering estrangement from her parents, causing a decline in her parents' stature, and bringing on the wrath of the ancestors, matrilineal or patrilineal, or of the refused mate.

In 1983 a grandmother of Maham, an outlying village of Bangangté chiefdom, pointed out some adolescent girls passing by along the road. Although they were "young and beautiful," the grandmother told me, they had an illness that would probably keep them from marrying. They were both epileptics. One of the girls had refused to marry an elderly man locally suspected of witchcraft. The grandmother surmised that this cantankerous fellow "gave" the girls epilepsy as revenge for their refusal.

Bangangté consider the sex that occurs in mismatched marriages, outside the control of elders, dangerous. Many Bangangté, including young women who wish for more choice for themselves as individuals, fear that the pairing of couples has escaped the regulation of their elders. They fear that marriage choice is no longer "inside," and that this increases the likelihood for such mishaps as incest, angering ancestors who then "seize" the kin group with the afflictions of illness and infertility. While either matrilineal or patrilineal ancestors can "seize" their descendants in their wrath, Bangangté most fear their matrilineal ancestresses who they believe are more sensitive and emotionally volatile. But even patrilineal ancestors can be dangerous, especially if incest has occurred, as we saw in the case of Paulette's disastrous marriage in chapter 1. Paulette's parents had been completely uninvolved in her choice of husband. Although the patrilineal connection between Paulette and the king was not discovered until after their marriage, from the moment the kin relation was discovered, the union became incestuous and needed to be dissolved. If the marriage had continued, the wife and her children would be no longer under the protection of her ancestors and could die (Kaberry 1969). Many informants observing Paulette's marriage to the mfen of Bangangté cited these rules and were convinced that only misfortune could result from a union now discovered to be incestuous. They assured me that Paulette's marriage could never produce offspring.

In addition to incest, Bangangté believe that extramarital sex, especially that involving a married woman, can cause infertility, serious illness, or death. Infidelity leads to a triangular relationship among the woman, her husband, and her lover. If any of these three falls ill, and sees or is visited by any of the others, they are believed to die. One wife of mfen Njiké Pokam, known to have had intercourse with a healer when seeking fertility enhancement medicine, was forbidden to visit her husband when he was hospitalized for cirrhosis in 1986. "It would be like murder," exclaimed the mfen's great-aunt, the corpulent and outspoken sister of the king's grandfather. Infidelity is particularly dangerous for women. They may be punished severely, such as when mfen Njiké II allegedly buried one of his wives alive after she had become pregnant by another man. Infidelity during pregnancy may cause fetal death, "when the two men's waters fight." It is also thought to lead to difficulties during childbirth.

With the exception of men who sleep with the mfen's wives, a heinous crime, only women are believed to commit adultery in Bangangté. In the context of polygyny, women are limited to a single partner; they are the only ones kept inside." Men not only can have many partners, they also are not sanctioned for sleeping with women other than their wives. Of course, this leaves their extramarital partners open to sanction. Women's sexual activity is limited to their single spouse because otherwise the father's paternity would be uncertain and the child's kinship affiliation would be in doubt. Beliefs about the relation of infidelity to illness support social norms limiting the range of sexual partners any one person may have. Bangangté men and women say that keeping sex "inside" marriage is *prudent,* a way of preventing misfortune.

In an environment of mutual distrust based on Bangangté gender images, Bangangté in rural communities incessantly lectured me, as the unaccustomed stranger, on prudent behavior. Being prudent means being able to control or contain aspects of daily life. These issues of control, however, differ for men and women. Men, as we have seen, seek to keep women inside the bounds of proper marital behavior: cooking and child-bearing. Bangangté women, by contrast, are more concerned with self-control, especially keeping information *inside* by not repeating hearsay and choosing their interlocutors carefully.

When Bangangté explain the causes of misfortune, they weave together a discussion of sexual relationships, emotional control or volatility, and insider versus outsider status. Bangangté men say that women's lack of emotional discipline leads them to commit adultery. Both men and women believe that adultery brings its own sanctions and also can lead to the practice of witchcraft by slighted, envious spouses. Thus, women are often blamed for causing sickness and misfortune through their jealousies, their spontaneity, and their lack of emotional control. Men suspect women of nefarious activities, especially if they perceive them as strangers or outsiders. Nearly all wives or sisters-in-law are outsiders since they move from their natal villages to that of their husbands upon marriage in the Bangangté system of virilocal residence. Many may even speak another language as their mother tongue. These outsiders are suspect because their families and their premarital comportment are little known and cannot easily be checked for evidence of sorcery, the biggest fear and greatest threat to the fertility of the entire residential group.

Concluding Remarks

Bangangté images of procreative processes and of gender differences reiterate important aspects of women's roles in the sexual division of labor, centering around the production and preparation of food. The image of ideal femininity for both Bangangté men and women is the married woman whose agricultural, household, and sexual activities are enclosed within the bounds of the marriage institution. Even her speech should be enclosed, for the good woman is prudent in her communication of feeling and information. Fields, cleared by husbands, have spatial boundaries, as does the wives' area within household compounds. The marital kitchen, a walled structure, is the dominant metaphor through which Bangangté express the containment within social bounds of the good woman's culinary and procreative skills. Bangangté believe that when a woman oversteps these social bounds by literally and figuratively cooking outside the procreative kitchen, social relations fall apart. Most particularly, the patrilineal and thus village belonging of a child born out of wedlock is always in doubt. This makes the ingredients of the social soup uncertain. Mixing and transforming specific, disparate ingredients into a new whole is the core image both of Bangangté concepts of procreation and of the constitution of society.

Cooking inside, *na nda,* when understood narrowly as marriage, is only one point in a long process that brings individuals together to procreate and reproduce Bangangté society. My discussion of the cooking imagery of procreation has followed the social and biological stages of the process of reproduction: mating, conception, gestation, and birth. Each of these stages calls forth specific social configurations. Human reproduction not only makes new biological beings, but also forms and transforms social relations as the key actors pass through its diverse biological stages and their immediate social contexts. The mother forms new social relations and the quality of her old ties change through the processes of maturation, mate-finding, marriage, sex, pregnancy, childbirth, and motherhood (MacCormack 1982). She is enclosed by her husband's compound and patrilineage, her claims upon her natal patrilineage persist but are weakened, and her matrilineal ties necessitate energetic work preparing and exchanging food. A young mother also actively shapes the social identity and web of relations of a new human being through the care and socialization she gives her new baby. In Bangangté these processes are regulated by beliefs about procreation, infidelity, and sickness, and by social institutions including marriage. Marriage, expressed as cooking inside, like birth transforms social relations and highlights actors' complementary and competing kinship ties. The activities associated with pregnancy, birth, and marriage, undertaken to treat illness or to maximize reproductive chances, are based on Bangangté understandings of good cuisine. Women put their metaphors into practice, using their experience in the kitchen to manage their social and sexual relations.

Cooking and commensality, central to Bangangté concepts of procreation, are also crucial forms of expressing and maintaining matrilineal kin ties in Bangangté's dual descent system, and of forming affinal ties through the symbolism of marriage oaths, exchanges, and ceremonies. The existence of these numerous ties of kinship affiliation supported by cooking and exchanging food shows that the Bangangté idiom of inside and outside expressed in *na nda* looks different from the various points of view of husbands' and wives' lineages (Feldman-Savelsberg 1995). The Bangangté socio-spatial dichotomy of inside/outside is linked simultaneously to kinship ideology and gender concepts (see also Collier and Yanagisako 1987:9). Bangangté define "inside" in patrilineal and virilocal terms, symbolizing enclosure in the husband's group through kitchen walls and compound fences. From the point of view of marriage and the (albeit seldom realized) ideal of patrilocal as well as virilocal residence, ties to nonresident kin are largely organized through women (by now a common theme in feminist rethinking of kinship studies).

But Bangangté talk about inside and outside in other contexts. With regard to the matrilineal ties of both husbands and wives, residence is not even loosely linked to descent, and lineages are not at all localized. They are definitely "outside" a patrilineal "inside." Pam nto', or uterine groups, are likewise dispersed; nonetheless, their core is matrifocal households. The mother's hearth is both the symbol and spatial center of these matrifocal households, the warm inside of the inside, with its special links to a patrilineally defined outside.

Through the way Bangangté explain procreation and marriage, they place kitchens, cooking, feeding, and sex in the same semantic field. This imagery emphasizes women's space, as defined by both women and men, and women's roles in the gendered division of labor.

These symbolic connections among procreation and realms of everyday gendered experience are not neutral. The gendered division of labor reflected and reinforced in Bangangté images of human reproduction is a vital part of being a Bangangté women, an important aspect of female identity. It is also part of relationships of domination and the ambiguities of power from above (the dominating) and from below (the dominated). Procreation imagery simultaneously reinforces a particular married-with-children identity that places women in situations of subordination to men's needs and control. But it also celebrates women's skills and their essential and unique abilities to make babies and to keep them alive. Procreation imagery serves as a source of female solidarity; when women invoke the metaphors of procreation, they emphasize the ties, through women, that hold together Bangangté society, socially as well as physically reproducing it.

Both men and women are vitally interested in matters of fertility, but in different ways. The segregation of men's and women's social experience, largely resulting from this division of labor, means that men and women vary in the material and social resources they can use to promote and protect their roles and interests in human reproduction. Both men and women try to use existing social institutions to guarantee their ability to reproduce and the well-being of their offspring.

Not all are successful. Bangangté in different social positions, experiencing different strains and opportunities in the changing social context of modern Bangangté, perceive threats to their reproductive capacities in varying ways and to varying extents. Actual threats, fears, and their distribution among different segments of the Bangangté population is the subject of the next chapter.

Chapter Four

The Kitchen Plundered:
Fear of Infertility

"Why do arguments prevent babies? If you shake the pot, the sauce sticks to the sides and can't come out right."

Bangangté women talk a lot about cooking—what sauce to make tonight, how to stir the *foofoo,* and who took the cocoyams. As exemplified in the preceding quotation, they also use cooking to talk about infertility. The symbolic construction of procreation, referring to hot sex, maternal hearths, and cooking-pot wombs, appears prominently in Bangangté women's explanations of infertility. This emic model of infertility causation uses culinary symbolism to illuminate why procreation works or fails in individual bodies. It also draws upon cooperative models of a gendered household economy to illuminate the impact of social relations on fertility. Contentiousness and a breakdown of reciprocity disturb the provisioning and sharing of food and likewise endanger fertility. When the king is metaphorically a bad cook, unable to manipulate social ingredients to prevent calumny, individual women's fertility is further endangered. Thus, the Bangangté culinary symbolism of procreation ripples out across several social fields, locating the causes of infertility in the individual body, the social body, and the body politic (Scheper-Hughes and Lock 1987) and linking them through a common set of idioms.

Strikingly, this common set of idioms is used not only to explain unfortunate *personal* events, the individual tragedy of infertility. Culinary symbolism also is invoked in tales of infertility, stories and laments that warn of physical and social dangers. While shelling peanuts or hoeing weeds together, I heard stories of bad cooking and the procreative kitchen being plundered by greedy witches. These everyday conversations, stories told around the hearth after the evening meal, and witchcraft accusations shouted in anger or brought to the mfen for adjudication were all peppered with laments about the inability to conceive, tales of fetuses stolen from the womb or "stuck to the sides of the cooking

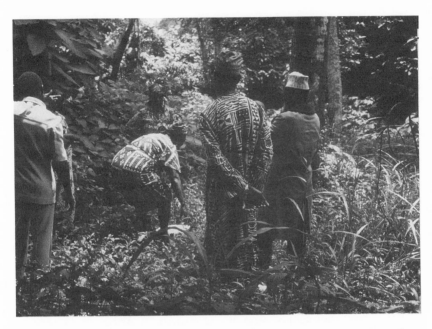

Fig. 11. In a rite of reconciliation to cure infertility, disputing kin wash themselves in raffia wine surveilled by the bandansi (ritual specialists of the palace). The "cooked" wine seals the participants' oaths. The rite is performed in the supernaturally fertile area downhill and behind the king's palace.

pot," and complaints that the king's family has too few children. The Bangangté women I came to know in the 1980s used culinary imagery not only to construct illness narratives of their individual bodies and afflictions, but even more frequently to express anxieties about the effects of social (or asocial) actions on fertility, and the political and cultural implications of population decline.

Bangangté women use infertility as an idiom to comment upon their lives. When Bangangté women begin their conversations with a lament about childlessness, they are expressing anxiety about a wide range of disorders of human and social reproduction. If not afflicted themselves, they have observed a sister, mother, or neighbor suffering from childlessness, secondary infertility, or child loss. They have personally felt the erosion of a distinctly Bangangté identity as their offspring have gone to school and/or left ancestral lands in search of urban wage labor. If Bangangté seem unduly anxious about infertility, it is because they are worried about their personal health, their poverty, and their weakening king. Women's complaints about infertility map areas of personal and social unease. Fertility and infertility are such powerful idioms in women's complaints because, in Bangangté and perhaps throughout Africa, fertility and infertility are the quintessential indicators of good and bad fortune.

This chapter explores Bangangté women's understandings of infertility in relation to women's feelings of vulnerability. Picking up on the themes of chapter 3, it examines the metaphors through which Bangangté express their notions of threatened procreation, a set of symbols that centers on kitchens, cooking, and theft. This symbolic explanation of infertility only makes sense in the context of beliefs about illness and misfortune. Explanation of misfortune, illness, and infertility are part of Bangangté thought concerning order, disorder, human agency, and personal fate. These beliefs help us understand women's feelings of vulnerability, at the root of their fear of reproductive illness. Through an examination of women's images of threatened procreation, we discover how importantly women relate procreation to social reproduction. They ponder the importance of the king and the kingship to their personal health and cultural identity, the changing meaning of reciprocity, the shifting hierarchies of status, wealth, and opportunity. Through their expressions, their explanations, and their grappling with the fear of infertility, Bangangté women develop an indigenous theory of the demographic and social implications of jealousy. The chapter concludes with a look at the social epidemiology of fear; social differentiation among women, especially direction of personal mobility, shapes who fears what aspect of procreative threats to what degree.

Bangangté Concepts of Misfortune and Illness

Misfortune (*li kebwo;* literally, "bad face") is a common topic of conversation in Bangangté. Individuals exchange the particulars of their very personal experience of unfortunate events that are all too common to others. "See how I suffer," they say, describing personal misfortunes of many forms, including persistent adversity, accidents, failure in school or at work, and illness (*ngokwet*). Illnesses that strike children, prevent one from working, or attack one's ability to have children are among the most vigorously mourned personal misfortunes.

When discussing royal institutions or the past, Bangangté bemoan the community misfortunes of wars, forced labor conscriptions, the "troubles" of 1955 through 1972,[1] widespread agricultural failure, and what many

Bangangté perceive as the increasing frequency and danger of witchcraft. Worry about declining population is by far the most commonly addressed community misfortune in Bangangté. Bangangté enjoy debating the causes of community-wide misfortunes, and arguing about the relative influence of colonization and the failing power of individual chiefs. They seek remedies in either royal or community group rituals of purification and through supplication to royal ancestors and to Nsi, the supreme being. Echoing a shift from group toward individual therapies in traditional African medicine throughout the continent (Chavunduka and Last 1986), such rites appear to have declined in the past half century, as both sufferers and ritual-healing specialists concentrate on individual misfortunes.

Illness is the most commonly discussed and the most threatening of misfortunes. It attacks the very being of the individual person, endangering her survival chances and preventing her from performing her social role and thus from being a whole (*bwo;* good, healthy, beautiful) person. The most consistently expressed markers of illness are the inability to work and the inability to bear children. Illness, a personal misfortune, thus also adversely affects group activities. When a sick woman cannot cultivate, her cowives must weed her garden, or her family will go hungry and her husband will have no food to distribute to his followers. When a woman is sterile, she not only misses the personal benefits of motherhood but also cannot help insure the physical continuation of the kinship group or of Bangangté society.

Bangangté conceive of two general types of illness, "simple" or "natural" diseases of the body (*pan pan*), and illness caused by custom (*ndonn*). These categories are similar to the distinction between disease of God and disease of man that Janzen draws in his classic analysis of Kongo therapeutics (1978a). Simple diseases, akin to the Kongo disease of God, are believed to originate in biological processes and to be caused by poor nutrition, fatigue, filth, infection, or accident. Such diseases include jaundice, malaria, and broken bones. Illnesses of custom are caused, however, by an array of human, divine, and ancestral actions. Illnesses thought almost invariably to be caused by custom include infertility and edema or a swollen belly.[2]

This distinction between simple or natural events and those due to custom is fluid. The cause of a particular unfortunate event is always open to negotiation. The biological processes of corporal illness can be visited upon the sick person because of ancestral wrath, breaking taboos, or witchcraft. As in the well-known case of the Azande seeking to explain unfortunate events (Evans-Pritchard 1937), Bangangté find it always possible to ask, "why me, why now?" The longer an illness or misfortune lasts, recurs, or increases in gravity, the more likely it is that Bangangté will seek explanations from the realm of custom. In a "dynamic" medical system, Bangangté theories of causality allow the same illness event to be explained with both "naturalistic" and "personalistic" concepts at different points in the ongoing process of being ill (Ndonko 1987b:49).[3] While experiencing a number of close calls on a motorcycle or with a machete in the fields may be attributed to a youth's carelessness, it could also be interpreted as due to ancestral wrath resulting from a breach of custom, or to the power of a fetish set by a malevolent sorcerer. A woman may burn her fingers while preparing food or cut her foot with a hoe in the fields because she was distracted by the antics of her child, but an annoyed ancestor may have created that distraction to send her a warning about her improper behavior. The malaria menacing the life of a child may be recognized as an illness that enters the blood of one bitten by mosquitoes, but simultaneously may provoke an examination of the behavior and social relations of its parents to determine the ultimate cause of the mosquitoes biting this particular victim.

Bangangté emphasize the cause of misfortune to define the problem, present symptoms, and seek cure for particular illness episodes. Definition and presentation are not neutral lists of the attributes of an illness episode searching blindly for a comprehensible cause. The way sufferers define and present their misfortunes anticipates the cause that will be determined by the specialist. Bangangté operate with a typology of interrelated causes (see fig. 12), each of which can be paired to almost any symptom. Assumptions or expectations about the cause affect how a person presents her suffering to others, and determine the therapeutic actions to be taken. When the chosen therapy works, the presumed cause is confirmed; when it fails, a new cause and new therapy are sought.[4]

The framework of the ritual system through which "customary" misfortune and illness are interpreted is provided on the one hand by relations of kinship and descent through ancestor and skull worship, and on the other hand through the idea of forces not specific to kinship: the powers of the supreme creator-deity Nsi and norms of sanctioned and tabooed behavior called *kan* (law), the mystical powers and responsibility of the mfen for the well-being of the population and land of his chiefdom, and the potentially nefarious activities of living people with special knowledge of mystical powers (including both healers and witches). Bangangté believe that ancestral wrath and, increasingly, witchcraft are the most important causes of misfortune, and that both are influenced by the general emotional climate. I discuss each element of this Bangangté typology of causes in turn.

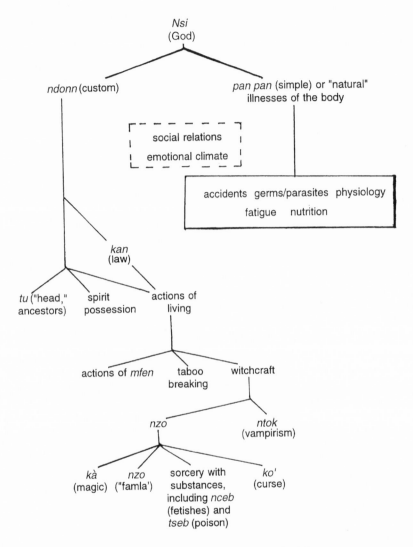

Fig. 12.   Bangangté typology of causes of misfortune

God, Norms, and Emotions

In the same way that Nsi (God), the supreme creator-deity, is ultimately the cause of conception (even if sexual intercourse and the mixing of male and female substances is also a well-understood prerequisite), Nsi is also the cause of all misfortune, including illness. When faced with a concrete event, Bangangté are most concerned to determine a more proximate cause of misfortune, but Nsi often remains an important actor in Bangangté efforts to ameliorate an unfortunate situation. Bangangté may perform propitiary rites[5] in the hope that Nsi will influence an angered ancestor in one's favor or set right a wrong done to the dignity of royal rituals.

In the Bangangté philosophy of illness causation, emotions take a mediating position between ultimate and proximate causes. Nsi, as well as ancestors, the actions of the living, and even physiological processes are affected by the general emotional climate. Bangangté view emotional climate and specific difficulties in social relations (e.g., an argument or envy between two cowives) as factors that can anger an ancestor, cause one to lose God's favor, or provoke a witchcraft attack. Bangangté believe that bad feeling multiplies, spreading among the living and even among the dead. This bad feeling needs to be "cooled" through mediation among the living and sacrifice to the ancestors or to Nsi. Tranquillity, animation, and being "of one heart" are the emotional conditions for good health and good government, and are promoted by sharing meals of cooked, vegetable-based sauces. Anger, jealousy, and selfishness prevent conception and lead to illness, crop failure, and political decline.

These indigenous theories of emotions take a slightly different shape for women of different positions and generations, and are invoked by the elderly to reprimand their younger, quarrelsome cowives. Because of the great amount of strife in the royal compound, the notion of the relation of emotional climate to one's state of health is of particular relevance there. Women who did not live in the royal compound expressed fear of going there and cited the unhealthy emotional climate of the palace as a reason why "no children are born there." Women in Bantoum contrasted the "tranquillity" of their village to both the royal compound and city life. All women attribute greater importance to these concepts than either traditional or biomedical health specialists.

The emotional component of health and illness infuses Bangangté ideas of *ndonn,* custom. Custom "catches" someone to cause illness because either Nsi or the ancestors have become angered. Acts that lead to this nonhuman anger include breaches of customary behavior, taboos, or etiquette (all part of *kan,* law). Humans also become angry or jealous and may use witchcraft to provoke illness in an opponent.

Kan (law), an abstract principle of norms, includes both articulable rules (e.g., a father should not take brideprice for his daughter if he did not pay brideprice for his wife) and a general notion of "the way we do things." Breaches of these norms, the negligent agency of living individuals, can cause misfortune. Kan includes all rules of descent, alliance, and uterine relation, as well as the proper way to join an association and rules governing male circumcision, seclusion, and female scarification. The care of sacred sites and the correct way to perform sacrifices are all governed by kan. We noted that Bangangté follow marriage and brideprice rules closely, fearing the supernatural consequences of breaking norms. Infertility may result from not following kan with regard to the mourning, purification, and inheritance of widows. Difficulties in childbirth can likewise follow offenses against kan, such as when a pregnant woman has sex with a man other than the father of her fetus or when she fails to name the father. The health of the resulting child may be threatened if the mother breaks alimentary and sexual taboos during pregnancy and lactation.

Rules governing the installation and behavior of the mfen are also kan; offenses against these rules are believed to have dire consequences for the well-being of the entire kingdom. The king thus has an enormous responsibility that would overwhelm any mortal. Installation rites fortify him to be able to withstand the task. When these rites do not follow kan, the proper way of doing things, the kingdom is just as endangered as when the mfen willfully offends against the rules of his office. The misfortunes resulting from breaking kan with regard to the king may render the women and the fields of the kingdom infertile, may prevent the royal family from producing offspring and thus continuing the dynasty, or may even bring retributive action upon the kingdom by outside political and military forces (be they the Bamoum kingdom of the nineteenth century or the colonial powers and Cameroonian state of the twentieth century).

Ancestral Wrath and Possession

Bamiléké, including Bangangté, believe their ancestors act upon the fortunes of their descendants. Ancestral wrath, expressed as "the head [skull] caught him/her" (*tû sheb i*), is the most common cause of misfortune (Ndonko 1987b:51). Ancestors may become angered when their skulls are not properly preserved or fed, or when the behavior of their descendants displeases them. These particular sensitivities of ancestors make sense in the context of Bangangté beliefs regarding what ancestors are and how they interact with the living.

Bangangté perceive death as a departure to an invisible world of unspecified location, reflected in verbal expressions announcing death (he is on a trip, has gone on) and of mourning (*o nen a ye, mama?,* where are you going, mama?). In becoming ancestors, the dead lose their corporality and thus their specific locus in space. Their *zwiak,* spirit or breath, is eternal, and as breath ancestors they can be everywhere, omniscient and watchful over their descendants' behavior and safety. Although breath, the ancestors need food and drink and shelter and participation in spiritual and celebratory life (for example, through the death celebrations put on by their descendants), just as the living do. These needs are at the center of their relations with the living, because only the living can satisfy them. When the living do not live up to their obligations to their ancestors, the ancestors become angered and send misfortune. Ancestors have emotions of anger, jealousy, and favoritism similar to living humans. Bangangté speak of their ancestors as cohabitants of their social and emotional world. Only when pressed do Bangangté specify that it is the zwiak of the ancestors that becomes angered and to which skull worship is addressed.[6]

Ancestors influence the lives only of those descendants who are morally obligated to sacrifice at their skulls. Just as ancestors watch over a number of clearly defined descendants, any individual descendant has obligations to numerous ancestors. Fear of ancestral wrath dominates Bangangté care of skulls and tombs. Duties are performed more or less rigorously to certain categories of ancestors, depending on expectations concerning the consequences of neglect. Not only do duties to ancestresses continue regardless of generational distance, ancestresses are also considered more emotionally volatile, vengeful, and sensitive to lack of consideration by their descendants than their male counterparts. While concentrating their efforts on ancestresses, the living invest much effort and resources into consulting specialists to "look" or to "see" whose anger has caused a misfortune.

The importance of ancestresses can put heiresses in a position of relative power with regard to their male and female relatives, by withholding or threatening to withhold their support of potentially curative rituals for a deceased ancestress. This manipulation of ritual access is considered unethical, but is an effective way for women to gain social support or to defend their rights over land (den Ouden 1980).

Possession by the divinity Nsi or by a general and undefined notion of "spirit" is a relatively rare cause of illness, cited by Bangangté only during sessions of sensational storytelling. Most often experienced by women, spirit possession reveals itself by a crisis with a specific recognized itinerary. The affected woman awakes on her bed mad, slaps the ground by the bed from which a muddy pool springs, and runs into the forest where she stays for hours, days, or even weeks. If the possessed person is not treated by a *minnyi* (spirit medium)[7] and initiated into spirit mediumship, she can suffer permanent madness. When properly managed, the crisis leads to the woman's profession as a minnyi. The crisis and its management by an initiate gives the woman a closeness to Nsi, special knowledge of plants and ancestors, and the "ownership" of a sacred grove that permits her to cure others. The minnyi's curative and divinatory tasks include treating spirit possession to prevent madness, ameliorating minor complaints such as headache, aiding conception, and determining the locus of needed sacrifices.

Actions of the Living: Witchcraft, Power, and Evil

Purposeful, nefarious activities of the living, and most especially the various forms of witchcraft, occupy the greatest part of the Bangangté imagination and storytelling regarding misfortune. Bangangté cite witchcraft second only to ancestral wrath as the most important and frequent cause of misfortune. In addition to witchcraft (the use of supernatural powers to harm others), Bangangté fear the malevolent activities of their fellow living beings in the form of poisoning and instigating strife (which may in turn lead to witchcraft).

All forms of witchcraft in Bangangté involve the misuse of powers held commonly by witches, the mfen, and ritual/healing specialists. While Bangangté in most situations vehemently and sharply distinguish witches from healers, their knowledge and control of supernatural powers are the same. *Kà,* medicine, also means magic or magical power.[8] It is activated by speech, whether through prayer, curse, or by calling forth the healing or poisonous properties of plants and objects. Kà can be used to heal or to harm, a duality of which healers are very aware. While almost all lay people call healers *ngak*à (person of or having kà), many healers reject this appellation for fear that it taints them as a magician-witch who uses his powers for evil ends. Whether one is witch or healer depends upon how one uses the supernatural powers one has gained through inheritance, initiation, apprenticeship, or dreams. Like other Bamiléké groups, Bangangté do not differentiate between "white and black magic," the distinction being based upon use (Hurault 1962:119). This fine line between witches and healers, dependent more upon their goals than upon their means, seems to be common to many African belief and medical systems. Wolff (1979:127) astutely questions the use of the term *healer* in the ethnomedical literature on sub-Saharan Africa. These "stock characters" must be viewed "primarily as power specialists who are capable of manipulating supra-sensory forces for the purpose of altering an individual's physical, social or mental state of being. It can be to heal, but conversely it can be to cause an affliction." As Bangangté express it, witch, healer, and king are all "complicated" (*kebwo*), somehow mysterious, possessing powers of unknown extent, and subject to restrictions and sensitivities in the running of everyday life. They are clever and can "manipulate the weight of their voice." What makes someone a witch is having "a bad heart," the potential and wish to do evil. While often committing their evil acts in response to being annoyed, witches require no excuses to harm their victims.

Bangangté conceive of two types of witchcraft, *ntok* and *nzo*. Ntok is practiced at night, when *ndum* (also called *gha ntok,* people with ntok or "vampires") leave their bodies and travel, transformed as animals, to harm their sleeping victims by slowly eating their organs. Most ndum are women, and only women practitioners can pass their powers on to their offspring.[9] Ntok witchcraft is an inversion of women's habitual and socially sanctioned activities. Rather than creating and serving food in good company, ndum feast alone on illegitimate food (human flesh). They are destructive and antisocial, as opposed to good women who are nurturing and social. Ndum perform their nefarious acts at night rather than in public daylight.[10]

Nzo, which involves both mystic powers and the manipulation of potions, powders, and fetishes, can be performed any time of day or night. Nzo is most often practiced by men, either alone or in groups. When *gha nzo* (witches) work together in groups, they appear as a rotating credit association, in which the contributions are sacrifices of the members' relatives. These "witches' *tontines*" are commonly referred to as *famla'* throughout the Bamiléké area. Their members are thought to enrich themselves through the labor of their victims, who appear to die from sudden illness or accident but actually toil on plantations in an invisible world.[11] Wealthy merchants and civil servants, the grand bourgeoisie, are often suspected of being members of famla'. Their wealth and power, lacking the legitimation of traditional title-holding, as well as urban life in general, are distrusted by rural Bangangté. Rural women, whose rotating credit associations involve considerably smaller individual contributions, are almost never suspected of membership in famla'.[12]

Other forms of nzo witchcraft include curses and instrumental, malevolent magic using such substances as herbal potions and powders, the victim's nail and hair clippings, fetishes, and poisons. Both *ko'* (curses) and sorcery with substances depend upon the power of speech. Curses, consisting solely of speech acts, are the flip side of prayers to the ancestors. Rather than "pronouncing someone's name" (i.e., invoking the name of an ancestor) to praise or to help someone, one may do so in spite to invoke a misfortune by naming it and its victim or by begging for the wrath of the ancestors. Fetishes, poisons, and other objects are not in themselves effective; they require the knowledge and the spoken word of a specialist to create their desired effects upon the victim. Fetishes, sometimes merely a bundle of three or four grasses tied together and placed on a log or path, are set with incantations. Learning these incantations is part of the initiation of witches and healers alike. In his discussion of fetishes causing epilepsy in the Bangangté village of Maham, Ndonko points out that the word is more important than the object itself (1987a:57).

Bangangté, confronted with a world inhabited by potentially malevolent neighbors, seek to understand the presence of evil among the living. They do so with three sets of concepts: the possession of power, the characteristics of body parts, and gender. All of these are part of a Bangangté philosophy of personhood and agency. Kings, healers, and witches gain mystical powers and capacities through their knowledge as ritual specialists. Bangangté assume that the possession of power at least tempts its holders to misuse it for personal gain. The tension between legitimate and redistributive use of power or fortune for the good of the kin-group or a wider public, and its illegitimate use for personal gain at the expense of others, is a recurring theme in Bangangté social thought. The rightful heir should succeed his father as lineage head, titleholder, or mfen, but he who can usurp him is admired for his "strength." The successful farmer or businessman is expected to house and pay school fees for his nieces and nephews, pay for health care for relatives in need, and organize flamboyant death celebrations for his ancestors, distributing huge quantities of food and drink to kin and neighbors. Nonetheless, if the wealthy man is "strong" enough to create a "complicated" reputation, he can keep demanding kin at bay without provoking accusations of witchcraft; he is then admired for his wealth and the possibilities it affords him. The extreme image of the selfish entrepreneur is the member of famla', who not only fails to redistribute his wealth but even sacrifices his kin for his private gain. Likewise a healer is expected to use his possession of kà to cure his suffering clients, but may use his power to harm others for his own or his clients' personal gain. The emotions a witch raises include not only disgust but also awe, a fearsome admiration of his "strength."

Bangangté also seek to explain the existence of evil through their understanding of the characteristics of body parts. Bangangté notions of the physical location of different faculties and emotions are linked to their concepts of power and agency. The belly is the seat of involuntary, inherited emotional characteristics. Witchcraft substance, ntok, is found in the belly and shared by those in a pam nto' kin group, who come from one belly or womb. Only with this special characteristic of the belly can one be a "vampire." In addition, all illnesses originate in the belly, which then becomes the focus of such curative procedures as purges and enemas. Not only patients, but also healers, witches, and the mfen ingest medicines that are understood to work from the belly outward to the rest of the body, radiating the power to fight or clean away disease or to perform magical acts. Thus, the belly can be the seat of a kind of fate, the involuntary possession of evil, while at the same time being manipulable via purges and medicines. These understandings of the belly are central to the ways women judge their reproductive capacity (and if and how they can manipulate it).[13]

The heart is the center of voluntary aspects of personality and sentiment. A person must learn to "hold one's heart," control one's sentiments, to become an adult who can safely manage the dangers of the social world. Weak people cannot hold their hearts and may therefore be overcome not only by such emotions as love or lust (which can lead to adultery), grief or pity (which may embarrass kin at a funeral), but also by destructive emotions of greed and envy. Those who give in to such sentiments may become "people with bad hearts," who are either witches or people who hire others to do their evil acts for them.

Bangangté images of gender likewise help them explain the presence of evil. Women are believed, especially by men, to be incapable of holding their hearts. Their emotional volatility leads them to directly cause misfortune by eating their fellows at night if they are "vampires" or by sending misfortune if they are sensitive ancestresses. Bangangté note that women's alleged emotional volatility also causes misfortune and evil indirectly through the creation of jealousy. Bangangté images of women as emotionally volatile support the perception of women as both a direct source and indirect cause of the practice of evil among the living, an evil that gives rise to that most feared misfortune—infertility. Ultimately, while women are the cooks who make procreation possible, they are often blamed for its failures.

These concepts of power, bodies, and gender contribute to understandings of the existence and cause of evil, misfortune, and illness held by nearly all Bangangté. Individual Bangangté of different social positions, however, tend to emphasize different parts of the preceding typology of causes to explain misfortune. An elderly woman who speaks no French, has had little contact with hospital-based medicine, and gains her status as wife of a polygynous Bangangté noble dependent upon the positive evaluation of royal institutions, finds most misfortunes to be caused by elements from the category ndonn, custom. A man of the same generation who holds an important position as evangelist in the local Protestant mission, by contrast, rejects the concept of ndonn causing illness and refers instead to the will of God and to the bacteria so vigorously fought in the mission hospital and in sermons.

Most Bangangté fall somewhere between these two extremes, admitting the entire range of causes found in the typology, but using varying hierarchies of resort in explaining misfortune. Which cause they first choose depends upon a variety of structural and circumstantial factors, from their closeness to traditional structures to the influence of kin and neighbors. Individuals concerned about succession disputes tend to first explain misfortune through ancestral wrath. Women fearing the envy of their competitive cowives tend to first think of witchcraft and other evil actions of the living when they explain infertility and other human suffering.

Citing infertility, population decline, economic crisis, and political upheavals, many Bangangté believe that the amount of witchcraft incidents has increased over the 1980s and 1990s. Some Bangangté even express a personal change in beliefs, such as a respondent in the outlying Bangangté village of Maham, who in 1983 claimed "we used to not believe in witchcraft, but now look. There is so much suffering here, it must be witchcraft."

This concept of increasing mystical misfortunes, of something going awry in the realm of custom, is part of Bangangté thought about the relation of order and disorder to personal fate (Feldman 1984). Based on research in the Western Grassfields kingdom of Kom between 1980 and 1985, Shanklin has noted that although belief in witchcraft has at least remained constant, the powers of traditional organizations that effectively manage witchcraft accusations have been eroded by national government authorities. This has left Kom villagers with a gap in their ability to deal with local malefactors and leads them to believe that the most witches are found in cities where governmental and not traditional authority is strongest (1988:27). The situation is similar in Bangangté. The experience of Bangangté villagers leading to the perception of increasing misfortune could be summarized as follows: the social order is becoming increasingly complex, confusing, and contradictory, so that one is no longer certain to whom one should show superiority or deference. This leads to strife between the living, and the anger of Nsi and the ancestors. Misfortune is then "sent" by ancestors and through witchcraft. In addition, people with bad hearts have "a taste for blood" since the civil war and seek to gain advantage from new opportunities through their nefarious activities. The ability of quarter chiefs to control local disputes has been attenuated since the resettlement of villages along the roads during the civil war. Thus, those with bad hearts are not only more bloodthirsty but also less controllable. This situation of societal disorder, seen from the perspective of the self-conscious traditionalist bemoaning bygone days, clearly leads to an unfortunate personal fate for increasing numbers of people. The examples Bangangté use to discuss the notion of increasing misfortune in Bangangté center around reproductive processes.

The Kitchen Plundered: Understanding Threats to Procreation

When Bangangté villagers complain that life is now harder than it was in the past, they refer not only to their unmet needs in an economy increasingly dependent upon cash but also to misfortunes and illnesses threatening their ability to bear children and, in the end, to reproduce their vision of an ideal Bangangté society.

This vision of an ideal Bangangté society is characterized by the balanced mixing of disparate elements, sought in the procreative kitchen as well as in other realms of social life. Families seek a balance of male and female children. The royal family, whose procreative kitchen should set an example for its subjects, performs rites to insure the birth of both male and female children to the newly coronated mfen and his wives. A commonly invoked Bangangté proverb, "it takes two hands to tie a knot," expresses the need for balanced cooperation between genders and among persons of disparate social statuses, including commoners, royal retainers, nobility, and royalty. Indeed, Bangangté and their neighbors alike joke about Bangangté's economic underdevelopment relative to other Bamiléké chiefdoms. Bangangté has too many nobles, who all sit around and drink, preventing "progress." These jokes emphasize a lack of balance among members of social categories and criticize the hegemony of titleholders and the wealthy.

The balance in this vision of an ideal Bangangté society is sometimes disturbed by individuals manipulating strength (supernatural power and physical force) and position for personal advancement. Siblings occasionally compete violently for succession, even leading to the theft of ancestral skulls. Many impoverished Bangangté believe that, while they work hard in agriculture or commerce to make ends meet, others gain economic success by joining witches' rotating credit associations. These witch-entrepreneurs mystically dispose of close relatives to insure economic gain. Echoing the culinary symbolism of procreation, the unfortunate relative is spoken of in terms of food, a goat sacrificed to share with one's comrades. This type of mystical food, however, inverts the legitimate order, becoming lethal rather than nutritious and procreative.

Bangangté women most often complain of connivance and usurpation with regard to marital relations and procreation. A woman who pushes herself before her cowives, or creates strife to diminish her cowives' chances to sleep with their husband, has already increased her own chance to become pregnant by usurping a place of dominance among her cowives. In contrast, the proper way to help one's fetus develop is through peaceful, repeated sexual relations with one's husband, the father of the fetus. Stealing another's fetus through witchcraft, to gain it for oneself or to destroy it to the disadvantage of one's cowife, disrupts the order of the procreative kitchen and is a means of usurping reproductive success for one's own gain.

As of the mid-1980s, many Bangangté felt that their young (39) but terminally ill king was not able to control the use of illegitimate means of personal advancement. Women felt that this disturbance of social relations prevented the process of procreation from working as smoothly as images of a well-functioning kitchen suggest. The threats Bangangté women perceived reiterate the images of bad cooking and the usurpation of another woman's hearth. These interferences in the good workings of the procreative kitchen occur at the various stages of the procreative process, from the pairing of couples (preparing the hearth and choosing the ingredients) through conception (mixing), gestation (cooking), and birth (serving), to proper socialization to insure the reproduction of Bangangté values and social forms.

Bangangté refer to a woman's faulty behavior that is believed to cause her own reproductive misfortunes (such as neglect of ancestors and disrespect for parents and husband) as her "bad cooking." Yet, Bangangté perceive *most* interferences in the procreative kitchen as coming from agents other than themselves. Their understanding of threats to reproductive health and success is best summarized as "the kitchen plundered." The looters of the procreative kitchen are witches and their patrons.

Nonarranged Marriage and Incest

Such outside threats to reproduction can enter the reproductive process as early as marriage; that is, "it is hard to build a good kitchen." In setting up the marital, procreative kitchen, Bangangté are concerned that it is stocked with the right ingredients, and thus with how pairs come together to make children. Bangangté women speak of a recent past when nearly all marriages were arranged between the parents of the betrothed. Arranged marriage resulted in beneficial political and economic alliance for the parents and also insured that the bride's and groom's genealogies were thoroughly checked, preventing the risk of incest for the new couple. With the spread of the "modern" ideal of romantic love, marriages are less often arranged by parents. Paulette, the unfortunate heroine of chapter 1, met the mfen socially and was quickly married without parental arrangement. A descendant of a previous mfen, she unwittingly married into an incestuous relation and was rejected by her family. "Paulette is *bagde'*, spoiled. She will never be able to bear a child," repeated many through the village gossip networks. Her nonarranged marriage was held up as a keen example of how carelessness and romantic liaisons can eventually lead to infertility as a supernatural sanction for breaking incest taboos.

While many young Bangangté women wish for more choice for themselves as individuals, they fear other dangers of nonarranged marriage besides incest. When parents are uninvolved in marital choice, bridewealth payments are often disputed, causing social strife. Bangangté fear that ancestors become angered and then "seize" the kin group with illness and infertility. Both arranged and nonarranged betrothals can be risky if a woman refuses a suitor's advances. As an elderly grandmother from the outlying Bangangté village of Maham recounted in 1983:

> Do you see those two young girls, scarred from the fire? They will never marry and have children, because they were too proud. That old grandpa wanted to marry them, but they refused. You know, the old codger was so mad that he spread a powder on the path. Now those girls have epilepsy.

In a society where women spend much of their time around open fires, epilepsy can prevent successful marriage and child rearing for risk of serious burns.

Adultery

Once properly paired, the new wife is expected to keep her cooking of food and babies within her husband's compound. Bangangté express their concern over a wife's fidelity and assuring paternity both directly ("the child needs to know his father") and in terms of their culinary analogy ("a good sauce needs carefully chosen ingredients"). These efforts to be certain about paternity are disrupted when the cooking of sex occurs outside the marital pair, allowing substances from more than two people to mix. Bangangté believe infidelity during pregnancy may cause fetal death, "when the two men's waters fight." It brings on numerous supernatural sanctions of sickness and death, affecting conception, gestation, and childbirth.

Bangangté claim that adultery is easier and more frequent now, because "since the white man came" adulterers are no longer threatened with death. They tell stories of how mfen Njiké II (reigned 1912–43) buried one of his wives alive after she had become pregnant from another man. A British adventurer-ethnographer, who visited Njiké II's court for several months in 1937, reports that Njiké II had an adulterous queen and her paramour thrown into a deep latrine to suffocate (Egerton 1938:241). The effect of the white man coming, that is, of colonial rule, was that the power of the mfen to kill his subjects was taken away. By the 1930s, punishment for adultery with a king's wife had changed from death to banishment (Egerton 1938:111–12). Likewise, the precolonial right of the father or husband to beat his pregnant daughter or adulterous wife to death was redefined from normatively expected social control to murder. The humanistic strivings of the colonial government to soften or eliminate punishment for errant girls and wives led in Bangangté eyes to a breakdown of sexual mores. This process continued during the postcolonial period, when Cameroonian legislators retained the statutes of the former colonial powers and further attempted to mitigate sanctions seen to discriminate against women. Nonetheless, liberalizations in Cameroonian family law, meant to improve the status of women, have had unintended, counterproductive effects at the level of implementation in the Grassfields (Geary 1986). Legal change has not, according to Bangangté, eliminated punishment for adultery. Now the punishment comes in a different form, via religious, supernatural sanctions resulting in infertility, miscarriage, disturbed fetal development, and difficult childbirth.

Cooking outside the sheltered procreative kitchen has other consequences, affecting conception. Husband and wife fight about their affairs and therefore do not have sex and do not mix their ingredients to cook the child. If the husband has affairs with women outside his marital compound, his wives complain of "lying fallow." The frustrated wives may also run away. All of this is perceived by Bangangté to be part of the breakdown of morals, which prevents conception by preventing sex and "mixing" within the marital pair.[14]

Conception in Bangangté is not just a matter of the mechanics of sex, abstinence, and the choice of partners, but also of emotions. Tranquillity and "being of one heart" within the marital relationship and within the wider community are the emotional conditions for good health. Anger, jealousy, and selfishness prevent conception and lead to illness. While Bangangté say the working of emotional climate upon a woman's fertility is mysterious, they express it in concrete, metaphorical terms: "when you shake the pot around too much the sauce cannot cook properly." Thus, when husband and wife no longer act toward each other as traditional Bangangté moral norms dictate, anger and infertility may result. Wives often express their anger by refusing to cook, or by cooking a pointedly unsavory meal devoid of palm oil. In contrast, sharing food is a crucial way of calming hearts and bringing couples together to be of one heart.

Female Envy, Witchcraft, and Theft.   Culinary skills, especially rules of hygiene in the Bangangté kitchen, also relate to concern about threats to conception from the setting of fetishes by "those with bad hearts" (e.g., jealous cowives or neighbors). The stirring spoon is always placed on the handle or rim of the pot, never on the floor where it could get dirty or pick up powders that had been set on the floor as a fetish. This powder-fetish would then be stirred into the food and enter its victims through the belly, the sensitive and dangerous origin of all illness. A woman must never walk over a pot or a plate of food, for fear of a fetish entering her vagina through the steam and aromas of the food. As I also learned by once unwittingly wasting the family's midday meal, a pot of food is thrown out immediately with the suspicion that a fetish may have been dropped into it if anyone strides over the pot in a cramped kitchen.

Bangangté women particularly fear sterility-fetishes that are placed in toilets, which "rise up into the woman's vagina" to prevent her from conceiving. For this reason there are no toilets or pit latrines in the two women's quarters of the Bangangté royal compound. Latrines in other compounds are often locked to prevent the setting of fetishes, the collection of excrement and other human wastes for witchcraft potions, and the theft of wood, yams, grain, or tools stored within the latrine hut.

The theme of theft of firewood and foodstocks from latrines is reiterated in Bangangté beliefs about reproductive illness threatening gestation. The imagery involved includes the theft of cooking ingredients necessary for healthy fetal development and the theft of the fetus itself. The fetus is described by Bangangté women as a sauce that must slowly bubble and thicken, a tiny animal or child that must grow in a protected environment, or a bean that absorbs water and swells. Several mishaps may occur that endanger or prevent the growth, thickening, or swelling of fetal development.

The visible physical changes of an expanding belly bring bad as well as good luck to Bangangté women. "Showing" can provoke the jealousy of cowives and neighbors who are not pregnant. While Bangangté consider motherhood "*wonder*ful" (emphasizing the miraculous nature of their joy) and the traditional Bangangté ideal of feminine beauty is to be rotund and shiny with oil, newer notions of beauty lead pregnant women to be concerned about their sexual attractiveness. More lithe cowives may lure their husbands away, preventing intercourse with the baby's father. Without fortifying water/semen and repeated mixing, the bean or sauce may dry up or the ingredients separate and crumble. The sauce may cease to bubble (movements and heartbeats can no longer be felt or heard) or may boil over (miscarriage). The sauce might stick to the pot (the woman's uterus or other organs), cease to develop, and fail to come out as a child.

If the water/semen is not "stolen" through interference in a woman's access to her husband, it can be spoiled by the pregnant woman's own bad cooking. In this case, Bangangté understand infidelity, described earlier, as a source of misfortune. When a pregnant woman has intercourse with more than one man Bangangté believe the mixing of two "waters" causes fetal distress. Bangangté say that rather than "fortifying" the fetus, the two waters "fight" and the fetus "may not know its father" or "may not like its father."

The most commonly, and dramatically, told accounts of threats to gestation reiterate imagery of theft and asocial eating wreaking havoc on the procreative kitchen. Women fear that "vampires," usually thought of as envious women, will eat or steal their fetuses or make them "stick" someplace within the mother where they are invisible and cannot develop.

My female informants said their cowives, mothers-in-law, and close neighbors were most likely to steal or destroy fetuses, motivated by envy. The actual stories I heard involved cowives (five cases), the wife of a foster father (one case), and a foster father (one case). Within the royal compound, the most commonly discussed case involved Josette, the *mabengoup* or "first queen," who accused a number of her cowives of destroying her alleged pregnancy.

Josette's Imagined Pregnancy

Josette's cowives often giggled and repeated stories about her imaginary, invisible pregnancies. They said she had claimed to be pregnant between the births of her two daughters (twelve and five years old in 1986), but after one year still had no baby. When asked by one of her cowives where the baby was, Josette allegedly answered that someone had hidden the child in her buttocks. When this case was brought up in Josette's presence, she always changed the subject.

Again in 1986 Josette claimed to be pregnant, contrary to the results of an examination at the mother–child clinic of Bangangté hospital and to any observable signs. While some wives ridiculed Josette or made clear they did not believe her stories of pregnancy, others gently hid their doubt and showed pity for their cowife queen. Josette ceased to talk about her pregnancy to those who expressed disbelief, but did not drop the issue completely. In March, Josette asked Jeanne to lend her money to buy clothes for the baby she claimed to expect. Jeanne put off this request by saying it was impossible for her to lend money at the time. Later that month, during a dispute over sexual access to the mfen, Josette expressed fear for the safety of her fetus if she should have intercourse with the king, who was ill. In April and again in June, she finally found a specific culprit for her previously vague accusations that her fetus had been bewitched, stuck to her back, or stolen. When Paulette, her weakest cowife, made sarcastic references about her motherhood,

Josette accused her of being ndum *(a vampire) and stealing her unborn child.*

In this case, Josette exhibited what a Bangangté obstetric nurse termed "hysterical pregnancy," due to the enormous psychological pressure many Bangangté women feel to bear children frequently, as well as a misunderstanding about irregularities in menstruation and menopause. Josette, officially the most powerful of the royal wives but in fact ridiculed by her cowives, blamed her cowives for damaging or stealing her fetus and thus denying her the pride of once again bearing a child.

Josette feared the effect of the king's illness on her wished-for pregnancy as well as the dangers of her greedy cowives. Like Josette, the mfen was officially powerful, the most important member not only of the royal family but of all of Bangangté; yet, he was occasionally ridiculed or criticized by his wives and subjects. During the year before his premature death at age 40, it was obvious to many, including Josette, that the mfen's authority and health both were dwindling. Like all her cowives, Josette worried that the mfen might die and leave her a widow. Unlike the majority of her cowives, however, this look into the future meant losing her position as queen as well as her house and fields, as a new "first queen" would be chosen for the new mfen. Josette also worried about the effect of the king's illness on the one thing she would be able to take with her from her final years as queen—her baby. She said she feared the mfen's waters would make her fetus crumble rather than fortify it.

Understanding Threats to Childbirth, Child Survival, and Children's Socialization

If a woman manages to get through the stage of gestation successfully and give birth to a child (serve the meal), the dangers of stillbirth or maternal death are ever-present. These tragedies are blamed on insufficient sex with the baby's father, leading to a small birth canal or to the child's "not knowing its father." Bangangté also believe that difficult childbirth is caused by extramarital conception of the child. Labor proceeds more quickly and less painfully after pronouncing the name of the heretofore unknown father. From the point of view of kin, especially male kin, these illness beliefs reiterate the importance of knowing paternity. For the birthing mother, the "theft" of her access to her husband or her own "cooking on the road," outside of the marital procreative kitchen, come back to haunt her.

Once this carefully prepared meal is served, once the child is born, Bangangté cease to use the analogy of food, cooking, and kitchens. The mysterious happenings occurring in the hidden depths of the human body are now over and no longer require concretizing, explanatory metaphors of the kitchen. The newborn (*men fi,* "fresh person") and its mother are subject to the misfortunes confronting any living human. In fact, Bangangté consider mother and child to be particularly vulnerable during the first months following birth. These dangers steadily decrease from the baby's first days, the most critical period, to the time when it can walk and is weaned.

Rural Bangangté mothers are rightfully concerned about their children's survival. Of the 31 informants in the Bangangté villages of Batela' and Bantoum who distinguished between children born and children living, only 54.5 percent of these women's children had survived to adulthood. Of the 14 children born to mfen Njiké Pokam during his reign, one died in infancy, a much better survival rate of 93 percent. The 1978 World Fertility Survey stated that one-sixth of all children in the Bamiléké area died before age five (1983:78), which means that only 83.7 percent survived beyond this critical threshold. The situation appeared to have improved by the time of the 1991 Demographic and Health Survey, when the under-five mortality rate for the Western and Littoral Provinces was calculated at 109.3 per thousand (Balépa, Fotso, and Barrère 1992a:135).

Of course, Bangangté mothers are not concerned with survival rates, but with the experiences they and their neighbors have with the tragic death of children. They express their sadness by emphasizing that despite giving birth (i.e., overcoming all the natural and supernatural dangers threatening marriage, sexual intercourse, conception, gestation, and childbirth), "all" their children have died. In the next breath they make clear that they still have a number of living descendants, but that the tragedy of losing children is felt as deeply as if all children had died.

> I gave birth to them and they are all dead, my dear. I only have five left. At Bazou I lost three children and here another . . . one said their deaths were problems of custom, but I always thought that God called them back. (Bwoda', Bantoum, born ca. 1920)

> I gave birth to many and they are all dead. Only some three are left to me. I miscarried four, and gave birth to four [before they died]. That may surprise you, but what can I do? (Ngassam, Batela', born ca. 1915)

> I gave birth and they are all dead. We have only three children . . . If one talks about giving birth, me, I would count twelve children. There

was not a single one who did not receive its name or who did not walk before dying. (Nyombab, Batela', born before 1910)

The common experience of facing the death of children has neither mitigated its pain nor led to attempts to create de-anthropomorphizing images (contrasting with Scheper-Hughes's account of child loss in Northeastern Brazil, 1992). Bangangté women grieve deeply for their dead children and continue to grieve into old age.

When sharing a set of photographs from the British ethnographer-adventurer Egerton's 1937 visit to Bangangté, Marguerite suddenly caught her breath. She showed me the picture of a little boy, and explained: "Nyombab's son was very beautiful, a good boy already bigger than Aimé [a 10-year-old boy in 1986]. You should not show her that picture of her son. It would only make her sad and would not bring him back to her." At the time, Nyombab was 65 years old. I never showed her the photo. In 1997, she was the only elderly wife remaining in the compound, an old woman with no descendants to ease her final days, apparently happy to be remembered by a long absent anthropologist.

Because one can only become an ancestor by having surviving, well-socialized descendents, Bangangté women's grief for their dead children is combined with anxiety about the future. Together these children, individually mourned, make up the backdrop of direct experience and teaching through telling that informs new and potential mothers of the dangers to child survival.

Bangangté mothers perceive some of these dangers to child survival in terms of specific threats. An angered ancestor may take the life of a child to punish its mother or father. An evil neighbor may give a child epilepsy through witchcraft; Bangangté consider epilepsy to be a form of death, mourned on the day of the child's first fit rather than on the day of actual death (Nkwi and Ndonko 1988:9). Rural Bangangté women recognize the symptoms of umbilical tetanus and deem this infection to be a common cause of neonatal death. Measles and colds are also recognized threats to child survival. Much attention is given to the sound of the infant's breathing, and this aspect of health is constantly monitored.

Bangangté women express concern about the mother's health during pregnancy (she is "menaced" by ailments ranging from malaria to witchcraft attacks), but do little to protect her during this time. In contrast, while Bangangté women almost never talk about maternal death or post-

partum illness, the new mother receives much attention in order to promote child survival.[15] She is bathed and massaged by her cowives, female
kin, and neighbors, "to make her feel good and make her belly take a nice
shape." Female kin and cowives take over all her household and agricultural work for anywhere from a month to, in the case of twins, one year.
The new mother is released from her housekeeping and sexual duties
toward her husband. She is fed rich foods and expected to get fat, have
plenty of milk, hold her baby constantly, and nurse it on demand. Only
extreme poverty and a deficient social network would leave a woman to
work and "remain thin" after the birth of a child, exhausting her and
putting her child at risk of malnutrition.

Beyond bringing a new being into the Bangangté world, Bangangté
are concerned with social reproduction via the socialization of this new
child. Bangangté parents want their children to become true Bangangté
persons. Their great efforts are wasted if their children do not respect
them, bring them honor, and care for their skull once they have become
ancestors.

Bangangté parents recognize a number of concrete social conditions
that can make this fear a reality. First, they recognize that their children
will not be able to get along even in rural Bangangté without knowledge of
French and familiarity with arithmetic and state institutions. Thus, parents, especially mothers, scrape together the means to send their children
to school. At these schools children learn about city life, monogamous
marriage based on romantic love, status, wealth, and power that can be
gained through formal education and participation in trade and wage
labor rather than in service to the mfen, inheritance from the father, or
through traditional titles. These children advance through opportunities
provided by the state and by mission schools, whose ideologies are
opposed to such "superstitious" practices as ancestral skull worship. They
sometimes quickly gain higher status and income than their parents by
nontraditional means. Younger children serve as translators for their
elders, possessing the power of knowledge in the face of their parents'
helplessness. None of these developments encourages respect for traditional hierarchies and religiously sanctioned honoring of ancestral skulls.

In addition, youth no longer find economic opportunities to practice
their new skills in the kingdom's territory. As noninheriting youth have
done since the 1920s (Tardits 1960), they migrate to the cities in search of
work and excitement, diminishing the immediate care and closeness they
can give to their parents. Parents become increasingly concerned about
this emigration because it captures more and more of their sons and even
daughters, whose aspirations can no longer be met in the rural milieu of
their parents.

Bangangté try to socialize their children in terms of traditional values to overcome these forces. They are at least partly successful, as even elites often travel frequently between their urban villas and their natal villages. Nearly all Bangangté, including strict adherents of the imported Christian faiths, carefully care for their ancestral skulls. The fear that future generations will cease to do so, however, is always present. Mothers' reminder to their children to "remember where their umbilical cord is buried," that is, not to neglect their duties to elders and ancestors and their identity as Bangangté citizens, does not always stand up to other social forces. Against this anxiety about what the future will bring for their children and for Bangangté traditions, Bangangté parents express helplessness in the form of laments of infertility and child mortality.

In sum, when Bangangté women worry about threats to reproduction, their fear concerns not only their ability to conceive and the physical survival of their children. Confronted with an increasingly complex world and a multitude of ways of being, Bangangté have an idea of what it means to be a "real Bangangté," a quality that those born Bangangté can lose. The estranged, deracinated Bangangté is a known character in the dramatis personae of current Bangangté social categories and is the antithesis of village women's image of the ideal Bangangté individual. Against the background of the Bangangté vision of society (i.e., made up of discrete parts, or individuals, in particular positions within the traditional hierarchy, all drawn together by their allegiance to the king), Bangangté extrapolate from the failure to continue the "ideal" individual in society to the failure to continue society. Thus, human reproduction and socialization become the focus of existential questions regarding an increasingly threatened way of life.

Threats to procreation, however, are felt first on a more personal, experiential level. The potential mother thinks of her own social standing within traditional, rural Bangangté life. She wonders who or what may want to harm it. When she and others look beyond themselves and notice the shared experience of dangers to reproduction, as many do, only then do they begin to worry about the present and future state of their kingdom.

The Poverty of Infertility:
Food, Theft, and Downward Mobility

Food, feeding, and commensality are central to the ways Bangangté think about how human beings are created and how they live together. On the one hand, as we have seen, certain foodstuffs such as palm oil and beans are symbols of fertility, and the process of procreation is likened to cooking. Eating together forges unity and a feeling of tranquillity, conditions

Bangangté believe enhance fertility. This social sharing of food occurs between husband and wife, mother and children, and among cowives, hosts and guests, and members of informal gift exchange networks among kin and neighbors. Central to the maintenance of communities, it is a particular kind of commensality; *ju,* which means sharing a soft, vegetable-based sauce, draws people together around the cook's hearth (symbolically her "womb") or at the host's table.

Bangangté also talk about another bad kind of eating. The solitary anthropophagic witchcraft of vampires (*ndum*) and evil commensality of witches' rotating credit associations are destructive rather than creative or procreative. This violent kind of eating is called *fed,* a special term used for roasted "snack" foods, the way animals eat, and the way witches eat. Bangangté emphasize teeth when talking about fed, and their sculptures of witches exhibit prominent, sharply filed teeth. This type of eating tears people apart rather than drawing them together. Fed interferes with the bonding nature of ju. In addition, when witches fed, the feasting animal or so-called goat that they tear apart with their pointy teeth is actually a sacrificed relative or another woman's fetus.

Food and eating, which can represent both sociability and the ultimate asocial behavior, figure prominently in the ways Bangangté women link their fear of infertility with a fear of theft and poverty. Since growing and selling food crops and establishing support networks through food exchange are the ways Bangangté women survive in an increasingly cash-oriented environment, food and commensality are also central to the experience of rural female poverty in Bangangté. This is even more true in the ongoing economic crisis of the 1990s than it was during the comparatively affluent times of the mid-1980s.

Both the fear and reality of rural female poverty in Bangangté are based upon the gendered division of labor, increasing needs for cash, and contemporary patterns of labor migration. The approximately 46,000 rural inhabitants of Bangangté are mostly farmers. Women gain access to land on which to grow their food crops (maize, beans, and peanuts) through their husbands and, occasionally, their natal families. Men who migrate in search of wage labor leave wives at home to fend for children, at least until they have found steady and lucrative employment, and often permanently. Even those who stay home have more access to cash than women do, but male and female incomes are rarely shared in household budgets. While Bangangté say men are supposed to provide meat, oil, salt, school fees, and medical care for their wives and children, women often find themselves meeting these "male" responsibilities. Bangangté women usually are strapped for cash.

Bangangté women now need cash to assure the health and proper socialization of their children, to pay for health care when they themselves fall ill, or seek treatment for infertility. Food, so closely associated with female labors, plays an important role in women's struggle for economic survival. When cash is short, women sell foodstuffs whether or not they have a "surplus." Thus, even though famine is rare, women worry about going hungry. Food is a social as well as a material resource for Bangangté women; when a health crisis strikes, these two types of resource are tightly interwoven. Women's support networks help manage and pay for therapies, and tend children and gardens during a woman's illness. The maintenance of these networks depends on the hospitable exchange of cooked food and sacks of beans or peanuts. No rural Bangangté woman can hope to survive without participating in this exchange of foodstuffs.

Infertility and child loss put a woman at greater risk of becoming poor and greatly attenuating her exchange and support networks. Childlessness can be the grounds for divorce in Bangangté, causing a woman to lose her access to land distributed by her husband. Even her natal family, angered at having to return her bridewealth, may give her only minimal solace. If she is able to avoid divorce, a childless woman receives fewer gifts from her husband than her luckier cowives. She has no children to help her cultivate her land, and no one to support her in old age. With this scenario in mind, Bangangté women have good reason to link poverty and concern about food to their anxieties about reproductive health.

Worried that theft will impoverish both their wombs and pantries, Bangangté women keep their doors and latrines locked. They are concerned about the theft of material goods, particularly of food and farm implements utilized to grow food, which could threaten their ability to give hospitality and participate in exchange networks. Bangangté women lock their latrines not only to guard their cocoyams and firewood, but also because they fear the theft of bodily wastes that could be used for fetishes and medicines to "block" fertility and "plug" fallopian tubes. Yet, no lock protects their fetuses from being stolen by envious ndum. Bangangté women's fear of theft is closely tied to the practical and symbolic roles of food both in procreation and in the ability to seek help when procreation fails (Feldman-Savelsberg 1994). The tenacity of infertility and the stigma and poverty induced by childlessness means that therapy management groups and social support tend to collapse over time (as in urban Egypt; see Inhorn 1994:8). Part of Bangangté women's fear of infertility is a fear of isolated poverty.

In sum, having and feeding children are marks of good fortune and competence for Bangangté women. Infertility and female poverty are linked in Bangangté conceptualizations and practice through the potential for a downward spiral in personal mobility. Infertility is thus an idiom of vulnerability to misfortune. Images of infertility involve the violence of anthropophagic witches, interference in good cooking (wrong ingredients, shaking the pot), and the theft of ingredients and fetuses. Bangangté infertility beliefs and their metaphoric expressions reflect material concerns of female poverty. They also reflect a concern that their dying king can neither control theft and witchcraft nor "feed" his populace with babies and well-being.

Diverging Views and Experiences:
The Social Epidemiology of Endangered Procreation

While I have described Bangangté perceptions of procreative threats as they are held, more or less, by all rural Bangangté women, not all perceive these problems in the same way or to the same extent. Women with differing social characteristics (e.g., age, formal education, type of marriage, extent of social networks) tend to emphasize one or the other threat to their reproductive success. Following Lindenbaum's exemplary study of *Kuru Sorcery* (1979), the distribution of the degree and kind of perceived threats to reproduction in Bangangté can be described as an epidemiology of fear.

Social differentiation among rural women, ultimately the result of significant power differentials between social classes and nations, creates differing risks for reproductive illness. Inhorn has named this conjuncture of political-economic and epidemiological models "the political epidemiology of infertility" (1994:10). I am less concerned with explaining patterns of infertility per se than with explaining the distribution of the *fear of infertility*. I examine the diverging tendencies of degree and types of concern about reproductive health and illness from two angles. First, I explore the views that medical personnel practicing in the Bangangté area in 1986 held on the medical threats experienced by different groups of rural Bangangté women. Second, I outline how the experience of status decline and relative disadvantage, for some, and the fear of envy, for others, both contribute to the shape and distribution of perceived reproductive threats in Bangangté.

Practitioners' Views of Medical Threats

While the personnel of the five biomedical institutions I studied (two hospitals and three predominantly ambulatory health centers) varied greatly in their perception of the extent of reproductive health problems, their views of the nature of medical threats were both consistent and limited. When biomedical personnel distinguished among types of women subject to these risks, they grouped women according to age, number of sexual partners, and form of marriage.

Biomedical institutions in Cameroon are complex hierarchical organizations, where each staff member has his or her own sphere of responsibility and competence, carefully guarded as one's own and carefully limited to prevent extra demands. Within this organization, personnel at the two extremes of the hierarchy consistently perceived reproductive illnesses that prevent women from conceiving or giving birth to living children as one of the four most important ailments facing their clients.[16] Physicians at hospitals and head nurses at health centers at the upper extreme of the hierarchy are confronted with all cases at their institutions and therefore have an overview of the relative frequency of various ailments. Helpers and attendants, at the other end, are in intimate, daily contact with patients and hear their complaints and worries that may have nothing to do with their current hospital visit. Helpers and attendants not only stress the importance of sterility in relation to other ailments, but also cite the highest numbers of requests for information about family planning (from eight per month to "many"). They claim to make more frequent referrals to traditional practitioners for disturbances of fertility than any other group of biomedical personnel. In the middle of the hospital/clinic hierarchy, only nurses and nurse's aides who worked in obstetrics and gynecology found women's problems having children one of the four most significant ailments. All biomedical personnel in Bangangté agree that many women come to their institutions complaining of reproductive difficulties. They all felt that the greatest proportion of their patients (ranging from 30 to 100 percent) consulted traditional practitioners for sterility rather than for any other complaint.

Not surprisingly, medical personnel emphasized sexually transmitted disease and other infections of the pelvic area as the single most important threat to women's reproductive success. They blame precocious sex, untreated infections of girls too embarrassed to seek help, promiscuity, and polygyny for the frequency of sexually transmitted diseases. They explain subsequent infertility through scarring, tubal blockage, and "congestion." Medical personnel complain of the difficulty of treating sexually transmitted diseases because of the multiple partners at least of the men in polygynous unions. Two physicians of Cameroonian nationality also believed young girls to have unbridled sexual appetite leading likewise to multiple partners and the spread of infection.[17]

Most staff expressed annoyance at what they perceived to be ignorance and uncooperativeness among their patients: husbands refuse to be examined for "their wives'" sterility, sexual relations are continued during treatment, and healers are consulted. Nurses at the two hospitals infer that the patients themselves are to blame for their plight, citing "promiscuity" and "prostitution" as the root causes of infertility. One physician complained that most cases are "women with five children who find a three year interval between pregnancies too long," thus dismissing women's fears as insignificant in the face of "true" infertility (primary sterility). Only one physician (a Dutch missionary) and one nurse mentioned that the biomedical focus on infection and the mechanics of reproduction are foreign to their patients' understanding of the problem. The nurse, characteristically curt, said, "what the people think [causes sterility] is custom, or God's will."

Local biomedical practitioners perceive different groups of women to be at greater or lesser risk of reproductive difficulties. Young women are at risk of contracting sexually transmitted diseases because their sexual activity is no longer guided by traditional morals regarding premarital sex and number of partners. Schoolgirls, often far from the control of their families and subject to outside influences, are believed particularly likely to be promiscuous. Likewise, biomedical personnel perceive that the mitigation of sanctions against adultery has opened the way to married women to have risky affairs. Among older and more traditional women, polygyny helps to spread sexually transmitted diseases and to complicate their treatment. Thus, biomedical staff find women in monogamous marriages with no extramarital sexual experience to best be able to avoid risks to their reproductive health. This woman fits both the ideal of the virtuous, but poor, traditional wife and the saintly modern wife as viewed by the largely Christian biomedical staff of all five institutions.

Physicians and nurses tend to focus on infection and overlook other factors affecting the reproductive success of their Bangangté patients. Poor nutrition, which can depress ovulation or delay the onset of menses, was mentioned by only one practitioner, a physician who pronounced that "famine is the root of all illness." In fact, underweight is rarely a problem among Bangangté adults, whose diet is rich in oils. While pregnant women are almost always anemic, nearly all Bangangté women have a high enough proportion of fatty tissue to support regular ovulation.

Even when a woman has enough body fat, a heavy work load can depress a woman's ovulation cycle even in the absence of any clinical indications (C. Lager, personal communication, December 1987). Bangangté women do in fact show clinical signs of irregular ovulation. My own impressionist observations and interviews indicate that Bangangté women frequently miss their periods and even cease to menstruate for months or years between pregnancies. This irregularity occurs frequently even among women who are not nursing. Physicians at Bangangté and Bangwa hospitals confirm these observations for their patients.

A heavy work load could affect the fertility of almost all rural women. A woman's workload is heaviest if her fields are far away, if she has many young children or wards, if her network of kin and neighbors who provide mutual aid with farm and household labor is attenuated, if her husband makes demands on her labor for his cash crop plantations, and if she has extra need to grow a surplus for ritual or redistributive purposes. This final addition to a woman's work load occurs only if she is the wife of the mfen or of his nobles and retainers, or at specific points in the developmental cycle of some households, for example, when preparing for a death celebration. Women whose work load is the lightest and therefore least likely to adversely affect her fertility, and who have fertile fields nearby their home, have maintained good relations with relatives who can help at times of crisis or labor bottlenecks, and have husbands with cash incomes who share responsibility for household needs, therefore have the best chances of reproductive success.

Finally, emotional stress can affect menstruation, ovulation, and hormonal balance, although the mechanisms through which this occurs are little understood. The sole physician in Ndé Division who raised the issue of emotional stress and infertility explained that secondary sterility is usually accounted for by scarring or inflammation in the fallopian tubes following an infection. Nonetheless, using sophisticated diagnostic equipment he found that many woman failed to conceive who showed no indication of tubal blockage. Some of these women succeeded in becoming pregnant once they had visited a traditional healer and solved "customary" problems. The physician felt that the traditional treatment eased psychosocial tensions within the family and allowed the woman to relax enough to restore normal reproductive functions.

Emotional stress is extremely high for new brides, who must prove their fecundity to become a full adult, and often to remain married. Women who have remained childless a number of years after marriage are also under extreme pressure to produce a child, pressure that may have counterproductive effects. Unless they have special redeeming qualities, childless women are disparaged by their luckier compatriots and lose the social support they need when they seek therapy. Finally, living in a large polygynous household with cowives competing for attention and goods from the husband and to produce an heir is an extremely stressful situation.

Social Differentiation and the Distribution of Fear

While nearly all Bangangté women are aware of the entire range of procreative threats discussed in this chapter, individuals of varying social positions tend to worry most about different threats and to emphasize different causes to explain these misfortunes. The interrelated factors that most clearly influence these diverging emphases include the woman's age (especially with regard to her place in the life cycle), education, and experience with modern institutions, the density and reliability of her social support networks, the place of her household in the developmental cycle of domestic groups, and the woman's material and psychological experience of status change.

These dimensions of a woman's social position help determine the reference groups from which she gains ideas about reproductive threats and what may cause them, and a standard against which she can judge her own fears and attempts at explanation. They also shape the social groups from which she gets advice and support in her attempts to prevent or cure attacks on her reproductive health. These social groups are conduits of knowledge about reproduction (Watkins 1987), but they are more than communication networks. They are part of the conditions under which reproductive life is lived (Greenhalgh 1995:6–7), essential to the distribution of fear of infertility in Bangangté, as well as to other reproductive issues such as decisions about obstetric care, birth spacing, and contraception.

Young Bangangté women worry most about threats to their ability to conceive and to bear children. They need children to help them gain full status as adults, and to protect them from divorce. A young, childless divorced woman loses the fields she has cultivated in her husband's territory, and thus her main source of livelihood. She also gains the scorn of her natal family, who must pay back the brideprice they had received for her. This diminishes the reliability of their support should she fall ill or wish to pursue treatment for infertility. Well aware of this probable fate should she remain childless, a newlywed Bangangté woman feels under great pressure to bear children. The young women I spoke with worried most about various threats that could interfere with their ability to conceive and to bring a pregnancy to term.

The more formal education a young woman has and the more contact she has had with biomedical institutions, the more likely she is to be concerned about infections and physiological malfunctioning. The more parochial she is in her village life-experience, the more likely she is to worry about threats from the realm of ndonn. The mfen's and noble's wives and sisters, the women closest to traditional politicoreligious structures, worried more than others about offenses against the traditional norms governing these structures. If the young woman's household is involved in a succession dispute, she may well be concerned that ancestral wrath will prevent her from conceiving. If she marries into a household with many wives leery of a new intruder into their world, a young woman will probably be afraid that her cowives will use witchcraft against her to keep her from becoming pregnant. Thus, a number of factors interact with age to influence a young woman's expectations of the most likely sources of threats to conception and pregnancy.

At the far end of the life cycle, elderly women worry most about having descendants. They are nearing death and concerned that they become ancestresses and their skulls be honored. Without descendants, a deceased person becomes a ghost, a homeless and harmful being. Elderly women may have seen many of their children die, and worry that any will survive them. They have also observed how their living children have moved to town, or to the large plantations and cities of southern Cameroon. These children have learned other values than the honoring of ancestral skulls and care of elderly kin. Their elderly mothers fear abandonment in old age and death.

Domestic groups at different stages in a developmental cycle have different needs with regard to personnel. Newly founded households need to establish a reputation of vigor, "having a full house," and to build up an agricultural labor force. The women of these households are under pressure to bear many children. Households with grown children and an aging husband, by contrast, need to have a reliable successor whose siblings respect the rules of inheritance. The wives of an aging or sick husband are concerned that their future status as widows under the care of their husband's successor is respected. All members of a household nearing succession worry about the proper unfolding of household and social reproduction, and thus about the "Bangangténess" of the household's children.

The Bangangté royal household in 1986 incorporated characteristics of households at both these stages of development. Young women newly married to the king needed to bear children to create a populous royal family and secure their positions as royal wives. They were confronted with occasionally hostile cowives, whom they feared would attack their reproductive abilities. The loosening of norms governing respect for status and dispute management often led to contentious relations among the royal wives and between the wives and the mfen. Unhappy in this situation far from meeting their expectations of royal marriage, many of the king's wives ran away. At the same time, the mfen was dying, making old and young alike worry about their future position as widows and about the peaceful unfolding of succession to royal office. In fact, none of their children became king following Njiké Pokam's death in 1987. That the royal household is viewed as the exemplary Bangangté family whose reproductive success affects the well-being of the entire kingdom made many within and without the royal family worry about indicators of royal decline.

Concern with royal decline is part of a far-reaching concern with social change and its effect on individuals in Bangangté. Not only does a woman's position within nexuses of social hierarchies, age, kin, education, and stage of domestic development influence what she most fears regarding her reproductive success, her experience of social change affects the amount and direction of her fears. Bangangté, ever concerned with prestige and reward gained through office and effort, experience social change most directly in terms of the rise, maintenance, or decline of their own status. Downwardly mobile women and those whose status expectations cannot be met within the new circumstances of contemporary Bangangté society perceive the most threats to their reproductive health. They feel these threats to come from competing equals. Upwardly mobile and newly privileged women fear the malevolent actions of their envious subordinates, but on the whole perceive fewer reproductive threats than their less fortunate compatriots. Both experience anxiety due to their change in status, which they express in the culturally appropriate idiom of dangers to procreation.

For women whose status was high in the past due to their relation to their husbands (e.g., wives of kings, nobles, and retainers) or to their own positions as titleholders in the traditional hierarchy (as mothers and sisters of the mfen), recent social changes have meant status decline. The feeling of decline and of confusion about the measures with which to judge one's self-perception and worth itself creates emotional stress that can impede reproduction from both indigenous Bangangté and biomedical views. In addition it leads to a perceived vulnerability to supernatural attack. The mfen is no longer strong enough to control these forces and protect his wives and subjects. Social relations are confusing and end in arguments and envy that lead to the use of witchcraft.

Those whose status has increased through taking advantage of new opportunities—for example, by becoming a politician, a successful business woman, or the wife of a civil servant—fear the envy of others. Likewise others suspect that these privileged women have profited through illegitimate means. At the least their privilege does not derive from a traditional "Bangangté" way of life. At the worst it has been gained through witchcraft, the asocial use of supernatural power. While a privileged woman may well suspect envy and witchcraft attacks upon her reproductive organs, as in the case of the wife of one of the highest civil servants in Bangangté, she certainly has more means with which to seek treatment than her neighbor experiencing status decline.

Thus, social differentiation shapes the means women of different positions can use to protect or cure themselves from threats they already perceive in divergent ways and to varying extents. Perhaps the most obvious of these means is being able to pay for health services. Renowned indigenous healers, private doctors, and even filling the prescriptions of the public clinics all require money. The new elite has access to health services denied to the poor (Doyal 1979:114–15). Consequently, all kinds of health care are not available to all women, as is discussed in greater detail in chapter 5. The relative social isolation these women experience means both that they have less material and social support, and that they feel more vulnerable than their more fortunate neighbors.

Equally important is the effect of social differentiation upon the material and social resources one gains from others. Feierman (1985: 83–84) notes that throughout sub-Saharan Africa, changes in labor and social organization during the colonial era have contributed to differentiation among women in their experience of illness. At the level of the family, household size has tended to decline along with the decline of polygyny, already decreasing therapy assistance networks. While polygyny is still common in rural Bangangté (63 percent of my Ntamleme-Batela'-Bantoum sample, $N = 35$), the scale of polygyny is decreasing. The polygynous households of women aged 35 and over averaged 3.07 wives ($N = 14$), while those of women under 35 averaged 2.5 wives. The majority of monogamous women are under 35. These women have no cowife to help them in case of illness. Mothers and sisters are no substitute, because they are generally too far away.[18] Sisters-in-law are rarely on friendly terms with their husband's wives. Although recognizing that fights among cowives are a major source of women's unhappiness and vulnerability to witchcraft attacks, many monogamous women in Batela' and Bantoum yearn for a cowife who could help when illness strikes.

Rural exodus further decreases the pool of kin from which one can seek help. When mostly men migrate to find wage labor in colonial and postcolonial economies, as is the case in Bangangté (den Ouden 1980; Tardits 1960), women are left behind as de facto if not de jure heads of households. Their networks may be cut through the absence of the husband (Feierman 1985:83) or through the economic burdens they experience that do not allow them to participate in gift exchange to maintain their social support networks (Dieckmann and Joldersma 1982). Thus, therapy assistance networks are currently attenuated for many women in rural Bangangté, leaving them stranded in case of a health or reproductive crisis. Among these women, specific constellations of factors make some more isolated and at risk than others. Those who move furthest from home at marriage have the hardest time creating and maintaining reliable support networks. This is especially so for royal wives, whose marriages were arranged to create political alliances among distant chiefdoms.

In addition, when husbands and fathers are absent, women lack the middlemen who watch over their land use rights, making unlucky women more impoverished if they do not have enough land on which to make a living. Disputes over land tenure are often sources of witchcraft accusations and counteraccusations in Bangangté. Since households were resettled in villages along the road during the 1950s and 1960s, the quarter chiefs are further from the fields and can no longer oversee the land they are supposed to manage. The ensuing disputes contribute to a perception among Bangangté that the rate of witchcraft, and therefore of threats to reproduction, is increasing (Feldman 1984). Fears of such threats are most relevant for women in households experiencing land disputes, women in resettled villages, or women with absent husbands.

Access to land is important to women because it is the basis of their livelihood, and the means with which to produce and prepare food. Women create and maintain their social networks and social status largely through their production, exchange, and serving of food. Differences among rural women's access to the means with which to grow, cook, serve, and make gifts of this food create divergent vulnerabilities among them. Those who have little food to offer have smaller social networks from which to seek help should a misfortune such as illness or infertility strike.

What is common among this variation is that Bangangté women fear the interferences in their procreative kitchens described here and often take steps to prevent them from threatening their own reproductive success. When misfortune does strike their procreative kitchens, they seek the help of their kin, neighbors, and the variety of health-care institutions now available in the Bangangté area. The next chapter explores how women seek cures—what different kinds of preventive measures and therapies they may choose from, and the processes through which they and those close to them try to ameliorate their woes.

Chapter Five

Seeking Remedies: Medical Pluralism and the Distribution of Fear

Why should I tell you about fu [medicine]? When you the white man first came, you asked so many questions about fu. Then you went home and put our medicines in bottles, came back, and sold them to us.
    —mfen Meshinke', elderly healer and subchief of Bantoum village

Don't tell, don't tell, Pamé. Why should they [my cowives] know that I am consulting a ngakà? They are the very ones who put something bad inside me. And they would tell our husband. No, no, it must be a secret.
    —Paulette, the unfortunate protagonist of chapter 1

These two quotations from a healer and a patient both refer to the power of knowledge and secrecy in Bangangté therapeutics. They confront us with social relations of domination in the exchange of knowledge about remedies, and knowledge about seeking these remedies.

To cure and prevent the infertility they fear so much, Bangangté search for remedies from among a wide variety of medical and social institutions. Most studies of medical pluralism are concerned with the underlying cultural and social logic of the quest for therapy, including the quest for obstetric care and the quest for conception (Inhorn 1994, 1996; Janzen 1978; Sargent 1982, 1989). Because this book focuses on fear of infertility and population decline more than on illness and cure per se, we build upon these works to ask another set of questions. How might the character of these institutions, the specific form of medical pluralism in the Bamiléké area, affect the way Bangangté women think about infertility? Does the treatment Bangangté women receive contribute to their anxieties regarding threats to procreation? Does the political and economic context of medical care help shape the uses of fertility and infertility as symbolic resources in negotiations over cultural identity in a changing local and national context?

In the previous chapter, we learned that the distribution of fear of

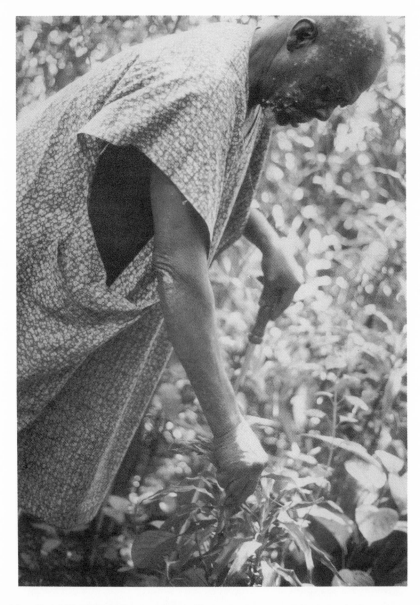

Fig. 13.   Mfen Meshinke', elderly healer and subchief of Bantoum village, cutting herbs for medicines. Mfen Meshinke' quietly chants an incantation to render his herbs powerful for healing.

infertility correlates with the material and social resources at a woman's disposition. Medical care is an important resource in treating infertility. It is also an important cognitive resource, playing a vital role in defining the problem, for example, as one of mechanical bodily failures or as the result of disturbed social relations.

As the elderly healer and subchief Meshinke' indicated, the history of health care is closely linked to processes of political and economic incorporation in Bangangté and Cameroon. Thus, there is a history to the way population and infertility have been defined as problems in the context of the Cameroonian Grassfields. This history includes the developing definitions of infertility and declining population by colonial, indigenous, and postcolonial medical practitioners, as well as by a host of other actors (including the king of Bangangté). The ways these actors have thought about population, and have affected Bangangté women's fears of infertility, are linked to other societal developments in Bangangté and in Cameroon as a whole, particularly those of labor migration, schooling, and the politicization of ethnicity.

These are the same actors whom Bangangté women must address when they seek cures for their reproductive complaints. The existence, organization, and premises of the health-care alternatives among which a woman must choose have been and continue to be shaped by the historical processes of the changing power and meaning of the kingship; colonization by Germany and France; regional, national, and international trade; the development of a national Cameroonian government; and the presence and guidelines of foreign aid agencies. As historians of health care in Africa have shown, government and missionary definitions, regulations, and policies have repercussions at many levels of health and health care (Comaroff 1981, 1993; Feierman 1985; Hunt 1993; Packard 1980; Vaughan 1991).

None of the health-care institutions in Bangangté treat exclusively reproductive problems. Some even combine the treatment and prevention of illness with other services such as providing mystical help for business deals, journeys, and school exams for individual clients, or serving the mfen and the royal court by identifying the place and timing of rites needed for maintaining agricultural success and social contentment throughout the kingdom. A woman seeking help for reproductive problems is often familiar with a particular healing institution or specialist from previous interaction regarding another type of service. This interweaving of medical, ritual, and pragmatic specialties underscores the integration of health care and health seeking with other domains of Bangangté social life. But integration and familiarity do not provide a sense of protection from reproductive threats.

Seeking remedies for reproductive complaints, an individual woman's quest for therapy can contribute to the fear of infertility. As in Paulette's case, practitioners may channel relatively vague physical complaints into categories of reproductive and social disorder. The vagaries of access and confidence in the many forms of health care (will I be able to find my healer? can I pay for transportation and consultation? can I trust that my treatment will be effective or at least not harmful?) further contribute to Bangangté women's frequent feelings of hopelessness and despair in confronting the risks of reproductive illness. The worries expressed by Bangangté women suggest that there is a cognitive parallel to the iatrogenic effects of infertility treatment pointed out by Inhorn (1994).

Remedy seeking goes beyond the quest for therapy in a strict sense. It is part of the management of social relations, as evidenced by Bangangté women's emphasis on discovering the cause of affliction (in relations with the living, the dead, and the divine) rather than with concern for therapeutic efficacy, for seeking conception. Here the Bangangté case differs from the plight of Egyptian women as eloquently portrayed in the only comprehensive account of non-Western women's experiences of infertility (Inhorn 1994, 1996). Inhorn cites many cases of women who vow never to end their peripatetic "search for children" (1994:xxvi). Through their quest for conception, these Egyptian women are managing their social relations, in their marriages, with their kin and neighbors, and in response to clerics and national policies (Inhorn 1996). The Bangangté women I know seemed less concerned with ameliorating social relations by finally achieving motherhood than with knowing how to recognize and avoid the danger of someone harming their reproductive capacity.

Janzen's now classic discussion of kinship therapy among the Bakongo clearly illustrates the management of kinship, marriage, education, and wealth in African healing systems (1978a). In a later work, he shows how intimately a specific therapeutic form, the Lemba "drum of affliction," is entwined not only in healing but also in managing market and political relations of those living in the interstices between African kingdoms (1982). The management of social relations through therapy seeking in Bangangté reaches beyond the scope of the therapeutic encounter among patient, kin, and healer. The public and social character of therapy management is peculiar in the case of infertility treatment. As Inhorn points out for Egypt (1994) and as evidenced by Paulette's plight portrayed in chapter 1, therapy management groups tend to collapse over time. In addition, the act of seeking remedies is itself a socially sensitive endeavor, bringing with it potential social costs. As Paulette indicates in the second quotation introducing this chapter, although patients may make enormous investments in time and money seeking cures for reproductive afflictions, secrecy and privacy play a tug-of-war with a wish for attention in the patient's management of therapies.

Remedy seeking also goes beyond the quest for conception because Bangangté women's concerns are broader. They worry not only about individual fate and individual fertility, but also about social reproduction. Their management of social relations includes a concern with internal and external threats from witches and from the complexities of local–state relations. They force us, as analysts, to place theses regarding therapeutic choice in medical anthropology in broader context, to see how individual variables interact and combine and how this interaction is conditioned by historical and political-economic forces.

The first part of this chapter investigates the historical processes over the past century that shaped the number and kind of health-care institutions in Bangangté today. The second section describes the health-care alternatives currently available for Bangangté women to consult regarding reproduction. It examines these health specialists' contending approaches to healing and their current attempts to adapt to a field of competing health-care alternatives. The third section analyzes the social relations of the therapeutic process, in other words how women and their kin go about managing crises in reproductive health, how they seek out health-care specialists and cures, and how their social situation affects their access to and use of various forms of health care. The chapter concludes with some propositions regarding the effect of social differentiation on access to health care and thus indirectly on the distribution of fear of reproductive illness in Bangangté.

The History of Health-care Alternatives in Bangangté

How did those white men described by the elderly healer and subchief Meshinke' come, learn about, and steal Bangangté medicine? At first European knowledge of Grassfields society and therapeutics was quite sketchy. The earliest colonial reports indicate an active indigenous attempt to counteract the disruptive effects of the establishment of colonial government and labor recruitment through the development and trading of "medicines" aimed at strengthening the kingship and counteracting witchcraft. As the colonial era progressed, first the German and then the French colonists attempted to establish medical hegemony, combining humanitarian and paternalistic good intentions with a wish for control. Government medicine was aimed mainly at insuring the labor capacity of African men, focusing on nutrition, epidemics, and enumerating populations. They viewed women's role as fertile producers of, variously, laborers, rural traditional order, and food (Guyer 1987; Vaughan 1991:22). Missionary medicine aimed to create a new type of African, an individual who would resist the collective will of "tradition" and "superstition" to embrace Christianity. Missionary doctors used dramatic surgery to draw converts and focused on mother–child health care in the long work of changing hearts and minds.

German Colonial Encounters with Grassfields Therapeutics

The earliest European inquiries into Grassfields modes of healing were based on reports on public ritual, herbal medicines, and foodways written by German explorers, researchers, and military officers at the time of direct European contact, on the eve of the twentieth century.[1] Working their way north from the port city and administrative center of Douala and from the plantation area of southern Cameroon, they focused on three areas. First, an interest in the role of sorcery and medicine in royal hegemony and interkingdom diplomacy emerged from concern with the ability of indigenous Grassfields to assist (or resist) labor recruitment efforts. Second, investigations into indigenous foodways were tied to colonial concerns with the suitability of Grassfields populations for labor. Third, the discourse on sexually transmitted diseases and infertility was likewise linked to the colonial need for labor for railroad construction and plantations in southern Cameroon.

German travelers and researchers on indigenous medicine were struck by indigenous attitudes toward death and fear of sorcery. They contrasted Grassfields "fatalism" to their own "rational" and "scientific" biomedical beliefs.[2] Fatalism, for doctors Preuss and Ziemann, was evidenced by the ways Grassfields peoples attributed deaths from pneumonia and other illnesses to the guilt of another party who has made a "fetish" (Preuss 1891b:143; Ziemann 1904:153). Behind this colonial criticism, we can hear the cries of a region suffering from the introduction of new microbes. We can also discern an indigenous theory of sociogenic etiology, that is, that disease is caused by disrupted or harmful social relations, now so familiar in contemporary studies of African therapeutics across the continent.

Conrau, author of the first travel report that includes the Eastern Grassfields, noted the relation between the fear of sorcery, royal hegemony, and the interethnic trade in indigenous medicines. Residents of the Noun River valley, which separates Bangangté and Bamoum,[3] bought medicines from neighboring groups to cure illness and prevent theft (Conrau 1898:196–197). In the Western Grassfields, a newly acquired medicine or "fetish" that was meant to strengthen the king against supernatural attack, again bought from a neighboring people, was displayed at the nobles' meetinghouse at the palace in Bangwa-Fontem during Conrau's 1898 visit (Conrau 1899:202). Both the king of Bangwa and his nobles complained to Conrau about "lawlessness" and the increasing incidence of witchcraft in the Grassfields. Such threats to royal hegemony were counteracted by rituals to maintain public peace and prosperity, including "blood friendship" pacts struck among prominent Grassfields kings (Hutter 1892:176–84). It appears that a concern for the safety of kings and the kingship, and thus with the maintenance and reproduction of a specific form of social order, arose at a time when the disruptions of colonialism were first being felt in the Grassfields. As we have seen, in systems of divine kingship social order is closely linked to individual health and fertility. Similar complaints arose during the 1980s, another period of changing power relations between Grassfields kings and larger, external political forces.

The context of these reports indicates that indigenous medicine at the turn of the century struggled to respond to the context of colonial labor policies. Labor shortages created by the competition among planters, traders, and colonial administrators for workers necessitated the use of migrant labor (Rudin 1938:316). During the earliest years of German colonization, workers were imported from other parts of West Africa. After the interior became subject to colonial control in 1898, labor recruiters sought plantation labor, porters, and public works laborers in the Grassfields area surrounding Bali, Bamenda, and the Bamiléké highlands.[4] Some local rulers seized the opportunity to solidify their hegemony over their neighbors, supplying plantation representatives and traders with laborers in return for colonial patronage; this system was formalized through labor contracts drawn between various Grassfields kings and the German colonial government (Rudin 1938:320, 322).

Working conditions and methods of labor recruitment were devastating to workers' health. Forced from their homes, workers were bound together by ropes and made to trek long distances, often through areas of smallpox epidemics, to reach their destinations (Rudin 1938:324, 326). Arriving in the hotter, wetter, lower altitude plantation areas, climatic change contributed to the suffering of Grassfields workers, especially from malaria and filariasis (DeLancey 1978:158, 160).[5] The death rate in the colonial plantations sometimes ranged from one-third to one-half of all plantation workers (Rudin 1938:328). Workers lived in barrack conditions, where crowded conditions and impure water were conducive to the spread of communicable disease, including dysentery, tuberculosis, pneumonia, and typhus (DeLancey 1978:162; Rudin 1938:328). Workers' one-sided diets of unfamiliar foods contrasted ironically with colonial investigations into indigenous Grassfields foodways; rather than seeking continuity in migrant workers' diets, researchers proposed changes in

Grassfields agriculture, encouraging peanut and black bean cultivation (Reichskolonialamt 1914:84; Wissenschaftliche Beihefte 1894:99–104).

When Grassfields laborers had finished their contracts, they often returned home "emaciated, [and] suffering from various diseases" (cited in DeLancey 1978:167) or died in the road. They brought the scourges of the labor barracks home with them, spreading disease beyond the immediate labor areas (Doyal 1979:111) with serious consequences for Grassfields populations. Dysentery and smallpox disseminated along trade routes and into the source areas of labor recruitment, scarring faces (Ziemann 1904:160) and devastating local populations. In 1910–11, 8000 people in Bamenda district died from a dysentery epidemic (Reichskolonialamt 1912:56). But the same page of the official report on the fight against disease in Bamenda discusses increases in the recruitment of indigenous labor for the Mittellandbahn, the railroad between Douala and Yaoundé (Reichskolonialamt 1912:56). The early colonial appetite for labor was insatiable and contributed to enduring local images of population decline.

It is probable that disease itself also contributed to fear of population decline in Grassfields polities such as Bangangté, as migrant laborers returned from the barracks with syphilis and gonorrhea. The areas and timing of the spread of sleeping sickness, influenza, and sexually transmitted diseases correlate strongly with pockets of low fertility in sub-Saharan Africa (Retel-Laurentin 1974). While no reliable data exists on fertility fluctuations among Grassfields populations during this time, indigenous fears of low or decreasing fertility were shared by several colonial actors, all with their own interests.

Reports of colonial officials express a repeated concern with reproductive strength in the Grassfields (Reichskolonialamt 1912:56, 58, 60; 1913:64; 1914: xii, 78).[6] Sexually transmitted disease and poor indigenous hygiene were most often cited as causes of the allegedly declining fertility of the Grassfields (Reichskolonialamt 1912:56, 60; 1913:64). Only one dissenting voice, a perceptive physician of the German navy, included the reduction of the male population via poorly regulated recruitment of laborers and porters for military expeditions in his report on low population in the Grassfields (Ziemann 1904:150–53). During the same time period, traders were concerned not only that enough laborers be guaranteed to carry their goods into the hinterland, but also that a large and prosperous population would exist to insure consumers (Diehn 1956). A daughter of the most prominent German trading firm, Woermann, offered a cash prize for the best study on ways to increase the native birthrate (Rudin 1938:346).[7] Missionaries were concerned with promoting the health of Grassfields populations in order to encourage and maintain followers, including medical evangelism in their efforts. The first missionary physician was sent to a Western Grassfields Basel Mission station in 1907, and to the mission's Foumban dispensary ca. 1908 (Basel Mission, Ärtzliche Mission in Kamerun, n.d.). But mission health care, later to focus on maternal and child health, did not become established in the Bangangté area until well into the French colonial era, during the interwar years.

The early colonial period brought a number of new diseases and an increase in the feeling of affliction even to Grassfields people who had had no direct contact with the colonizers. Not only disease, but the social effects of labor recruitment and colonial rule disturbed the health and fertility of Grassfields populations. Young Bamiléké men were absent, doing forced labor or emigrating to the urban centers to escape labor recruitment in the countryside. This led to the neglect of native farms (DeLancey 1978:157). The involvement of the Bamiléké kings, including mfen Njiké II of Bangangté, in labor recruitment weakened the mfens' hold on some of their subjects. Those most affected by labor recruitment were commoners and those from royal retainer families, and many young men from these social strata sought to escape the mfens' realm of dominance in order to escape forced labor recruitment. The women from these groups lost access to land gained previously through now absent husbands. They suffered more than other women from lack of resources, shrinking support networks, and malnutrition. In the absence of reliable population data, we can surmise that the wives and sisters of labor recruits suffered lower fertility due to separation from their husbands and potential mates.

As sexually transmitted diseases became endemic to the Grassfields, and as more and more migrant workers returned home sick, local forms of caring for the afflicted became strained. New social conditions may therefore have contributed to changes in healing practices in the Grassfields during the early decades of the twentieth century. The intergroup trade in "medicines" (i.e., buying herbal recipes or instructions for amulet- and fetish-making along with the skill to apply them) observed as early as 1898 by Conrau may have been stimulated by the indigenous health-care specialists' increased need to find cures for new and more frequent afflictions. Labor migrants, like mfen Meshinke' who complained so heavily about whites stealing indigenous medical knowledge, incorporated new ideas (e.g., "measuring" sickness) from their encounters with biomedicine. But at the same time that they sought new medicines to cure new diseases, they were hindered in their endeavors by a repressive colonial administration. In Bana district, then including Bangangté, punishment "with arms" was used against the "evil influence of so-called medicine-men, who got the population into an upset state following a murder by poisoning trial" (Reichskolonialamt 1914:70, my translation). An official report argues that low fertility and high maternal and infant mortality in the Grassfields was not to be fought with health education, but by combating "bush medicine and wise women" (Reichskolonialamt 1912:60, my translation). To this end, plans were made toward the end of German colonial rule to train indigenous midwives in biomedical techniques of birth attendance (Reichskolonialamt 1914:80).

Bamiléké encounters with colonial biomedical practices was negligible for all but the migrants to the cities and plantations. Colonial medical services reached the Grassfields only at the very end of the German colonial period and were delivered in a sporadic and repressive fashion. Grassfields populations first encountered biomedical treatment through mobile troops delivering smallpox vaccinations (Reichskolonialamt 1911:65–67). On the eve of World War I, one official report records that a number of Grassfields kings were punished for their resistance against the vaccination campaigns (Reichskolonialamt 1914:70).

The German colonial period led to real and perceived threats to Grassfields fertility and numbers. A labor reserve area, the Grassfields were drained of young men. Those who were not recruited often fled to the bush, away from both colonial and chiefly authority. The repressive nature of early colonial biomedicine, military expeditions vaccinating against dread diseases and punishing resisters, further contributed to the flight of young men and fear of disease. Women, particularly of those social strata contributing most heavily to the colonial labor pool, suffered sexually transmitted diseases, secondary infertility, and decreased opportunities to become pregnant. These conditions set the stage for continuing indigenous images of population decline during the French colonial period, images that were exacerbated by French fears regarding population.

New Actors: French Military Medicine and Medical Missionaries

While the 30 years of German colonization affected patterns of health and most likely influenced the practices and demand for indigenous health care in the Grassfields, the availability of biomedical treatment and its impact upon the Bamiléké in general and Bangangté in particular remained negligible. After the Germans lost Cameroon in 1916, two groups of new European actors entered the field of health care in Bangangté. Although they shared the biomedical model of germ theory, specific etiology, and the notion that medicine treats the physical problems of individual patients, the French colonial military medical staff and Protestant medical missionaries had divergent goals and different relationships with the local population surrounding Bangangté.

Colonial Medical Efforts. The Service de Santé de la France Outre-Mer, a part of the French army, ran public health care in Cameroon under French mandate and trusteeship. At the beginning of French rule, public biomedical units expanded rapidly into the Bamiléké region. The French were very concerned to eliminate Cameroonians' identification with their former German colonizers (Ngongo 1982:16–23), and increasing their presence through health services was one way to *franciser* (Frenchify) their new subjects. In addition, the League of Nations decision had split the Eastern and Western Grassfields between French and British mandates. The Germans had concentrated their nascent infrastructure in the Western Grassfields, while still drawing on Eastern Grassfields (Bamiléké) labor. The new French masters could draw only on Bamiléké labor, and the Bamiléké plateau thus increased in importance to its colonial rulers.

Continuing the aims of their German predecessors, French colonial military medicine sought to insure a sufficiently healthy indigenous population as a potential labor force. The Bamiléké plateau was mentioned as an important source of labor as early as 1917 (Tardits 1960:65), even before the territory was officially ceded to France under a League of Nations mandate in 1920. The value of the Bamiléké plateau as a labor reserve area became even more significant throughout the period of French rule. Influenced by the need for labor in central Cameroon, colonial medical officials were particularly concerned about (1) the devastating endemic diseases trypanosomiasis (sleeping sickness) and leprosy, and (2) an allegedly declining indigenous population.

Throughout the colonial period, the state of health of Bamiléké populations in the countryside remained a problem for labor recruiters. In 1944 the French administrator at Bafoussam, Relly, reported that he habitually demanded twice as many laborers as needed for plantation work since 50 percent were rejected by the plantations' health service (Tardits 1960:67).[8] In the same report Relly complained that 90 percent of Bamiléké youth fled the labor recruiters, either temporarily to the forest or for longer periods (even permanently) to urban centers. The heavy-handed recruitment policies of the French administration thus contributed to uncontrolled rural flight and an imbalanced demographic structure within the territories of the Bamiléké kingdoms.

One step in improving the health of labor source populations was combating endemic disease. Colonial military medicine organized the fight against sleeping sickness and leprosy, well-advertised medical campaigns that brought some positive recognition to France's efforts in the mandated territory. In 1922, Eugène Jamot, a military doctor in the service of the French administration, began his campaign against sleeping sickness (trypanosomiasis), a disease threatening the lives and productivity of central Cameroonian populations and colonists alike (LeVine and Nye 1974:59–60). Jamot established mobile treatment centers that surveyed the population for cases of both sleeping sickness and leprosy.[9] Bamiléké contact with mobile medical services increased during epidemics; in 1945 21,095 Bamiléké were vaccinated to prevent the spread of a smallpox epidemic then raging in the Western Grassfields of British Cameroon (Farinaud 1945:3, 113). From the point of view of the Bangangté and their neighbors, these contacts were far from benign. Mobile teams rounded up local populations for vaccinations, and those infected with targeted endemic diseases were isolated in treatment colonies.

The work of the mobile teams of the Service d'Hygiène Mobile et de Prophylaxie (SHMP) that aimed to insure the native labor supply was at the same time linked to French concerns about population (Feierman 1985:121–22). Statements regarding Bamiléké population occur as early as 1928 in reports to the League of Nations. In the mid-1940s, the medical-colonel Farinaud expressed concern about the increasing rate of gonor-rhea and its deleterious effect on Bamiléké fertility (Farinaud 1944:79), but felt that solving the problem of low fertility among the Bamiléké was less a medical than a social task of education (1945:204). Nonetheless, medical officers expressed concern when Bamiléké use of biomedical gyne-cological care diminished; a decrease in Bamiléké deliveries in government health services in 1947 was attributed to the political climate (Vaisseau 1948:66, 69).[10]

The French were particularly sensitive to questions of population in equatorial Africa and in the metropole, but their concerns were often based on misunderstandings of social and demographic processes. Kuczynski introduces his extensive demographic study of Cameroon and Togo by criticizing French concern with population decline in the Cameroonian Grassfields as unfounded and revealing the "administrator's lack of sense for figures" (1939:xvi). Not only was most census data based on estimates, but people also fled into the forest to avoid census takers, fearing taxation, labor conscription, and violence. Those who were actu-ally counted had to assemble at designated points on designated days (Egerton 1938: 177–79). In addition to depending upon unreliable census data, the French occasionally frightened themselves unnecessarily about demographic threats to their Grassfields labor supply because they were ignorant of the effect of Bamiléké and Bamoum history on population dis-tribution. The Noun valley, on the frontier between the Bangangté and Bamoum kingdoms, had been depopulated by the last Bangangté-Bamoum war at the end of the nineteenth century. A French military physician, Cartron, was concerned with the effect of low fertility and low population densities among the Bamoum on the economic exploitation of valuable agricultural land. He suggested resettling the more populous Bamiléké as agricultural laborers in the Noun valley, never realizing the historical reason for low population in the Noun valley (Cartron 1934).

The actual effect of French rule upon Bamiléké population change seems contradictory. On the one hand, labor migration and the flight of young adult men from labor recruitment to the cities contributed to the neglect of farms and the overburdening of women with both men's and women's agricultural tasks in the production of food crops. It also separated husbands and wives for long periods of time, created a shortage of young men, and helped spread sexually transmitted diseases—all factors that can potentially lower fertility. In addition, now de facto female headed households were socially more vulnerable should disease or misfortune strike (Feierman 1981). These social processes began during the German colonial period and intensified during the French colonial period. Particularly after World War II, Bangangté was more affected by labor migration than any other Bamiléké kingdom (Tardits 1960:86). Current Bangangté concerns about declining population refer not only to birthrates but also to the ongoing pattern of labor migration that got its impetus during French rule.

On the other hand, certain aspects of biomedical care reduced mortality from epidemic disease, according to some reports resulting in rapid population increase (DeLancey 1978). This led to land shortage and increased labor migration, decreasing fallow periods, and declining soil fertility. When the cash crops cocoa, tobacco, and especially coffee were introduced in the 1930s, and when their production was liberalized around 1950, land for food crops became ever scarcer and the diet more one-sided. These aspects of "overpopulation" and economic change created both economic and health stresses upon rural Bamiléké populations during the period of French mandate and trusteeship. They also created the conditions for differential risks to fertility indicated by the distribution of women's fears in contemporary Bangangté. Some households may have expanded their numbers and land use, while others were broken apart by the enforced labor migration of noninheriting males.

During the greater part of French rule, colonial health care aiming to prevent demographic decline and devastating disease in the Bangangté area was limited to the mobile teams of the SHMP. Through these mobile teams, Bangangté encounters with the medicine of their new rulers were often intermittent and overshadowed by the repressive nature of medical police. The forced vaccination of healthy individuals brought no immediate, visible benefits and made little sense to Bangangté patients. The first government doctor treating Bamiléké patients was sent to Dschang in 1920, where a hospital was opened in 1930 (Debarge 1934:7).

In Bangangté itself, the first government medical center, an ill-equipped dispensary built of wattle and daub construction, existed during the late 1930s and early 1940s.[11] A new dispensary was constructed between 1940 and 1943 of permanent materials and staffed with nurses trained at the colonial school for indigenous health workers at Ayos, in south-central Cameroon. The dispensary received its first physician in 1953, although by 1951 it already had an inpatient capacity of 57 beds (Rapport . . . à L'Assemblé Générale 1951:212). According to oral testimony, the present Bangangté provincial hospital was built in the 1940s on the former cite of the "Hausa" (including Hausa and Fulani) settlement in Bangangté town. It appears to have been opened only in 1960 with the arrival of the French Médecin-Lieutenant Lassauvagerie. As with the mobile teams of the Service d'Hygiène Mobile et de Prophylaxie, these stationary biomedical establishments of the Action Médicale Indigène (AMI) were run in the authoritarian manner of the military medical services.

Protestant Missionary Medicine. As Vaughan points out in her study of missionary medicine in East and Central Africa, "throughout most of the colonial period and throughout most of Africa, Christian missions . . . provided vastly more medical care for African communities than did colonial states" (1991:56). This was true in the Cameroonian Grassfields surrounding Bangangté as well, where the bulk of biomedical care of indigenous populations was provided by the Protestant mission. The Société des Missions Evangéliques de Paris (now DEFAP) took over the work of the Basel Mission in French Cameroon in 1916 and began reporting on its Cameroonian activities toward the end of the war, in 1918. The French Protestant mission quickly expanded its medical work, beginning with a dispensary (clinic run by a nurse) in Foumban. The energetic Josette Debarge joined the Foumban dispensary in November 1926 as the first missionary doctor in the Eastern Grassfields (Debarge 1934:8). Two years later a dispensary staffed by two nurses was constructed in Bafoussam (Debarge 1934:10). Joining the Bafoussam dispensary in 1930, Debarge opened a dispensary at Bangwa near Bangangté in 1931 (1934:11). The construction of Bangwa hospital, still the most important and famous biomedical establishment in Ndé Division, began in 1934.

The mission's medical work was explicitly tied to the goal of evangelization. The missionaries hoped to convince the local population of the power of Christian faith through demonstrating the power of European drugs and surgery. Daily practice at Bangwa dispensary began with the admonition that the "tutelary spirits" would not seek vengeance on patients visiting the mission doctor (Debarge 1934:88). When the medical missionary teams arrived in a village during treatment and evangelization tours, hundreds of patients and escorts would be waiting. The missionaries preached a sermon about the virtues of Christianity and its power to heal, and the evils of polygyny, nakedness, alcohol, and "bush medicine," to the crowd before beginning the individual consultation of patients (Debarge 1934:74). Dramatic surgical operations were explicitly used to convince royals and the Bamiléké nobility, resistant to evangelization, of the immense power of Christianity and its medicine (Debarge 1934:78).

The premises underlying missionary healing were those of traditional biomedicine of the time. The physician felt privileged to deal with the concrete body; she complained that her patients found her questions about the body's physical symptoms incomprehensible (Debarge 1934:51). Because Bamiléké patients and their indigenous healers deal with custom and notions of angered "spirits" that are "moved by the subconscious," Debarge concluded that they are interested in completely different information regarding illness and that it is best not to interrogate but merely to physically examine the hopefully passive patient (1934:51). For the Franco-Swiss physician, surgical operations were "an oasis of calm," with "their ritual technique, their silence, their obligatory isolation" (1934:75). One can only imagine the deep impression the ritual of surgery must have made upon patients and their kin, and the fear the isolation of the patient from her family must have awakened.

The isolation of the patient via the practices of missionary medicine occurred in other ways as well. The largest group of patients during the 1930s, the formative years of mission medicine in the Bangangté area, was women.[12] Debarge found sterility, infant mortality, and tuberculosis to be the most serious problems (1934:112). Bangwa's mission doctor attributed sterility and infant mortality to the spread of sexually transmitted disease (1934:61, 62) and recognized that they were devastating to women, who suffered since "children are their reason for living" (1934:28). Building upon this felt need, midwifery, fertility, and child care became a focus of Protestant mission work in Bangwa and, by the 1940s, in Bangangté. As elsewhere in Africa, Christian missionaries found that African ideas about fertility, childbirth, and child rearing were "the locus of the reproduction of many strongly-held beliefs" (Vaughan 1991:66), the very "superstitions" or non-Christian social and moral controls that evangelization sought to change. Gradually, childbirth at mission hospitals and dispensaries became ever more common. Debarge and her colleagues focused much of their attention on infant feeding and child rearing practices, encouraging habits of regularity more fitting with the early-twentieth-century European model of self-discipline. Infants became patients isolated from African families, first in the form of an orphanage in Bangwa. In 1946 Charles and Yvette Bergeret founded a school of home economics for girls, instituting an elaborate system of reeducation in which the students were isolated from their families, their customs, and their "pagan superstitions" (Njiké-Bergeret 1997:23).

Reports in the mission archives from the opening of Bangwa Hospital in 1934 through the mid-1960s reveal a long tradition of a well-staffed and expanding missionary health-care system in the Bangangté-Bangwa-Bafoussam area. Concern with evangelization continued, citing that the role of God's disciples is to "chase demons" and that this is best done by serving the sick in the mission's hospitals, dispensaries, and leprosariums (Société des Missions Evangéliques de Paris 1960:19). Maternal and child health care, long neglected by the colonial state, became a notable element of the medical mission and furthered the goal of evangelization.

The French mission gradually ceased to have exclusive control of Protestant medical work in the Grassfields. The missionaries had to share power with the Cameroonian church they themselves had called into being, the Eglise Evangélique du Cameroun (EEC), autonomous since 1957. Starting in 1961, the professional staffing of Bangwa and other Protestant hospitals was also shared between the French mission and that of the Dutch Reformed Church. The civil war of the 1960s, and a related incident in which two French missionaries were murdered in 1965, initiated a number of years during which French missionaries were totally absent from Ndé Division. The goals of the missionaries slowly changed from that of proselytizing to doing good works through health care of the poor. With this change in mission policy and attitude, some tension developed between officials of the Cameroonian church (EEC)—who are most interested in evangelization, curative medicine, and privileges for church members—and foreign missionaries dedicated to primary health care and the disregard of the hard-won status of higher level church members.

Medical Pluralism in Bangangté: The 1980s

The arrival of French military and missionary medicine and their coexistence with the various forms of indigenous health care present in Bangangté in the 1930s created a field of divergent ways of organizing health care and contending ideologies of illness and curing. Even before the permanent establishment of biomedical dispensaries in Ndé Division, indigenous medicine was characterized by its variety and innovative response to social change.[13] At the time of my initial fieldwork, 50 years after the founding of Bangwa Hospital, Bangangté women still had to manage complex alternatives when seeking remedies for reproductive ailments.

To understand how the form of medical pluralism in Bangangté affects the ways Bangangté women think about threats to their fertility, we first must grasp the entire field of health-care institutions and how they are classified and perceived by their practitioners and clients. Each of the health-care institutions in and near Bangangté kingdom has its distinctive form of organization, methods and specialties of healing, medicines, premises, ways of training specialists, and modes of interacting with patients. Each of them by and large has the characteristics of a medical system, a "patterned, interrelated body of values and deliberate practices, governed by a single paradigm of the meaning, identification, prevention and treatment of sickness" (Press 1980:3). They differ from this classic definition of medical systems in two respects. First, they are particular organizations and may share paradigms of meaning, identification, prevention, and treatment with other health-care institutions. For example, the public biomedical hospital and the public rural health clinic share the same premises regarding illness and health care, but differ in their degree of functional differentiation. Second, any one institution may refer to more than one illness/treatment paradigm, although each institution tends to emphasize what Press would define as a particular medical system.[14]

When seeking remedies, Bangangté distinguish among different types of healing institutions and among individual practitioners (see table 1). Most village women refer to all biomedical institutions as providing the same type of health care and working according to a single set of premises. They call biomedicine *la médecine moderne* (modern medicine) or *fu mekat* (white man's medicine). Often a woman will have a preference for a particular biomedical institution, based on reputation or personal connection to a staff member.

Likewise, these same health seekers refer to the majority of indigenous health-care practitioners as *ngakà* (person of power/medicine) or as *guérisseur* (healer). Indigenous practitioners make finer distinctions among themselves: *ngafu* (persons of herbs) cure primarily with herbs, *ngakà* (persons of *kà*) combine the control of magical power with herbal treatments and, occasionally, with divination, and *ngazenu* (sages, clairvoyants) use their wisdom or their power to "see" to recommend therapies and perform small treatments using herbs or manipulative techniques.[15] Both indigenous healing specialists and lay Bangangté distinguish two further types of traditional health-care institutions or specialists: the *ngangame* (diviner), who performs divination with the earth spider oracle; and the *minnyi* (spirit medium), a person, most often a woman, who is

TABLE 1. Inventory of Health Care Specialists and Institutions

French Term	Lay Bangangté Term	Differentiated Bangangté Term	Characteristics
I. Specialists			
A. Biomedical			
médecin	dokta	dokta	physician; sometimes nurse; both can write prescriptions
infirmier	dokta	dokta	
aide-soignant	infirmier		nurses's aide
fille/garçon de salle			aide, generally with formal training
B. Indigenous			
guérissuer	ngakà	ngafu	man of herbal medicine; uses only herbs
		ngakà	man of medicine/magic; uses herbs as well as divination and spells
		ngazenu	sage; can "see" causes, recommend therapies, and perform minor treatments
	ngangame	ngangame	man of the earth spider; performs spider divination to find causes and predict the future; rarely cures
médium	minnyi	minnyi	usually female, divinely inspired or possessed; can diagnose causes, indicate which ancestor needs to be appeased, and give herbal treatments for minor maladies and to enhance fertility
II. Biomedical Institutions			
hôpital (publique, privée)	waswita		hierarchical organization with many departments and role sets
centre de santé	waswita		rural or urban clinic staffed by personnel of varying rank, none higher than nurses; low specialization
CDMP	waswita		Centre Départemental de Médecine Preventive; functions as urban clinic
pharmacie	famasi		private pharmacy

alternately described as possessing divine inspiration or as being possessed by a "spirit,"[16] ancestor, or *Nsi* (God). Minnyis have special powers of clairvoyance, and prepare medicines to enhance their clients' fertility or cure minor complaints such as headache.

In contrast to the attitudes of biomedical personnel and to national and international health policy makers, this inventory shows that indigenous medicine in Bangangté is neither uniform nor static, but is constituted by highly diverse and dynamic forms of healing. Furthermore, individual practitioners within each type of indigenous health institution are highly, and often purposefully, individualistic.

Some Bangangté who are specialists in other fields, such as dispute resolution, perform curative or preventive health-care roles. The *bandansi,* the people of the house of Nsi, perform rites of washing and oath taking supported by drinking "cooked" (mystically transformed) raffia wine[17] for litigants in suits brought to the mfen. Often these cases involve the reproductive difficulties of one of the litigants. The following case was brought before the mfen, and resolved through the action of the bandansi.

Infertility as a Legal Case

The plaintiff had been married to a young woman for a number of years. She bore him two children, but one died. Since then, she has borne no more children and has been in bad health. The plaintiff "has spent just too much money" (mfen) trying to restore his wife's health. Through his vain attempts with biomedicine, he discovered that his wife could not get well by modern medicine alone; the cause of her affliction was in the family.

In October 1986, the plaintiff accused two relations of his sick wife— her "tuteur" or guardian before she was married, and the heiress of one of her maternal kin—of making or keeping her sick. The mfen listened to the stories of each of the four parties concerned: the plaintiff, his sick wife, the tuteur, and the maternal heiress. He found no one guilty, but ordered a rite of reconciliation to be performed under the guidance of the bandansi.

The rite took place two days later, at the intersection of two paths in mâfen, *the sacred forest of the lower part of the royal compound. Members of bandansi, including a high ranking royal retainer, oversaw the rite, quietly instructing the four participants in turn how they should wash their face, forearms, and feet in "cooked" raffia wine (* nâ ndu*). Each of the four participants then handed some money into the palm of the royal retainer and made a speech of around three minutes. Approx-*

*imately twenty-five bystanders, most of them women, looked on (see fig.
11, chap. 4).*

*All participants and onlookers then returned to the palace and stood
around the edge of the palace living and reception room. The four participants addressed the mfen, who was sitting on a leopard skin on the
sofa, with a few words. The mfen then gave a brief speech about the
necessity of living in peace together. The crowd applauded, and the mfen
ended the event with the announcement "a mî" (it is finished).*

The mfen and bandansi become involved in cases of reproductive illness most often when the participants have previously pursued a long and
complex but unsuccessful therapeutic itinerary. The longer an affliction
remains uncured despite the intervention of health-care specialists, the
more likely the case will be transformed into a legal dispute involving
accusations and counteraccusations of kin. Only then do "legal" experts
become health-care providers.

Among all disorders, infertility is most likely to remain uncured; its
cure is most likely to cross outsiders' conceptual categories of medical, religious, and legal remedies. Therapeutic efficacy, defined in biomedical
terms as the elimination of disease and in sociological terms as the termination of the sick role (Csordas and Kleinman 1996:9), is rarely achieved
by any form of health care in cases of infertility in Bangangté. A successful outcome in these terms is even more unlikely for sufferers from the fear
of infertility. Bangangté women who fear attacks to their reproductive
capacity are most concerned with diagnosis, with finding the many layers
of the causes of their affliction, causes both physical and social. For them,
diagnosis is an important part of the healing process, as it guides women
in understanding and responding to crises in their bodies and in their
social relations. They often seek their remedies-cum-diagnoses from a
broad range of health-care institutions, each potentially uncovering a different layer of the causes of reproductive threats.

Contending Approaches to Healing Reproductive Disorders

In seeking to uncover the causes of affliction and to cure reproductive disorders, Bangangté recognize distinctive premises and areas of competence
for biomedical and indigenous care-giving institutions. The varying ideologies and specialties of health-care institutions in Bangangté communicate different messages about the nature of infertility and the ways reproductive health and illness are connected to or divorced from their social
context. The organization of space, personnel, and practitioner–patient
interaction in biomedical and indigenous health-care institutions further

contributes to what counts as "authoritative knowledge" in assessing reproductive threat (Jordan 1993; Sargent and Davis-Floyd 1997).

Bangangté patients seek out biomedical institutions to treat the specific, visible symptoms of illness and immediate, acute conditions. They consult biomedical practitioners to obtain injections or prescriptions for antibiotics and other manufactured drugs they hope will cure or diminish symptoms of pain, hypertension, accident, or infection. They seek biomedical treatment for such well-known conditions as malaria or wounds involving loss of blood, and for childbirth, which they understand as the "simple" part of procreation. In addition, patients view surgery as the undisputed monopoly of biomedical practitioners. Bangangté women consult biomedical physicians and nurses for prenatal consultations, physical complications of pregnancy, and delivery. They also seek relief of pelvic pain, radiographic diagnosis to "see blocked tubes," and occasionally surgical intervention to correct anatomical causes of infertility. In the limited purposes they attribute to biomedical care, women respond to biomedical definitions of reproductive illness as caused by germs and mechanical failures of reproductive anatomy, and to biomedical definitions of the role of therapy as the elimination of organic disorder.

Biomedical practitioners believe they are treating causes as well as symptoms of concrete organic conditions. Biomedical personnel of varying rank and experience identify specific infections (bacterial, viral, or parasitic) and physiological processes or conditions as the ultimate cause of illness. They understand their task and special skill as diagnosing these infectious and physiological causes and prescribing or performing treatments that eliminate them and thereby cure the condition. They view their clients' interpretation of social and mystical causes as superstitious ignorance. Most biomedical practitioners rarely explain their own diagnosis of illness etiology to patients. Several stated that explaining their diagnoses is harmful both to treatment and to their own position as medical expert. This systematic lack of communication supports the beliefs of Bangangté patients that successful biomedical treatment of symptoms is not a complete cure of their afflictions.

By contrast, practitioners of indigenous medicine claim to address the ultimate causes of affliction. Most Bangangté believe that specific afflictions are caused by the presence of evil in human relations and are the consequence of human and supernatural action. The anger of ancestors or the spells and fetishes of living evildoers "seize" and therefore become "attached to" the afflicted, causing illness, sterility, and other forms of misfortune. A number of indigenous healing procedures "detach" the patient from the bad influence ultimately causing the affliction. Mfen Meshinke' and Nana, two elderly healers, both use water with herbs floating in it to "wash" patients suffering from the ill wishes of others. This washing rinses away the bad feeling or spell, and thus opens or frees the patient to receive further treatment or to conceive. Felix, Paulette's younger and more syncretistic healer, ties and unties of tiny bundles of grasses, feathers, and black thread to "detach" his patients from others' spells. Perfoming rites of protection, Felix also ties a bundle of grasses and feathers to "attach" his spell of mystical armor, thus reversing the "detaching" necessary to begin healing. In the case of the disputing family, the bandansi had the litigants "wash" away their bad feeling. At the same time, the use of "cooked" raffia wine sealed or "attached" to their persons the participants' oaths of good intentions, creating the conditions that would allow the young women to once again bear children. The implicit message communicated to patients is that the anatomical changes evident in reproductive illness (e.g., blocked tubes or amenorrhea) result ultimately from disturbed relations with one's fellow beings. Only reestablishing tranquillity with the living, the ancestors, and the unseen will effect a lasting cure and the good fortune of fertility.

Not only the ideologies and specializations of health-care institutions, but also the organization of space and personnel affects practitioners' interactions with women and their escorts. Space and functional differentiation in health-care institutions communicate messages about what and whose knowledge counts regarding the cause and cure of reproductive illness.

The locus of caregiving in different institutions affects the patient's experience of social distance from the physician, nurse, or healer. Hospital patients wait in long lines in outside corridors, if they are lucky on benches.[18] The patients of indigenous practitioners also wait separated from the healing scene, on benches or stools along the edges of the compound courtyard. In all settings, high status patients rarely need to wait in line. Only the healer or physician determines how soon a patient is to be examined and treated. Waiting patients are passive; the physician or healer is the powerful actor in this interaction dyad, and patients fear that upsetting the potential caregiver may prevent the desired cure. Social distance is dramatized by the symbolic use of space and rank in all healing institutions, but in different ways and with different effects for interaction style. Later we examine several examples of health-care providers in and around Bangangté, representing a continuum of styles and innovations between what most Bangangté informants identify as "modern" and "indigenous" medicine.

Biomedical Institutions.   Biomedical hospitals in the Bangangté area are hierarchically organized, reflected in the division of hospital buildings into pavilions by types of illness and function (e.g., a reception and walk-in clinic area, internal medicine, pediatrics, maternity ward, isolation ward for tubercular patients), arranged around a central courtyard. The two most imposing buildings, at both Bangangté Divisional Hospital and Bangwa Protestant Hospital, are those for administration and for surgery. Each member of the hospital staff has an assigned place within one of the pavilions, and an assigned rank within each functional unit of the hospital. Within each pavilion, ranked differentiation among staff members is expressed not only in the activities they are assigned but also in the space in which they may move. Nurses and occasionally nurses' aides often have desks and tables with medical equipment around which their healing activities center. Orderlies at most have chairs where they may sit; they must usually walk around from patient to patient or from the pavilion to water source.

Smaller biomedical clinics, usually under the administration of one of these two hospitals, are less differentiated both in the tasks assigned to different staff members and in spatial organization. The pavilions (wards) of the hospitals translate into corners of one-room buildings, or into small rooms off the largest central waiting room. An examination room with an examination table may double as a delivery room, and a room or separate one-room building for the few inpatients, mostly women waiting to give birth or recovering from birth.

Verbal communication between biomedical practitioners and their patients is minimal. Sometimes biomedical personnel share no common language with their patients, and lower level staff or the patients' escorts must be used as interpreters. Often nearly half the consultation time is used to fill out the register (Hours 1985:22). Part of the brief remaining time that physician or nurse and patient have together is taken up by a silent physical examination. Biomedical practitioners inform their patients of their diagnosis and recommended treatment in the form of authoritarian pronouncements with little or no explanation. Biomedical practitioners sometimes merely scribble a prescription in the patient's health booklet and send the patient away without a word. Some regret having to do this, excusing themselves with the time pressure they are under to see as many patients as possible and with their lack of local language competence. Other biomedical practitioners, especially nurses, express dismay at the thought of explaining a medical diagnosis to a patient. They claim the patient would not understand, would worry unnecessarily, or would use the diagnosis to seek care from someone else (e.g., to self-medicate with prescription drugs or herbs bought at market).

This biomedical interaction style reflects organizational hierarchies, material constraints, and, perhaps, the role of competition in a highly pluralistic medical setting. No staff member will answer a question or perform a service for a patient if they believe the task falls in another staff member's sphere of responsibility and competence. These sharp delineations of spheres of therapeutic action protect biomedical personnel from accusations of incompetence, and help to limit the demands made upon their time and material resources. In addition, resistance to revealing the diagnoses may reflect practitioners' fears of losing clientele. Information would free their patient from dependence upon the practitioner, allowing her to go with the diagnosis to another, competing practitioner, whether biomedical or indigenous.

Bangangté patients I observed present their problems to biomedical caregivers in a way diverging greatly from the stories of familial relations and "spirits" described by Debarge in the 1930s. Fifty years later, patients presented detailed descriptions of symptoms without superfluous commentary. They described pain and recalled the date of their last menstrual period with almost unbelievable exactness. Patients occasionally proposed a diagnosis; physicians and nurses made clear their annoyance at this short-circuiting of their competence and authority.

Felix's Practice: A Creolized Medical Style. The spatial organization of healer Felix's healing compound and practice is an example of the present-day possibilities in a continuum between biomedical and indigenous practice and the impossibility of identifying which forms of practice and organization are truly "traditional" and when new forms emerged. Felix actively combines the symbols and practices of several healing traditions in a vibrant example of what Hannerz has termed "cultural creolization" (1987). Felix understands himself as a traditional healer, a ngakà who combines knowledge of herbs with divination and dramatic ritual to cure or protect his patients from the evil machinations of their enemies. His practice is in between indigenous and biomedical forms in terms of its organization as a business (he more than other indigenous healers is paid in advance) and its spatial and hierarchical organization as a "hospital" compound.

Felix's healing compound is one kilometer distant from his residential compound, like that of physicians but unlike the compounds of other indigenous practitioners. Felix imitates the pavilions and largely functional spatial distinctions of the hospital, including a separate "pharmacy" building where herbs are dried and mixed by his apprentices. The hierarchical relationship among healer and various apprentices, expressed also in the location of their major activities within the healing compound (Felix in his consultation hut, certain apprentices in the pavilions, others in the pharmacy), parallels on a small scale that found in biomedical hospitals and clinics.

Felix combines these "modern" elements of spatial and staff organization with signs of self-conscious traditionalism: the bush location of his healing compound, the herb garden in back of his consultation hut, and a low, dark and mysterious-looking consultation hut (of "traditional," i.e., palmfrond-spine and thatched-roof construction) mixing a sense of the mystery and power of an indigenous healer's sacred grove and the organization of a biomedical physician's office. The objects within Felix's consultation hut also combine signs of modernism (a stack of health booklets, an X-ray photograph stuck into a space in the palm-spine wall) with rattles, horns, herb-filled calabashes, feathers, and a "tree of peace." Felix's practice appeals particularly to Bangangté's more educated elite and to younger Bangangté patients. Both groups of clients are concerned with the cultural authenticity of things "black" and the supposed reliability of things "white."

Felix's practice combines the health booklets (*carnets*), prescription writing, and rubber stamps of biomedical institutions with the dramatic seances, diagnostic divination, and ceremonies of the attachment and detachment of spells known from indigenous practices. He has set consultation hours, seeing patients one after another, referring them to his "pharmacist" or asking them to wait or return for divination and healing requiring the presence of kin. When Felix treats patients for infertility, he uses the "biomedical" vocabulary of blocked fallopian tubes rather than speaking more generally about blocked passages and bad water, as do other healers. In his negotiation of ethnogynecological reality, however, these fallopian tubes are often blocked not by infection and scar tissue but by the nefarious activities of mean-spirited kin. Thus, he focused Paulette's anxieties about her social position in the royal compound upon the alleged havoc her cowives could wreak upon her ability to conceive.

Nana's Practice: Healing as a Family Enterprise. Unlike the young and flamboyant Felix, Nana in 1986 was an elderly, modest man who has since passed away. Also a ngakà, or healer performing both herbal treatments and divination, Nana received his patients in the living compound he shares with his five wives and numerous children. One of Nana's wives or children led newly arrived patients and their escorts into the central courtyard of the compound, the space between the main living house, the kitchen for medicines, and the kitchen-houses of his wives. Nana most often consulted his patients in his medicine-kitchen, a bare mud-brick room with a fire in the middle and a number of low stools. Lacking the cooking pots of a woman's kitchen, Nana's medicine-kitchen instead contained some bottles and calabashes filled with ground, dried herbs, and a colored picture of Pope John Paul II. Objects evoking the power of royalty were displayed, but not protected from the playfulness of Nana's children;

next to one wall a small wooden sculpture of a male noble wore a hat of an upside-down plastic bag. The kitchen's hearth was used to "cook [herbal] medicines" (*nâ fu*), often ground by one of the younger wives or occasionally by one of Nana's sons serving as apprentice.

Nana listened to his patients' illness narratives in the medicine-kitchen, eliciting information through a parlay of questions and answers among himself, the patient, and her escort. Occasionally one of the healer's sons or daughters, acting as informal apprentices, would be present at these consultations. After a nod from healer Nana, the patient introduced the question-answer period with a brief narrative of symptoms or disturbing events that led the patient to seek the healer's help. These narratives usually left out visits to other healers but included visits to hospitals.[19] Some consultations then ended when Nana gave the patient some ground herbs wrapped in a scrap of paper and described how to take the herbs and when to come back for the next consultation. The patient then paid Nana in cash for his services, a voluntary amount without discussion. Nana claimed he would argue and ask for more if dissatisfied.

Nana performed hands-on healing practices in a small enclosure surrounded by palm-frond screens at the rear of the entire compound. He referred to the enclosure as a sacred grove, a place of privacy and imbued with spiritual power, similar to sacrifice spots under large trees in the "below" of the royal compound. Within this enclosure, Nana washed his patients in an herbal bath, massaged arms, legs, or abdomen, and drew poisons or objects out of the body. For women complaining of infertility, Nana drew a blood clot, hair, or small pebble out of his patient's vagina. Nana accompanied this action with an explanation of how the woman's fertility was "blocked" by an ill-wisher, and that now at least part of the blockage was removed. Nana's patients were passive, submitting silently to his procedures and initiating no actions themselves. The following case illustrates the interaction between Nana, an infertility patient, and her escorts in a single therapeutic encounter.

A Case of Infertility and Marital Strife

Miteu, a 21-year-old woman, had been married three years but had never been pregnant. She lived in Douala and came to Nana accompanied by her sister and their paternal aunt. The two sisters were orphans and claimed that their father's sister could guide them and keep them from being fooled by charlatans. Nana nodded at this acknowledgment of the aunt's trust in his authenticity.

Before Miteu was married, her husband had proposed to another woman and then changed his mind. Miteu suspected that her husband's former fiancée had paid a sorcerer to put poison in her belly, preventing her from conceiving. Miteu had been to the hospital in Douala. There the doctors had asked to treat her and her husband simultaneously. Miteu's husband refused, and he also refused to pay for his wife's treatment. Instead, he took a Bamiléké woman from the provincial capital of Bafoussam as a lover and made her pregnant. Miteu said her husband wanted to marry the Bafoussam woman "and chase me from the house first." Miteu was not sure if she wanted to return to her husband. What she wanted most from Nana was to have a baby to make her life "complete" and to leave someone after her so that she would not "disappear from this earth."

Nana led Miteu to his enclosure, where she undressed. Nana washed her in an herbal bath, groped around Miteu's crotch, and "removed" a wad of black pubic hair surrounding a tiny piece of bright red plastic. Nana said this was the "poison" that someone had put in her to keep her from getting pregnant. He then took a razor blade and made seven small incisions on Miteu's belly, which he then painted with an herbal mixture. The consultation ended in the medicine-kitchen, where Nana prepared an herbal mixture for Miteu to take home. Miteu's paternal aunt paid him 2,600 CFA francs (about $5.00 U.S. in 1986), wordlessly.

Miteu found herself in Nana's vicinity and in the supportive company of her sister and aunt because all three were caring for yet another relative at Bangangté Provincial Hospital. Nana's healing compound was only a ten-minute walk from the hospital, and Nana was well-known among the hospital patients and the scores of kin who cared for them, cooking meals, washing clothes, and fetching medicines. Miteu and her kin encountered a familiar form of therapy and interaction with the healer at Nana's compound. Despite differences in specializations, most indigenous practitioners treat cases of infertility and suspected attack to reproductive capacity in a strikingly similar fashion.

Similar to biomedical practitioners, indigenous healers like Nana mainly pronounce their diagnosis (or even merely the necessary treatment) in an authoritarian manner with little or no explanation of the cause or progression of the affliction. Treatment for infertility, however, almost always requires more explanation than herbal treatment for a "simple" illness. Women consulting a ngakà assume an element of "custom" in their reproductive afflictions. Diagnosis is part of the treatment; it goes beyond the naming of a particular disease to identify the cause of the patient's troubles in wrongdoing, ancestral wrath, or witchcraft. The ngakà usually expresses this diagnosis in vague enough terms that it is likely to be further interpreted by the patient and her escorts in such a way that it fits a particular situation, applying his knowledge of stereotypical social conflicts to the information contained in the patient's opening narrative.

Healers like Nana run their practices like a family enterprise. The consultation space is located within the healers' residential compounds, little differentiated from other areas of the compound. The differentiation of tasks among the healers' helpers is the same differentiation that occurs between family members. The medicine-kitchens, the central location of consultation, are visible monuments to these healers' emphasis on and skill with herbal medicines. Despite the familiarity of the household compound, both the doctor's office and the healer's medicine-kitchen are rather mysterious to the patient; who knows what power lies in the various medicine-filled vials and equipment displayed on white tables in the hospital and along the walls on the floor of the medicine-kitchen. The doctor's office, however, is even more mysterious, having no similarity to the patient's own home or kitchen. A large desk, covered with papers and books the patient cannot read, separates patient and doctor during most of the consultation. By contrast, both healer and patient squat on low stools around the medicine-kitchen's hearth, beginning the consultation with involved narratives about the social background to the sufferer's affliction.

Despite an emphasis on social relations and ancestral sanction in the causes of infertility, indigenous healers increasingly treat isolated illness episodes of individual clients. This tendency parallels recent transformations in social and family organization and economic realities. As Bangangté more frequently choose their own marriage partners and/or migrate far from their home villages, extended kin ties become loosened. This tendency toward narrower group ties and nuclear families finds its extreme among the rural poor, especially among those wives of absent labor migrants who can no longer participate in informal economic exchange networks. These women, relatively socially isolated, have fewer people to offer them social and material support in the event of an illness crisis. Likewise, the healer of such a woman is less likely to draw her already few social relations into therapeutic procedures.

Space, Secrecy, and Therapeutic Choice in Infertility Treatment. The consultation areas of biomedical and indigenous practitioners dramatize differences in caregiver/patient competence and thus help shape interaction during the consultation. Expectations of what is relevant to various kinds of practitioners shape the way patients present their afflictions. Because infertility patients seek to uncover different layers of the sources of their afflictions by consulting multiple kinds of health-care providers, therapeutic choice is not wholly guided by the typing and pairing of afflictions and healers. In addition, choice of therapy for reproductive disorders is rarely discussed openly among an extended therapy management group. Instead, a woman's wish for discretion powerfully shapes the timing and locale of her quest for therapy. The location of different types of health-care institutions affects the degree to which a patient can fulfill her wish to keep her quest for a cure secret. The bush or neighborhood location of most indigenous practitioners allows a patient to visit this specialist more or less discreetly. A visit to the hospital or clinic is, by contrast, much more public. It requires an appearance in the town or village center or waiting time at the taxi park if the patient is to travel to the mission hospital 15 kilometers away.

Discretion is especially important to women seeking cures for reproductive difficulties. They do not wish to publicize the shame of infertility. They may suspect the very people from their potential support networks of threatening their reproductive potential. Thus, unlike with other health problems, they often try to keep their search for health care secret from potential escorts and other supporters. This discretion is almost impossible to maintain if the afflicted woman visits a biomedical hospital or clinic. In addition to women's assumptions about biomedical lack of competence in matters of infertility, the public nature of visits to biomedical institutions contributes to their almost total avoidance by women for all reproductive matters excluding prenatal and delivery care.

The separation of obstetric care and the treatment of infertility is an interesting case of patients and healers defining areas of expertise and utilizing biomedical and indigenous care for different aspects of reproductive health. Indigenous healers treat problems of infertility, believed by most Bangangté to be illnesses of custom (*ndonn*) and thus improperly understood by biomedical practitioners. Nonetheless, Bangangté women go to these "unseeing" biomedical specialists and not to indigenous practitioners when they give birth. Some women vaguely mentioned getting charms to ease birth from healers. Their reference to childbirth "medicines" as "those little things" may have been women's attempt to limit information about their most private visits to healers. On the other hand, the analysis of Bangangté women's fears regarding reproductive processes in the preceding chapter indicates that while the stages of conception and gestation are full of dangers that could be mitigated by an indigenous practitioner, childbirth itself is threatened by custom only if the woman has committed adultery. Women's concerns regarding childbirth therefore address problems they feel are best treated by biomedical institutions: pain, loss of blood, and infection.

All of the Bangangté women who reported receiving childbirth medicines insist that they always go either to hospital or clinic for delivery. As early as 1937 Egerton noted the gradual disappearance of traditional midwifery in Bangangté (1938:236). He and current commentators on Bangangté health care (ranging from patients to biomedical personnel) attribute the decline of traditional midwifery to the high density of biomedical facilities in Bangangté and its surroundings.

Visits to new mothers who have just given birth provide women the opportunity to become familiar with biomedical obstetric facilities, equipment, and procedures. While all visitors comment on the baby's size, skin color, and hair (the more the better), much of the conversation focuses on the creams, powders, linens, and baby clothes the mother has brought to the hospital. Visitors also ask the mother about biomedical neonatal care, and the mother is proud to demonstrate her new knowledge. In this way, a woman's social network provides her with sources of information on which to base her own decisions regarding indigenous and biomedical gynecological and obstetric care.

Therapeutic Choice and the Rhetoric of Affliction

When a Bangangté woman fears some disturbance of her reproductive health, she now has a wide array of health-care institutions from which she can seek cures. When health planners discuss therapeutic choice, they emphasize traditional–modern differences in specialization on particular afflictions, distance, and shared beliefs between caregiver and patient. Bangangté women tend to delineate reproductive problems as a domain for indigenous healers, and medical care of childbirth as the responsibility of biomedical institutions.

But Bangangté women do not manage their reproductive health crises as isolated individuals. In choosing health care they are affected by the kind of social and material support they can expect from others, their knowledge of health-care alternatives, and the social dynamics of their therapeutic management group (the fluid association of kin and acquaintances who help decide about the choice, timing, and allocation of resources to her therapy [Janzen 1978a, 1987]).

In the next chapter we will explore the ways the rhetoric of reproductive affliction is a symbolic resource in negotiations over gender relations and cultural identity. Here I view therapeutic choice as a symbolic resource. Patients and their therapy management groups negotiate who has social control over reproductive behavior and ideological control over values through the way they define an unexpected timing and number of pregnancies. But patients and their therapy management groups choose therapies within the constraints of broader social and economic conditions. Women fearing infertility or seeking reproductive health care bring differing resources of knowledge and wealth to their quest for therapy.

Some Bangangté women have the knowledge and resources to patronize the most renowned healer and simultaneously receive treatment in a private room at the Protestant Hospital in Bangwa. Other women only have the resources to consult a single institution, know of only few alternatives, or cannot afford to bring any single therapy sequence to conclusion. Such differences in access to health care contribute to divergent qualities of women's fear of infertility and their ways to deal with this fear.

While the anthropological literature on therapeutic choice addresses these issues, it tends to concentrate on a series of single variables in developing hypotheses regarding the social relations of care seeking. These variables include: shared illness beliefs, support networks, kinship and jural or moral responsibility, the duration of the health crisis, material resources, and forms of face-to-face interaction between caregivers and their clients. I examine each of these variables in the light of how Bangangté women seek care and cures for their reproductive difficulties. These variables interact in a field shaped by the history and political economy not only of health care in Bangangté, but also of relations between men and women, nobles and commoners, and the local polity and the state.

Beliefs. One body of the medical anthropology literature finds the most salient determinant of therapeutic choice to be that patient (or patient and kin) and health care giver hold common beliefs or assumptions regarding health and illness. This approach emphasizing the cultural or meaning aspects of therapeutic choice is applied by Sargent (1982) in her study of obstetrical care choices among the Bariba of Benin and is at the center of the early work of Kleinman (1980) on explanatory models and caregiver/patient interaction in the medically pluralistic setting of contemporary Taiwan.

When Bangangté talk about the past, particularly the early years of Protestant evangelization and medical care, they describe clear lines of choice based on belief for certain segments of the Bangangté population. Members of the royal family followed the mfen's wishes and completely rejected the Christian missionaries and their healing. They sought cures for their afflictions from those indigenous healers whose healing powers were closely tied to notions of royalty and its magical strength. The early converts, largely descendants of slaves and members of other groups marginal to royal power, were zealous in their rejection of all witchcraft and magic. They strictly sought care only in biomedical institutions where the model of illness causation, including germs and God but excluding the malevolent actions of others, fit with the sermons of their religious leaders. This strict rejection of certain types of health care is one way to simplify the field of choice. With changes both in the royal compound and the sermons of the missionaries, such clear distinctions of religious belonging, shared medical ideologies, and therapeutic choice no longer exist.

In Bangangté of the 1980s, few people chose their health care primarily because they shared the same model of illness and healing with their caregiver. Some beliefs, general ideas about reproductive processes and the sources of their evil disturbances, were learned over a long time and were explicitly Bangangté. In this sense, most Bangangté women shared the kitchen and cooking metaphors of reproductive processes with nearly all indigenous healers. Indigenous practitioners used elaborations of these ideas both for their own healing and when they wish to refer a patient to a biomedical institution. When mfen Meshinke' of Bantoum diagnoses a woman's reproductive difficulties as the presence of *ntse kebwo* (bad water), the patient can understand his explanation in terms of her notions of the need for proper, unspoiled ingredients in her reproductive cooking. But mfen Meshinke' often refers such patients to the hospital to have this bad water removed. The biomedical practitioner does not share the healer's or patient's beliefs regarding procreative ingredients. He may nonetheless perform a dilation and curettage, a procedure that the patient thinks is cleaning the bad water away. Patient and caregivers thus approach this procedure with completely different assumptions about the causes of reproductive disturbances.

Most young Bangangté women consult biomedical practitioners during their pregnancy, in the framework of regular prenatal consultations, although their main concerns during pregnancy involve problems of custom that are out of the range of the physician's or nurse's competence. Women feel that certain practitioners can best perform specific caring or curing tasks, regardless of their understanding of what the woman believes is going on in her body or in the social relations that can affect her health.

More importantly, a patient's beliefs and knowledge regarding health, illness, and reproduction are not set and unchanging, but at the time of crisis are further formed in interaction with the health care giver and with others who become involved in the care-seeking process. Some of what appears to be new knowledge formed during the healing encounter may be impression management on the part of patients, going along with a healer's diagnosis but not believing it. However, Paulette's case in chapter 1 demonstrates how her "knowledge" regarding her affliction, its causes, and the sources of illness in general developed in the dialogue between her first fears and selectivities and the information she received from Felix's diagnoses during her series of visits.

In addition, seeking cure involves not only the suffering woman, but also her social relations, people who act as brokers, helping her learn about health-care alternatives and choose among them. These people act as go-betweens, forming preliminary diagnoses, making appointments for the patient, and escorting her to various health-care institutions (Boswell 1969). Thus, it is not only the patient's illness beliefs that must be taken into account in choosing therapies, but also those of her support network.

Support Networks.   Janzen (1978a) suggests that most patients in Africa take a passive sick role, and that the timing, arrangements, and choice of consultations among multiple alternative forms of health care are managed by those in the patient's social network. This network forms the basis for the more or less temporary therapy management group. Group dynamics within this therapy management group determine whose suggestions will prevail in actual therapeutic choice and timing.

Bangangté refer to the opinion leader in a therapy management group as a person whose voice has "weight." For Paulette, her cowife "mother" Claude had the "heaviest" voice since she was the only person whom Paulette knew in Bangangté who expressed an interest in her problem. The other Bangangté women I knew perceived the sporadic advice they received on reproductive and medical treatment according to the "weight" of their interlocutor's voice. Since therapy management in Bangangté operates as disjointed conversations among a dispersed network of people with varying relations to the care seeker and to each other, it is difficult to actually observe group dynamics within therapy management groups. These groups rarely meet all together unless the case goes into the realm of customary law. In addition, Bangangté women are very secretive about their search for cures when they are still involved in a health crisis.

Bangangté materials indicate that women in different positions have support networks of different extent and reliability. The ability to reciprocate at a later time is important in encouraging help from others at a time of need. Thus, geographical proximity and some degree or combination of prestige and/or material resources help gain support from more people. Almost no one in contemporary Cameroon has the means to care for themselves in the event of a health emergency. Maintaining social ties through affection and exchange is the best "investment" or "insurance" should misfortune require a person to consult one or many health-care specialists. The poorest women, whose social ties loosen because they cannot fully participate in informal gift exchange networks, have a more limited pool of kin and acquaintances from which they can receive advice and aid when illness strikes or when they fail to bring living children into the community. Women who live far from the households in which they grew up are relatively geographically isolated from their pam nto' relations, those with whom they have established close ties of affection and on whom they can most certainly depend for aid.

In many cases of illness, a woman's cowives are closest to her and most available to help.

> When you are two [wives] in the house, if you are ever ill she [the co-wife] can fetch you a little water before she even goes to tell your husband that you are ill. (Bwoda', an elderly woman of Bantoum)

> I like polygyny. Even my mothers numbered twelve in their compound. It is good because if I fall ill, one of my cowives must give me water or even bathe me, another will prepare food for our husband so he won't starve during my illness. (So'nju, aged ca. 60, Batela')

> To be in polygyny is good. For example, you can be sick and it is your cowife who helps you. In a monogamous marriage you are only part of a pair with your husband. If you fall ill and your husband falls ill, who will give you water to drink? That's what it is. If your husband works [for wages], he can't leave his work because you are ill. It is even thanks to this job that he can buy the products [medicines] they will prescribe for you at the hospital. And to leave you like that without caring for you, it's bad. A cowife could take care of you. (Ncanko, aged 28, Batela')

Nonetheless, Bangangté women rarely turn to their cowives in seeking cures for reproductive illness. Cowives might help with food preparation or childcare if one is bedridden or absent. Reproductive difficulties rarely render a woman bedridden and dependent upon this aspect of her cowives' help. They may also fear that their cowives have caused their reproductive illness.

> Me, I tell myself that a woman who lives alone doesn't profit from it. I think that when you are two or three, that's good. And even if it's good, there is a 'but'. It's that if you are sick, the other could fetch water, for example. But when there is no understanding between you, it becomes difficult. It's the big misfortune that has already come to earth. (Kokwa, older than 73, Bantoum)

> I have lost one child. And I then had problems to have a second child. Because I was in a polygynous household, there were too many problems. I was sometimes told that it [the reproductive difficulties] is because of my cowives. (Jacobine, aged 23, divorced, Bantoum)

Because most women at one time or another suspect their cowives of evil machinations threatening their reproductive health, they rarely inform their cowives of their difficulties or ask them for advice and support.

Kinship and Jural Responsibility.   In contrast to cowives, it is kin and those who have jural responsibility for the patient from whom Bangangté expect help in case of reproductive difficulties. Bangangté women may suspect certain categories of kin of being implicated in the cause of their reproductive affliction, for example a foster parent (tuteur) or an errant husband. But those same and other kin may also try to insure the afflicted woman's reproductive success, out of interest in adding to their matriline or patriline or out of affection and solidarity with the woman. The composition of women's therapy management groups (Feierman 1985; Janzen 1978a, 1987) reflects the multiple forms of jural and affective ties in Bangangté kinship. Not all members of these often fluid groups have the same amount of interest, responsibility, and authority in relation to the patient and to the other members of the group.

Different members of Bangangté therapy management groups have diverging amounts of influence and authority within the group. Bangangté refer to their power to convince others and to determine the course of action as the "weight of their voice," an expression also used to describe degrees of "complicatedness" with reference to political and economic power and witchcraft. Being "complicated" may give someone power, but differs from moral and jural authority.

Bangangté recognize differences in group members' moral and jural responsibility toward the afflicted person. In contrast to cowives and neighbors, Bangangté feel that both agnatic and uterine (*pam nto'*) kin are the most reliable supporters in case of reproductive illness. Bangangté often call on agnatic kin, and particularly the father or his heir, in the context of *jural* responsibility. Husbands, and sometimes their agnatic kin, are thought to be jurally responsible for the well-being and care of their wives and children, but this responsibility is most often expressed in terms of complaints when not fulfilled. Miteu, who consulted healer Nana for infertility, accused her husband not only of neglect but also of involvement in causing her reproductive failure.

While Bangangté believe that agnatic kin and husbands hold jural responsibility for the afflicted, pam nto' kin hold moral responsibility. Women often seek recommendations about indigenous and biomedical healing specialists from their maternal kin. Jeanne, a wife of the mfen, traveled to her maternal family in the three hours distant kingdom of Bapi to receive her mother's advice on fertility enhancement medicines. The trust she had in her mother's advice and the discretion she could expect in this sensitive subject of fertility outweighed the cost and inconvenience travel posed to Jeanne.

The use of kinship ties and the jural responsibility of certain categories of kin within Bangangté therapy management groups varies according to the afflicted woman's social position. When a woman has become estranged from her kin, as in Paulette's case, the jural responsibility of agnatic kin and even the moral responsibility of pam nto' relations may no longer count. In addition, members of a therapy management group may not be able to give the support required by their responsibilities, either because their position within the group is too weak to influence decision making or because they do not have the knowledge or material means to truly help the patient. These distinctions refine our view of social differentiation among those who surround, support, and/or impede a sick or infertile woman's efforts at cure and solace.

Duration of the Health Crisis.   In addition to social relations among members of a therapy management group and between them and the patient, the duration of the health crisis affects the choice and range of explanations and therapies they attempt. Referring to his Tanzanian data, Feierman (1981) points out that the longer a crisis lasts, the more people become involved in therapy management. Through this process, the group either grows in size, which changes group dynamics, or some members drop out while new ones become involved in the case.

In Bangangté, fertility problems are particularly long-lasting, and thus often require long-term and broad support networks. Because these problems are of such long duration, women may have a difficult time gaining or retaining support when seeking cures for reproductive difficulties. In addition, reproductive difficulties almost never appear as a crisis requiring immediate care. A woman's complaint about childlessness may not awaken potential supporters' sense of urgency. De facto female heads of households, women whose husbands are absent due to wage labor migration, often have a smaller pool from which to draw supporters in times of crisis (Feierman 1981). For a health crisis of long duration, this may put such women at particular risk. Isolated women like Paulette have an even harder time mustering cure-seeking support for their long-lasting and rather unclear misfortunes. Thus, as Inhorn points out for infertile Egyptian women, therapy management groups tend to collapse over time for poor, infertile women. Nonetheless, many women continue their lonely search for cure and explanation, consulting healer after healer, doctor after doctor.

Material Resources.   As with the demographic literature on reproductive decision making, the public health literature on health-care access and choice assumes that patients analyze the divergent costs and benefits of indigenous and biomedical treatment when seeking cures (Bannerman 1982). The anthropological literature on therapeutic choice also refers to costs and benefits, but includes social as well as strictly material calculations. For example, Boswell (1969) analyzes the social costs and benefits of associating with certain escorts. Mullings (1984) discusses how a lineage head will direct a patient to a health-care institution that supports his own view of social relations and his interests in maintaining his position vis-à-vis the other members of the therapy management group.

In Bangangté, the mode of payment, costs, and the certainty of the fee for service in different types of health-care institutions affect Bangangté women's access to and choice of various curing alternatives. Consultations at the public hospital were free in the 1980s, but costs of attending this institution were incalculable because patients must buy their drugs at what was then the only private pharmacy in Bangangté. (In the 1990s, fees were introduced in public health institutions, and two private pharmacies were in business in Bangangté.) In contrast, both consultations and the filling of prescriptions at Bangwa Protestant Hospital were made on a fixed-fee basis. The costs of indigenous healers were less calculable for patients and often ended up being higher than those of either hospital. At hospitals and clinics, however, payment was always in cash. For some patients it was easier to consult a healer who might eventually demand higher payment, but who could be paid in kind.

Patients and therapy management group members must also calculate the cost in time that visits to various institutions entail. Visiting the healer is sometimes more costly in time because healers are frequently absent from their compounds. Their treatments also generally require many visits. Patients have long waits at whatever type of institution they choose, although the wait is always less for very prominent patrons. Distance and transportation are among the most important cost factors considered by Bangangté patients. Getting to and from the caregiver is figured into the cash outlay, as is the debt of a personal favor should one receive a ride from an acquaintance. Distance and the available modes of transportation to various institutions are also part of Bangangté patients' time calculations when they choose between different forms of care. The experience of distance and transportation has changed considerably through time. Elderly Bangangté express that going to Bangwa hospital was very difficult in the past; "it did not exist for us." Now, with paved roads and rather frequent bush taxi service, traveling the 15 kilometers from Bangangté town is much easier, although it still requires cash.

Interaction Styles.   Bangangté patients choose to consult different health-care institutions or particular practitioners within them according to their perception of how they are treated by caregivers and their institutions. While they expect demonstration of superior knowledge and authority from caregivers, especially from biomedical staff, Bangangté prefer attending those institutions where they find solace and feel they are treated with dignity. Some biomedical physicians exhibit condescending mannerisms toward the "uneducated"; for patients who cannot express themselves well in French, this effectively denies them a needed sense of consolation. Those who admit having visited indigenous healers are often reprimanded and humiliated by biomedical practitioners. Patients with much experience or with knowledgeable escorts find the type of interaction they prefer by attending specific healers, the mission hospital (which has a good reputation for humanitarian treatment), or the local public or mission clinics where they know the staff personally and can use particular staff members as escorts. At Bangangté Divisional Hospital, patients often go directly to the pharmacist or a known pediatric nurse, or they wait in a long line in front of a particular physician's office, rather than being served immediately by another physician perceived as less friendly. Jeanne, a young wife of the mfen, prefers to make the longer trip to the mission hospital in Bangwa rather than seeking care at the public hospital in Bangangté. As a mfen's wife, Jeanne should receive free care and drugs at the provincial public hospital; she claims, however, that hospital personnel always dispute whether she is really a royal wife, which she finds humiliating.

A Bangangté woman's social network is her most important source for learning about the different interaction styles of various health-care institutions. Such knowledge is crucial in women's decision making regarding therapies for their reproductive problems. In addition, previous knowledge of interaction styles allows the patient to adjust her way of presenting symptoms according to her expectations of the warmth, communicativeness, and expertise of different health-care specialists.

Single-factor hypotheses attributing the process of therapy seeking to shared beliefs, to economic calculations, or even to the social dynamics of decision making over the definition of illness and choice of therapy, do not capture the complexity of social, cultural, and historical dynamics in plural health systems. Current conditions in Bangangté offer varieties of health care, but also confront women with a field of uncertainty in their ability to address fundamental problems of reproductive health.

Access to Care, the Therapeutic Process,
and the Distribution of Fear

Over the past century, the already varied and dynamic field of health care expanded dramatically in Bangangté. New illnesses, including sterility-producing sexually transmitted diseases, and such changes in social structure as the introduction of labor migration on a grand scale and the mfen's loss of political autonomy during the colonial era led indigenous healers to seek new medicines and forms of healing. The continuing decline of royal power and the diversification of the hierarchies within which Bangangté could strive for personal advancement led to innovations and shifts within the field of indigenous medicine. Specialists whose healing activities were closely tied to concepts of royalty and its magical influence on health declined in importance for patients seeking cures. Healers who concentrated on herbal treatments of isolated disorders, whether caused by physical agents alone or through the activities of ancestors and witches, increased in importance. Many present-day healers have adapted to their current cash needs and require forms of payment barely distinguishable from those of biomedical institutions. They have become entrepreneurs, competing with other indigenous and biomedical institutions in the expanding field of Bangangté health care.

The growing kinds and numbers of health-care institutions in Bangangté give Bangangté women suffering from reproductive difficulties greater choice when they seek care and cure for their afflictions. This choice, however, does not exist equally for all women. The existence of certain forms of health care does not guarantee that all have access to these alternatives. Such access requires that a woman know of a particular institution, can get to it, and can pay for the treatment she hopes to receive. The few Bangangté women with significant cash incomes (civil servants, wives of civil servants, and successful entrepreneurs) can consult more types of health-care institutions more frequently than the majority of poor, rural cultivators. Among the group of poor rural women, significant differences exist in their ability to take advantage of health-care alternatives. Their social and material resources depend most on the size and reliability of their support networks, including cowives, neighbors, and agnatic, affinal, and maternal kin. Their choice of health-care alternatives depends on these resources as well as upon group dynamics within the woman's support group, and the duration and apparent urgency of their illness. A woman whose limited social and material resources do not allow her to seek all the cures she needs feels truly vulnerable to reproductive threats. Should reproductive misfortune strike, she would be less able to deal with it than her wealthier neighbor.

When a woman seeks cures, she may try to manage differing aspects of her fear of reproductive threats. Her main concern may be with her physical infertility, and thus directly with her wish for a child or, in the case of secondary infertility, with additional children. Nonetheless, seeking cures may fulfill other functions for this woman. The process of seeking cure may dramatize the woman's social and medical plight to others. By becoming the center of a good story, even if her "infertility" is shown to be due to her own shortcomings (as in Paulette's case), the woman may hope to gain social recognition (Bleek 1976). For a particularly poor woman, being ill and seeking cure may be a way of increasing social support. When she works on her tiny fields, she may never grow enough crops to allow her to pay for her children's school fees. But when she falls ill, a number of cowives and neighbors may help her out to make this medically unrelated goal possible.

Finally, a woman may secretly consult a diviner to solve an inner conflict for herself (Shaw 1985). While she may keep the diviner's diagnosis a secret, her fears about the social relations causing her difficulties will be given a concrete answer. The diviner's opinion that her cowives are evil, or on the other hand that she has nothing to fear from them, allows her to adjust her interaction with her immediate social environment.

Bangangté women's expressions about reproductive threats indicate that disturbances in their immediate social environment, and in the state of the kingdom as a whole, are as important as actually curing a state of infertility. Women talk about not being able to bear children, keep them alive, or keep them faithful to Bangangté traditions. Nonetheless, they often seem to seek explanations for their suffering instead of cures. Is this because cures cannot be reached? Or, is it because infertility is merely an idiom expressing other problems that confront rural Bangangté women? If so, does the idiom of infertility provide a vocabulary of affliction and explanation with which to understand these problems?

Chapter Six

"Then We Were Many": The Search for Vitality in a Changing Context

The sun slanted toward us one late afternoon in mid-October 1986. Che'elou, the oldest woman at the palace and a mfen's wife for nearly eight decades, sat on a small grassy hillock. Two younger royal wives and I stood around her, our backs to the banana grove and forest now growing in large areas of the palace grounds. We were attending the burial of one of Che'elou's deceased cowives. Like Che'elou, the deceased woman had married king Njiké II during the 1910s and had been inherited by his son Pokam Robert in 1943, then by his grandson Njiké Pokam François in 1974. It was an unusually sad week for Che'elou, as three of her cowives had died within three days. Two had been brought back from their current residences to the royal compound in their last hours to allow them to die near their house sites. The third of Che'elou's recently deceased cowives had no living children and had resided in the royal compound at the time of her death. Che'elou was exhausted after "crying" (publicly mourning)[1] her cowives for the past three days. She held her bamboo staff as she sat and watched her younger cowives and female kin of the deceased dance slowly around the fresh grave (see fig. 14).

Che'elou said quietly, half to herself and half to the small group around her, "Then we were many, as many as the blades of grass that now grow in the royal compound." Che'elou was contrasting the past of her own childhood and vigorous young adulthood in the royal compound of Bangangté with the scene now before us. At the time she married mfen Njiké II, probably within the first years following his enthronement in 1912, Che'elou was one of some 150 royal wives. At happier times she often described the royal compound of her youth as a lively village, filled with more inhabitants than one could get to know well. In the royal compound of her old age, half of the 14 royal wives were elderly widows. Many younger wives either failed to perform all the duties of a wife of the mfen or ran away. Instead of being a crowded village, only 16 adults (including myself) and 23 children lived in the royal compound. The compound also

175

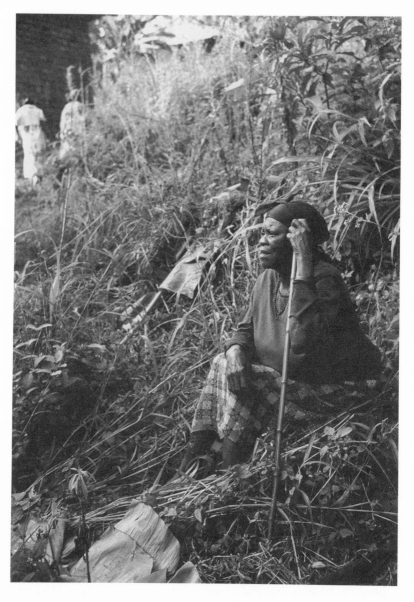

Fig. 14.   Che'elou, ca. 85 years old, watching the burial of one of her cowives at the royal compound of Bangangté, October 1986. Sad and exhausted after several deaths of her elderly cowives, Che'elou remembers the more vital palace life of her young adulthood.

looked quite different from Che'elou's memories of years past. Few of Che'elou's cowives in 1986 were as fastidious as she in cleaning their houses or keeping their yards free of weeds. There were so few royal wives in 1986 that sites inhabited during Che'elou's youth were overgrown with grasses or reverting to forest. The burial dance was being held right on the edge of one of these overgrown sites full of savanna grass and young forest.

The grave site was directly in front of the deceased wife's former house, one of a row of three abandoned one-room kitchen-houses in Josette's quarter of the royal compound. One of these houses had belonged to Che'elou until she moved up the hill to be closer to her younger cowives. Suffering from rheumatism and fearing snakes and witches, Che'elou had moved closer to her younger cowives. In November 1984, only two years before the burial of Che'elou's three elderly cowives, mfen Njiké Pokam's original *mabengoup* (first queen) had been mortally bitten by a snake in the grass near the grave site. This woman had been admired by all, especially by Che'elou, and the memory of the tragedy attached itself to this place of abandoned kitchens and invading weeds.

Che'elou's lament about the many blades of grass was thus a poignant indication of an elderly woman's feelings about the physical and social decline of the royal compound. Her nostalgia, both socially and bio-graphically structured, was expressed by many Bangangté citizens. Nearly all Bangangté shared concerns about the state of the kingship and the kingdom, rural flight, and reproducing Bangangté citizens physically and through socialization. Depending on one's position and interest in polity and population, each concentrated on different aspects of human and social reproduction ranging from having babies to political allegiance and representation.[2]

The impetus for this book began early in fieldwork with a flood of bewildering statements about infertility and child loss that contrasted sharply with standard demographic indicators showing Bangangté to be part of a fecund region within Cameroon and within the central African "infertility belt." This apparent paradox led me to search for the meanings Bangangté women give to their experiences. My investigation of expressions about infertility and threats to procreation led to the discovery of indigenous conceptions of fertility and vitality, of illness, vulnerability, and decline, and of the intimate relation between culinary skill and reproductive capacity. I learned that in Bangangté cosmology women's role in human reproduction is linked to the role of royalty in social reproduction through a shared symbolism of food, cooking, and provisioning. It became clear that, although fertility and infertility are issues of the health of women's and men's bodies, complaints about these physical matters reach far beyond the medical realm. Women's discourse on reproductive illness comments upon rural female poverty and struggles over the survival and meaning of a distinctive cultural identity within a multicultural state.

The following three explanations of the apparent paradox between Bangangté anxieties and demographic indicators describe the situations of ever-wider groups of Bangangté women. First, Bangangté women suffer real infertility or depressed fertility due to changes in male–female relations and increased economic and psychological stress. Second, even if rural Bangangté women are not infertile, they may fear reproductive threats more than men or better-placed women do because the consequences of infertility would be so grave. Third, Bangangté women use infertility as an idiom to comment upon other difficulties, regardless of their own fertility.

This final chapter focuses on the third explanation, the use of reproductive threats as an idiom to discuss social processes perceived to be just as threatening as infertility. It explores the implications of women's perceptions of dangers to their reproductive health for attitudes toward social change and polity in Bangangté. Because rural Bangangté women feel personal, reproductive, and social vulnerability, they search for vitality through creating and adjusting to new social forms, through a nostalgic view of times gone by "when they were many," and through attempts at therapy to make oneself and one's kingdom rich in people.

A close examination of how rural Bangangté women talk about the vulnerability of their reproductive health shows that women's fears are much broader than their initial expressions of infertility anxiety. Only a small segment of Bangangté women either are incapable of conceiving and bearing children or fear they are infertile in its narrowest, biological sense. Shaped by a number of factors, including a woman's place in the life cycle, Bangangté women's fears include the range of processes from pairing to child rearing and socialization, in other words both procreation and social reproduction. Through the idiom of complaints about infertility and threats to their reproductive health, women express anxiety about status decline, impoverishment, uncertainty in social roles and gender relations, and the kingdom's loss of political autonomy. These fears are grounded in social insecurities specific to the experience of social change among certain groups within Bangangté society. These social insecurities, expressed via a rhetoric of infertility, center upon ambiguity regarding social differentiation and the politics of identity.

The set of anxieties plaguing rural Bangangté women during a period of increasing impoverishment are expressed via infertility due to the symbolic complex within divine kingships, beliefs linking procreation with the state of the polity. Che'elou's nostalgic lament about the bygone days of a kingdom governed by unambiguous royal power, of a palace rich in wives and children, is set against the background of the declining status of royal wives. But it is also an expression of concern about the physical, spiritual, and political future of Bangangté. Che'elou's lament includes a poverty of babies as well as other woes because the collective productivity of Bangangté women's wombs and the strength of the king are mutually dependent. They are expressed in a common symbolic language, through metaphors of measuring, mixing, cooking, and eating. Women measure, mix, and cook male and female ingredients to make new human beings, while the king measures and mixes diverse social elements to constitute a social whole and reproduce social order.

This ideal royal social reproduction was always challenged both by the internal threats of succession disputes and the asocial use of occult power (witchcraft) and by the external threats of war, migration, and traffic in slaves among the Grassfields polities and their neighbors. It is even more threatened now, through global social change and the impact of the state on local affairs. Rural Bangangté women fear not only external threats to their kingdom's vitality (and thus to their own fertility and well-being), but also cooptation of their king and their men by the Cameroonian state and the lures of modernity. They fear that, in the pursuit of economic survival and individual success, their husbands, brothers, and king are not doing their job of preserving a "true" Bangangté cultural identity and holding the cosmological and social order together.

Thus, women's expressions of fear of infertility are shaped by the impact that the incorporation of the Bangangté polity into the modern Cameroonian state has on people of varying social positions within Bangangté. Within this ever-changing Bangangté society, there are contending visions of reproductive vigor, Bangangté kingship, and the ideal society. These multiple visions regarding population and identity emerge in the situation-bound nature of much of knowledge production (see, e.g., van der Geest 1988). They also result from variations in life experience and perspective shaped by individual personality and, especially, social differentiation in Bangangté. Rosaldo (1989:7) refers to the "positioned subject" to describe these psychologically and socially shaped distinctions in perspective and knowledge. In feminist anthropology, gender is one of the most salient dimensions of a subject's positionality or standpoint. Women, because they are systematically excluded from positions of dominance in most societies, are best able to see the contradictions of a social system (Abu-Lughod 1993; Haraway 1988; Raheja 1995; Stacey 1988). Such positions outside of dominant structures vary widely among and within cultures, negating any possibility of a universal category "woman" (H. Moore 1994:9). Such positions are not fixed, as each individual negotiates life not from the position of a single social role, but from that of a multiplicity of roles, each one gaining relevance in different contexts (as in Merton's now classic role set theory).[3] While there are many positioned subjects in Bangangté, my main interest is in how political and economic changes occurring through the incorporation of Bangangté kingdom into larger political and economic units are experienced by rural Bangangté women, poor smallholding cultivators whose life experience is largely shaped by their gender, their status as wife and mother, their level of education, and their access to land.

By looking at the context of fears of infertility, and the varieties of perspectives from which these fears are expressed, we note that Bangangté ideas regarding procreation and society are both culturally and historically specific and internally differentiated. Nonetheless, the political, social, and economic changes feeding local concerns about infertility and declining or at least stagnant population occur not only in the Cameroonian Grassfields, but also in various permutations throughout much of sub-Saharan Africa.

The idiom of infertility gives meaning to the way women's lives and health are affected by social change and expression to the role that ordinary female farmers play in envisioning their past and future society. But the rhetoric of reproductive threat is not merely an idiom, an expressive modality. It shapes social action, and therefore demographic outcomes. Rural Bangangté women's socially structured experience is interpreted through a symbolic system organized around culinary images of human and social reproduction. These images emerge from and are reinforced through mundane activities and royal rituals alike. Observable conflicts over royal power and a feeling of failed reciprocity and disrupted social order lead women to fear reproductive illness because of the practical and symbolic connections between social order, royal allegiance, and human fertility. This fear of infertility affects women's decisions regarding marriage timing, marriage partners, sex, childbearing, and gynecological/obstetric care. These decisions have demographic consequences, including a Bamiléké fertility rate higher than models based on economic rationales would predict (Wakam 1994).

While their expressions about plundered kitchens, empty wombs, and absent children may be personally, culturally, and historically specific, Bangangté women are not unique in their use of a procreative idiom to talk about broader social issues. Delaney (1991) has argued cogently that the metaphors of seed and soil describing procreation in Anatolia reveal the gendered nature of Turkish village cosmology and help shape and reproduce gender inequalities. As in Bangangté, where procreation and notions of kingship and allegiance are closely linked, the way procreation is represented structures the identity of both persons and peoples in

Turkey, who belong to concentric circles of social context: the house, the village, the nation, and the world. Inhorn's work on infertility among the urban Egyptian poor shows how profoundly the failure to procreate can disrupt a woman's relationships to her husband, kin, and neighbors, and how she disappoints the expectations of nation and of Islam by "missing motherhood" (Inhorn 1996). In these two Middle Eastern communities, as in the west-central African kingdom of Bangangté, the contradictions between shared identities and conflicting interests and representations intersect in the social arena of reproduction (Delaney 1991:17). Despite the very different politicoreligious settings of the Turkish village, the Egyptian slum, and the kingdoms of the Cameroonian Grassfields, the parallels of the salience of procreative metaphors for organizing social life are astounding.

In Bangangté, the procreative metaphors through which women comment upon broader social processes are expressed through culinary imagery. Among the Hua of highland New Guinea, discussion of food taboos delineates an ideology about procreation, nurturance, and gender relations (Meigs 1984). Just as I was struck by Bangangté women's apparent preoccupation with reproductive illness, Meigs's own research agenda was shaped by Hua preoccupation with the symbolic evaluation of food (1984:ix). While she concentrates on other aspects in the body of her book, Meigs raises an intriguing question regarding the historical depth of Hua ideological focus on food. She suggests that this preoccupation may have been less intense in precontact times, and that in the context of a decline of other aspects of Hua male culture (such as initiations and men's houses), "Hua males . . . use these [food] rules as a tool for talking about traditional culture and remembering the past" (1984:xi–xii). I try to actively engage the question Meigs has raised. I suggest that, regardless of how rhetoric about procreation may have been used in the past, Bangangté women currently use procreation as a way of lamenting a bygone era of fertile wombs and plentiful granaries and of expressing their anxieties about their present health risks, poverty, and social status.

Anthropologists interested in the social role of metaphor have pointed out that metaphors of both successful and failed procreation reveal tensions and contradictions in social organization. Sapir's analysis of a Kujamaat-Diola folktale uncovers notions of consanguinity and personal legitimacy, and their link to Kujamaat gender roles through the metaphors of beehives and cooked rice (1977). Two studies of folk illness plaguing Haitian women show a direct link between the metaphoric descriptions of the illness categories *pedisyon* ("perdition" or pregnancy loss), *move san* ("bad blood"), and *lèt gate* ("spoiled milk") and these women's experiences with the constraints and emotional stress of poverty

(Farmer 1988; Singer, Davison, and Gerdes 1988). Ott, writing about the cheese analogy of conception among the Basque (1979), and Beidelman, concerned with "the imagery of social and physical being" among the Kaguru (1986:30), both point out that key metaphors concretize otherwise abstract or difficult to understand processes (e.g., procreation) and relations (e.g., gender and social organization). These concretizing metaphors are drawn from the mundane aspects of daily life, the activities of hearth and bed, of food preparation and eating.

In Bangangté, the culinary symbolism of procreation, while centered around cooking and eating, does not merely stem from the mundane actions of domestic experience. Bangangté culinary imagery is also more than a reflection either of the gendered division of labor or of parallel experiences of cooperation and conflict between Bangangté men and women. In a divine kingship such as Bangangté, procreation and politics are closely linked through the symbolism of cooking and feeding, and through a cosmology that guides citizens' actions. Procreation and social change are also inseparably linked in Bangangté, both in practice and thought. Since African monarchies such as Bangangté have found themselves embedded first in colonies and now in independent states, the social context in which metaphors of procreation are used is changing.

The Context of Change in Bangangté Kingship: Vitality, Vulnerability, and Multiple Centers

Bangangté believe that the health and wealth of the mfen's subjects and territory are dependent upon the health, wealth, and reproductive vigor of the king. As in other divine kingships, the mfen is, or should be, the principle of vitality in the inseparable domains of social, religious, political, and physical life. If the king and his polity are enfeebled, human life and its reproduction are put in danger. In this light, female fertility is a sign of the strength of the divine king, and infertility is a barometer of social ills. Women are the crucial link in male power within divine kingships, through their roles in human reproduction, in determining inheritance through the house property complex (Gluckman 1950), in interkingdom diplomacy, in food production, and in hosting assemblies of the king's followers. The rhetoric of declining and expanding population, dependent upon women's healthy wombs as well as their reproductive decisions, is intimately linked to the rhetoric of declining and expanding allegiance to the king. This study of Bangangté women's concerns about fertility and infertility, vitality and vulnerability, throws a new light upon notions of gender and social change in contemporary African monarchies.

Postwar studies of divine kingship focused on the integrative and regenerative functions of African kingships and royal ritual (Beidelman 1966; Fortes 1968; Gluckman 1954; Hocart 1936; Kuper 1947, 1963; Richards 1939, 1969). Since then, little attention has been paid to divine kingships in postcolonial, modernizing Africa (Kuper's more recent work on the Swazi [1978, 1986], Feeley-Harnik's investigation of labor and loyalty in the Sakalava monarchy of Madagascar (1991) and Goheen's study of the relationship between the Cameroonian state and the local polity of Nso' in the western Grassfields [1996] are exceptions). Likewise, while the symbolic connections between procreation and kingship are recognized in the divine kingship literature, there are—surprisingly—no explicit analyses in terms of gender relations. Perhaps this lack of attention to gender in the fertility symbolism of African monarchies has come about because this symbolism is rarely examined outside the immediate events, for example, coronation rituals, in which it is articulated.[4] By examining the use of culinary symbolism in everyday life, I have been able to show the links between women's labor, their cosmology, and the ritual expressions of royal power to feed, rule, and engender.

For the approximately two centuries preceding German annexation of Cameroon in 1884 Bangangté was one of some one hundred expanding and contracting, newly founded and dissolving, consolidating and fissioning Grassfields kingdoms. One of the major features of colonization was the consolidation of kingdoms and the freezing of their borders. Both the German and the French colonial rulers chose particular kingdoms as favored client states through which they hoped to rule these and subordinated kingdoms. They built monuments to their consolidation and patronage in the form of European-designed palaces. *Bwopa',* the palace ruins from Njiké II's reign (1912–43), and the current palace, respectively, are memorials to German and French patronage of Bangangté.[5]

Political incorporation was accompanied by economic incorporation into wider spheres of trade and control of production. The introduction of coffee and cocoa as cash crops and the commercialization of food crops during the French colonial period caused deep changes in the agrarian Bangangté economy. The political and economic incorporation of Bangangté has been an ongoing feature of postcolonial life in Cameroon. Current Bangangté concerns with the decline of the institution of kingship are historically specific, stemming from colonial history, the effect of the modern state on social differentiation and multiple centers of reference and allegiance, and the historical contingencies of the 1980s and 1990s.

Beginning with the colonial era, the mfen and his kingdom have experienced a continual loss of political autonomy. The mfen in the 1980s and 1990s was even less a middleman between the centralized state and his subjects than under colonial rule. He was denied power over the life and death of his subjects or the judging of criminal cases and could no longer arbitrarily demand tribute in the form of wives or goods from his subjects. Both his economic base and his activities in guiding his subjects had declined. New forms of economic mobility and prestige, depending upon academic education and positions in the civil service or the cash economy, compete with royal forms of wealth and prestige. Even the mfen's "wealth in people," his ability to gain and maintain a followership, was much weaker than in the past since his subjects now had alternative modes of action and mobility available to them.

While retaining a sense of allegiance to their kingdom, Bangangté citizens of the 1980s also felt that they belonged to the Cameroonian state, their branch of the political party (RDPC, Renouveau Démocratique des Peuples Camerounais), their professional group, their economic class, their religious community as Protestant, Catholic, or Muslim, and their local émigré community. Bangangté citizens were no longer primarily differentiated according to their ranks in the system of commoners and nobility; educational and economic status gained (and continues to gain) ever-increasing relevance. In any given context, several collective and personal identities were at issue. Bangangté people's attempts to manage these multiple identities contributed to their perception of population decline (see also Kreager 1997:139, 142).

The meaning of old social distinctions (e.g., kingship and title-holding, gender hierarchies) has changed. Previously, holding titles such as *nkam* (noble), *ngwala'* (mfen's representative), *che' mfen* (royal retainer), or *mamfen* (queen mother) was tied to recognized responsibilities and prestige. Now being a titleholder is, alone, usually not enough to guarantee an individual's prestige or to determine his or her social standing. Titles are sometimes bought by the new, educated elite to add legitimacy to their positions (Blank 1985; Fjellman and Goheen 1984). The position of women in Bangangté society has also been transformed. In the past a Bangangté woman's life course progressed within a limited range of possibilities. Presently the expectations Bangangté women hold of male–female relations have changed and are confronted with the reality of increasing male–female segregation for *rural* women.

New social distinctions have been added to the range of Bangangté diversity. These include new elites, new state and commercial structures, and people from other regions of the country and the world. Bangangté was always composed of peoples of varying origin united by allegiance to the mfen. Through colonial rule, missionization, and through postcolonial state building, others not owing fealty to the king became an integral part of the Bangangté landscape. During the last third of the twentieth century Cameroonians from many groups and regions have been assigned to Bangangté territory as civil servants in governmental and parastatal institutions. Throughout these decades of nation building, the Cameroonian state purposely assigned civil servants, especially those at higher levels, outside their home areas to promote national unity and prevent ethnic-based corruption. In the years just following President Ahidjo's resignation (1982) and President Biya's constitutional crisis (1983), ethnicity was particularly politicized in the Western Province, the homeland of the Bamiléké and Bamoum. Beti and Bulu groups perceived the Bamiléké as a tight group pursuing hegemony in the financial and intellectual life of Cameroon, condemning the "ethno-facism" of the Westerners (Bayart 1993:45). This climate of barely hidden animosity has contributed to the trepidation with which rural Bangangté women approach these "foreign" (non-Bamiléké) civil servants. The state and commercial institutions within which non-Bangangté work were added to, and sometimes challenged, traditional Bangangté political and economic institutions.

One of the biggest challenges to the Bangangté social order, however, (because of their very ambiguity) comes from the new, educated, and commercial Bangangté elite, citizens who owe allegiance to the mfen but who find their sources of power and authority and their major reference groups outside of the kingdom context. They take advantage of new economic and political opportunities in a sphere extending beyond the kingdom. Although shrinking dramatically in the 1990s due to an extended political and economic crisis, in the relatively prosperous years of the 1980s new economic and political opportunities offered Bangangté, especially men, a number of strategies to advance their interests and to mitigate the personal vulnerability brought about by the insecurities of recent social changes. Men increasingly migrated, using lineage and kingdom ties to establish themselves in urban centers. Youths used the institution of the *tuteur,* or foster parent, to permit them to go to secondary school.

Bangangté believe that *kà* (supernatural power necessary for both success and witchcraft) is often misused to take advantage of these new opportunities (den Ouden 1987; Rowlands and Warnier 1988). Indeed, some try to improve their socioeconomic and political situation through a "strategy of terror" (den Ouden 1987:27), the manipulation of a reputation of being "complicated," that is, possessing supernatural powers that could be used as witchcraft. Bangangté assume that power tempts its owner to misuse it for personal gain and often cite examples of the misuse of power by healers, witches, and members of an imagined witches' association called *famla'*. Rural Bangangté women are largely blocked from new opportunities, but gain a reputation of misusing occult powers, especially ntok, in the realm of reproduction, stealing fetuses to weaken the competition of other women.

Bangangté (in the mid-1980s as well as currently) feel that the misuse of occult powers, particularly kà, and other forms of strength has increased in the context of recent social change, leading to social disequilibrium. Witches were formerly kept in check by the balance of occult powers; the mfen and his ritual experts were equally strong as the witches. One new element in the social fabric, the centralized state, has been crucial in disrupting the balance of occult powers by undermining the mfen's power and by outlawing established brakes on the malevolent use of occult power, failing to distinguish healers and antisorcery specialists from witches and fighting all three in a struggle against "superstition."[6] Bangangté, and many other Grassfields peoples as well, feel that the suppression of checks on witchcraft has led to the multiplication and increasing brashness of witches in contemporary Cameroon. Youth migrate to cities to flee the threat of witchcraft in their home villages, and elites' fear of witchcraft prevents investment in the natal kingdom (Rowlands and Warnier 1988:121, 128). This has contributed to rural perceptions of population decline and economic weakness.

Bangangté perceive that the new educated and commercial elite are an additional contributor to the increasing misuse of kà. The elite seem to side with the state against royal authority and the institutions that keep witchcraft in check. It is difficult for villagers to understand how members of the elite could become so wealthy and powerful without using strong kà. They are suspected of having profited by mystically taking from poor village compatriots and kin through a new form of witchcraft called *famla'*.

Since Edwin Ardener's seminal article (1970), a number of scholars studying Cameroonian societies have pointed out that the unequal and changing distribution of wealth brought about by economic incorporation and development leads to new and changing witchcraft beliefs (den Ouden 1987; de Rosny 1981; Geschiere 1980, 1982; Notué and Perrois 1984; Rowlands and Warnier 1988). Bangangté suspect elite compatriots of forming witches' conjuries under the guise of rotating credit associations. Rather than contributing only money, members of *nda nzo* (the house of mystery, or *famla'*) contribute a victim, usually a close relative. The victim appears to die a sudden death, but actually works in an invisible world for the famla' member. The profit from this invisible labor makes the investments of the *nganzo* witch sound and makes his money grow and fill his bank account. Famla' beliefs contain many elements associated with the very different world of the new elites: rotating credit associations requiring costly contributions, geographically distant labor, profits from another's labor, bank accounts and the growth of money (e.g., through interest).[7] The idea that one person's plenty is another's loss is expressed, in Bangangté and elsewhere in Cameroon, through a cannabalistic metaphor:

"someone has 'eaten' the life, the health, the crops, the wealth of his neighbour" (Rowlands and Warnier 1988:123, summarizing Geschiere 1982).

Many Bangangté villagers also view distant political struggles in the national and international arena as a contest among occult powers, piecing together coincidental events as evidence of occult fights among prominent politicians. The Lake Nyos disaster in 1986 brought the following story back into memory, and it was discussed for months in Bangangté.

> . . . on the 16th August 1984, the Monoun, a volcano in the Foumbot area (close to the Noun river [where the royal wives had their farms]) released a gas that asphyxiated thirty-seven people including a Catholic priest, and many animals . . . Two weeks later, on the 31st of August, a Boeing 727 of the national company, Cameroon Airlines, was destroyed by fire as it taxied before take off at Douala airport. One person died and many were injured. The name of the aircraft was 'The Noun'. Three weeks later, on September 22nd, a bridge collapsed on the Noun River, cutting off the Foumban and Foumbot area from the main road network. All three events were interpreted by public rumour as attempts by former President Ahidjo (a Muslim) to regain his position against President Biya (a Catholic) through a demonstration of the superiority of his occult powers in the region of one of his erstwhile enemies, the Bamiléké. (Rowlands and Warnier 1988:128)

The rural Bangangté men and women I lived with perceived the existence of social groups outside the reach of mechanisms controlling the use of kà as meaning that the balance of occult as well as political and economic powers had been seriously disturbed, increasing the vulnerability of Bangangté citizens to misfortune.

This social imbalance was interpreted by many Bangangté as a sign of the incompetence of their mfen. While they still honored his office, the kingship, they criticized certain aspects of the mfen's health and behavior as the failings of an individual that could have terrible consequences for his subjects. Mfen Njiké Pokam, in 1986, appeared ineffective in keeping the disparate elements of Bangangté society in balance; he seemed incapable of controlling occult and state forces to maintain Bangangté unity. For one, he was sick (only 40, he died in early 1987), physically declining in a way that worried his subjects and particularly his wives. Second, he was caught between wanting to promote modern development and maintaining his prerogatives as mfen. Unlike his successor, he did not have the formal education to be an equal partner with the local representatives of the state. His attempts at modernism were interpreted by some as insults to the dignity of the kingship, from shaking hands, eating, and dancing with commoners to granting sacred land to a non-Bangangté merchant to build a factory, as illustrated in the following case.

A Dispute over Sacred Land

Mafam *is an area of land on the border between Batela' and Banekane villages, not far from the original site of the royal compound in Batela', which Bangangté deem sacred. It is allegedly the site where the invading Bamoum army was once turned away through the last-minute defense of Bangangté magicians (*ngakà*). As part of the complex of beliefs and practices connecting the kingship and the fertility of the land, mafam should be cultivated by* njwi mfen *(royal wives),* mâ mfen *(queen mothers), and sisters of the mfen. After the death of a mfen, mafam is supposed to lie fallow for seven years. Its recultivation is opened through ceremonies initiated by the mfen.*

Following the death of mfen Pokam, mafam was left fallow as kan prescribes. However, in 1986, already twelve years after his father's death, mfen Njiké Pokam had not yet reopened cultivation of the sacred fields. This was one point with which his competence as mfen was criticized.

Once the new Yaoundé-Bafoussam road was planned by the Italian firm COGEFAR, mafam was suddenly at an important crossroads of the new highway and the old Bangangté access road. The mfen granted four hectares of the now commercially valuable mafam to a merchant from the neighboring kingdom of Balengou (also in Ndé Division, and much smaller than Bangangté). This merchant owned a store on one of the main streets in downtown Yaoundé, and rumor had it that he planned to build a factory on mafam. This granting of land led to an exchange of letters and meetings in which the mfen was unusually aligned with state representatives against the Bangangté elite, new and old.

In late September 1986, a member of the Bangangté elite sent a letter to the mfen in the name of his fellow Bangangté from Yaoundé, protesting the granting of a piece of mafam to the Balengou merchant. The essential points of the letter refer to the historical and cultural importance of mafam, plea for the maintenance of its integrity, and suggest that rather than leaving the now valuable land as a "historical monument lying fallow" or transforming it into a place for individual profit, it should become a center of Bangangté culture and life. Finally, the elite promised to invest in the development of mafam as long as it remained in Bangangté hands.

Early in October, a meeting was held to discuss the matter, attended by the mfen, his sister the parliamentarian and mamfen, and three highly placed representatives of the central government in Bangangté, including the prefect. One of the civil servants attending the meeting expressed consternation at the elite's concerns. He felt that the Bangangté were working against the development of their own territory and were too "tribalistic," calling a neighbor from their own division a stranger. He claimed the mfen had denied that the land was sacred. Back at the palace, the mfen encouraged his titled wives to testify that the land had not been cultivated even before mfen Pokam's death, but they instead recalled situations when they had worked mafam soil at the end of Pokam's reign.

By the end of 1986, when the field research for this study ended, the outcome of the case of mafam was still inconclusive. Six weeks later mfen Njiké Pokam suffered a tragically early death, after a long illness. On a return visit to Bangangté in June 1997, it appeared that this land was under commercial use.

The multiple centers and forms of power in the kingdom, the economy, and the state (see Arens and Karp 1989) are a challenge that all contemporary Bangangté citizens must manage. They have led to contending views of belonging and of cultural authenticity. Those Bangangté who benefit or hope to benefit from the incorporation of their kingdom into national and international structures have adopted a rhetoric of development. Originating in French writings about the *mise en valeur* (exploitation) of the colonies (e.g., Sarraut 1923), this rhetoric has taken its own shape, combining adaptation to the goals and constraints of international lending organizations with mild pan-Africanist, pro-natalist overtones. Heavily pushed by the Cameroonian government through state-controlled media, this rhetoric of development is shared by high school students and the urban elite. Its vision of the ideal society is a dynamic, changing one, dichotomizing actions, attitudes, and communities into progress and development on the one hand, and decline, backwardness, underdevelopment, superstition, and poverty on the other.

The rural Bangangté with whom I spent most of my time made a similar dichotomized distinction, but shifted the moral evaluation; they preferred "black" over "white," "ours" over that "from the outside" (see also den Ouden 1987:3). Rural Bangangté women are particularly sensitive to such issues, experiencing daily their ambiguous insider–outsider position as in-marrying wives "cooking inside." Rural Bangangté complained to me that new social differentiation disturbs the sense of Bangangté unity and leads people to be not of one heart (*nchu' ntu*). They believed that not being of one heart helps create a disturbed emotional climate, lethargy, and divisiveness, all conditions antithetical to good health, high fertility, and good government. These Bangangté created sharply distinguished pictures of a past ideal Bangangté society and a present disturbed, declining kingdom, illustrated by Che'elou's moving lament of times when "we were many."

For those with the closest ties to royal authority and traditional hierarchies, new social differentiation, the loss of political autonomy, and speculations about new and increasing forms of witchcraft contributed to a general feeling of vulnerability to misfortune. During the two periods of fieldwork for this study, 1983 and 1986, a drought, the construction of a new paved road, and the beginning of a long economic recession further increased rural suffering and uncertainty. Suffering has increased dramatically in the following decade, as evidenced by a return trip in 1997. Most importantly, in 1986 the mfen, a young man, was dying. The mfen of a healthy kingdom should not be sick, and a young man should not die. The mfen's illness symbolized the disorder of the political and spiritual worlds for the majority of rural Bangangté citizens. Many cited population loss and failures of procreation as evidence for this disorder; Bangangté women, in particular, felt their vulnerability in their wombs.

Women's Vulnerability and the Politics of Procreation

The rural women I knew in the mid-1980s felt particularly close ties to the kingdom and what they viewed as traditional Bangangté lifeways. Their farm and kitchen labor contributed to royal festivals and helped the mfen maintain his followership through the redistribution of food that his wives and the wives of his retainers had grown and prepared. They likewise contributed to the maintenance of their husbands', fathers', and mothers' lineages through the cultivation and preparation of food for family gatherings such as funerals and weddings. The rhythm of women's farm and kitchen labor was determined by the traditional eight day week, commemorating past Bangangté kings through select days prohibiting the use of the iron hoe. Rural Bangangté women gained a positive sense of self and security from this rhythm and from the recognition of their labors. As other criteria of prestige and advancement intruded upon the rural life of the kingdom, Bangangté women in particular worried about the transformation of the institution of kingship. They were concerned with the fate of the kingship as a positive force on fortune and fertility, and with the impact the decline of the kingship had on their own social mobility. Both symbolically and in terms of interests, the link between procreation and kingship is strongly shaped by gender relations in Bangangté.

Then and now, both Bangangté wives and the mfen are enveloped in parallel symbolism of their roles as feeders (of families and of the kingdom) and reproducers (of children and of social organization and the conditions for fertility). Women's skills in cooking are recognized in the elaboration of culinary metaphors of procreation. Bangangté ideas about cooking and procreation provide a model for Bangangté perceptions of the mfen's responsibility for maintaining the proper measurement and mix of social "ingredients" (gender balance, ranks, and powers). Royal control over Bangangté social organization reiterates women's control over the "cooking" of procreation. They are linked through the mfen's role in creating appropriate social and spiritual conditions for women's fertility. A weak mfen can only weaken women's reproductive success.

Bangangté women are also particularly concerned about what they perceive as the mfen's diminishing control over witchcraft and the nefarious use of kà. Gender stereotypes of women as contentious, believed by both women and men, contribute to women's anxiety regarding witchcraft. Changing gender relations provide a social context further contributing to this anxiety. As male and female roles are shifting, husbands and wives fight over their mutually disappointed expectations, and cowives compete for attention and material support. The relations between brothers and sisters are also being transformed by increasing individualization and the economic constraints of a recessionary cash economy, weakening women's claims on their brothers' support and land. These developments contribute to domestic strife and wear on extra-domestic exchange and support networks as well. Rural Bangangté women feel vulnerable, fearing they will find insufficient support in case of reproductive illness, and fearing supernatural attacks on their wombs and children brought about by envy and calumny.

While rural Bangangté women initiate conversations with laments about infertility, they go on to discuss not only their own health and procreative success but also their concerns about belonging, identity, and the continuation of a Bangangté way of life. Women experience the ambiguities of belonging as daughters who will marry outside their patrilineage, as wives who are drawn from outside into their husband's patrilineage and the kitchen of his domestic compound, and as the essential links holding together spatially dispersed matrilineages. This experience makes the rural women I worked with particularly sensitive to the changing nature of Bangangté identity in face of the increasing complexity of notions of allegiance, authenticity, and orientation. They were particularly concerned with the socialization of their children. Women invested enormous effort in giving their children the education that would allow them to take advantage of new opportunities, or just survive, in a new context. They recognized, however, that these efforts contributed to their children's estrangement from an "authentic" Bangangté life-style. Rural women worried that their children would abandon them in old age and fail to honor them as ancestors.

As we saw in the previous chapter, the amount and quality of rural Bangangté women's anxieties regarding threats to procreation and social reproduction varies according to a number of dimensions, including their exposure to alternative health beliefs, their place in the life cycle, the developmental stage of their household, and their upward or downward mobility. The distribution of Bangangté women's fears parallels the material and social resources with which women can manage crises and use Bangangté's many health-care alternatives.

Among all rural women I spoke to, the vast majority of their concerns centered around witchcraft-induced infertility and infant mortality. How these women expressed their fears depended upon the ways recent social change had affected their social status. Downwardly mobile women perceive witchcraft dangers to come primarily from competing equals. This is particularly true for the downwardly mobile royal wives, who suspect their cowives of laying "fetishes" in latrines, of hiring witches to harm them, and of slowly and magically eating away at their vital organs through "vampirism." Upwardly mobile women mainly fear the witchcraft of jealous subordinates, most particularly less fortunate kin.

The cases of Josette, the magengoup, and Justine, the civil servant's wife, introduced in chapter 4, illustrate these two scenarios. The first queen and officially the most powerful of the royal wives, Josette was not well-respected by her cowives. They often ridiculed her, a clear sign of downward mobility for a queen. Perhaps seeking to gain some respect through bearing a child (her youngest daughter was already five years old), Josette repeatedly claimed to be pregnant although she had no physical signs of pregnancy. To explain her invisible pregnancies, she accused a number of her cowives of having stolen or hidden her fetus. Paulette, the socially weakest, most vulnerable of her cowives, was the most often accused. Josette's accusations of her cowives did not lead them to fear or respect her, but rather increased their disrespect and even led them to disregard some of her positive qualities such as taking the initiative to care for the mfen's otherwise neglected sheep. Josette's tragedy was that her respect-gaining strategy of accusing her approximate equals of witchcraft, typical of downwardly mobile women, neither helped her to conceive nor improved her social situation. It rather increased her isolation and, at least for the brief remaining period of Njiké Pokam's reign, accelerated her downward mobility and her loss of prestige.

In contrast, Justine, the wife of a highly placed (Bamiléké) civil servant in Bangangté, expressed the fears and therapeutic strategy of an upwardly mobile woman who suspects jealous kin of rendering her infertile through witchcraft. A mother of five children, her youngest child only two years old, Justine felt herself to have a problem with her fertility because she had never before had a two-year interval between pregnancies. Her symptoms began with dreams in which her *tuteur* (foster father) appeared and had sex with her. She identified her tuteur as a villager jealous of her luxurious life who put poison into her body during these dreams. Justine later felt "things" moving in her legs, accompanied by weakness and depression. She said these "things" felt different from *filaires,* microfilarial worms that cause swelling and itching. These "things" moving in her, she claimed, had also attacked her vagina and blocked her tubes, resulting in her perceived fertility problem.

Justine consulted Felix, the healer who had also treated Paulette. With his help, and much expense for medicinal objects and healer's fees, Justine tried to send her foster father's poison back to him and thus to heal herself. Referring to her own case, she made the following assessment of the risks facing the new elite.

> People fall ill and even die more now than in the past because of a conflict between modern, city life and village life, a conflict between haves and have-nots that erupts in jealousy. Villagers say of their city relatives, "Now you live like the whites. You do not even like to eat our village food or drink our water." And, still knowing the traditions, unlike their deracinated urban relatives, the jealous villagers can perform sorcery, do evil things to make one fall ill. The city dwellers have been made vulnerable by . . . their ignorance of custom. The illnesses they catch are undetectable by hospitals and of long duration. If one is unlucky, the cause is never discovered and one dies.

Justine's answer to her vulnerability caused by ignorance of custom was to use her superior economic resources to "buy" the use of counter-witchcraft, to turn the perceived advantage of her opponent against him.

While women voice a variety of concerns regarding threats to procreation, taken together rural women's expressions are one voice among many in Bangangté discussions of procreation, social reproduction, and social change. Creating future generations of "authentic" Bangangté citizens and a "truly Bangangté" way of life, that is, social reproduction, is a concern of those with an interest in maintaining this Bangangté life-style. My use of the terms *Bangangté* and *Bamiléké* here is not meant to reify a timeless ethnicity, but to serve as a shorthand for representing people's own construction of these categories. Rural women's (as well as many royals') idea of being Bangangté is largely nostalgic and conservative. They wish and strive to preserve a comprehensible and recognized, historically deep, relatively encompassing scheme of identities and networks of social relations among these identities. It is exactly this "all-encompassing scheme of identities" that is challenged, in Bangangté and throughout the world, in the modern era (Calhoun 1994). At the same time that ethnic distinctiveness is losing clarity in practice, "identity" becomes a marker of difference. Not only are identity and difference "correlatives, one unthinkable without the other" (Tyler 1987:13), but ethnic lines are drawn ever more sharply and become ever more politicized in Cameroon of the late 1990s, "engraving ethnicity into the constitution" (Nkwi and Nyamnjoh 1997:10).

Bangangté women and holders of traditional office do not have a monopoly on talk about being "truly" Bangangté. The interest in differing forms of social reproduction and transformation is shown in how the idiom of Bangangté unity is used by those with differing interests in development. The rhetoric of Bangangté unity and cohesiveness in the face of disunity, diversification, and changing social structures is simultaneously a conservative response of self-conscious traditionalists and an interest-promoting and idealistic response of new elites. By maintaining a strong, if transformed, Bangangté identity, the latter can use ethnic networks to promote their personal interests without having to redistribute much of their wealth.

These differing thoughts on "Bangangté-ness" have their parallel in Bangangté discussions of demography, especially regarding the politics of pro-natalism, infant mortality, and child survival. Again, rural women form one voice among many. In discussing desired family size and the widespread rejection of voluntary limitations on births, some Bangangté refer to the relation between the mfen and fertility, and how a "full house" or many children is an indicator of personal well-being and of the well-being of the kingdom. Other Bangangté, particularly schoolchildren and politicians, adopt the rhetoric of the state media, stating that "children are the motor of development."

Within the context of their divine kingship beliefs, Bangangté see population as an indicator of the king's and the kingdom's vigor. A fertile royal family extends its fortune to the wombs and fields of Bangangté citizens. Most rural Bangangté, including all but two of the women I interviewed, say that limiting births through contraception or abstinence is both something shameful (interfering with the gift of fortune from the mfen and one's ancestors) and an unreasonable risk (since many children die in infancy). These Bangangté view the royal family, in its narrow sense as the household of the mfen, as the exemplary reproducer. Ideally, within the royal family the most wives are found and the most babies of both sexes are born. The mfen's children grow up in close proximity to the persons, institutions, and events considered the epitome of traditional Bangangté life. The activities and rituals of kingship draw Bangangté subjects into this compound and family and help continue the Bangangté-ness of the territory.

In 1986, Bangangté worried that the physical, reproductive, and political misfortunes of the royal household disturbed the conditions for human conception and even for the creation of agricultural wealth throughout the kingdom. The exemplary reproductive system of the Bangangté royal family was no longer perceived as setting a good example. Wives of the king ran away, few children were born, and the mfen himself did not act like a Bangangté king but shook hands and shared food with strangers. As we have seen, he even ceded sacred land to a non-Bangangté entrepreneur, provoking letters of protest from the urbanized Bangangté elite. To women who perceive limiting births as a shameful shirking of duty and refusal of a gift, these vagaries of a king and changes in kingship were very threatening.

Most rural Bangangté women feel that limiting births is a risk they cannot afford because of their fears regarding child survival. It is likely that infant mortality was high during the precolonial and early colonial periods. Reports of first European contacts with the Grassfields contain alarming assessments of high infant mortality and the threat it and low fertility posed to maintaining this important labor pool (Reichskolonialamt 1912:60). As late as the 1930s, the foundress of Bangwa hospital cited female sterility and infant mortality as two of the three most common and serious health problems facing the Bangangté and Bangwa populations (Debarge 1934:28, 62, 112), although she could discover "no dangerous practices accompanying childbirth" (1934:65). No statistics are available to reliably assess the effect of the major shift from home to hospital births in Bangangté kingdom over the past fifty years on infant mortality in general or on the control of specific diseases such as neonatal tetanus. I assume this expansion of biomedical health care, with its unusually dense coverage in Ndé Division compared to other rural Cameroonian areas, has somewhat reduced infant mortality in Bangangté.

Nonetheless rural Bangangté mothers' anxiety about their children's survival is justified. Bangangté children's rate of survival to adulthood is shockingly low (54.54 percent of children born to mothers in the small sample of interviewees in Batela' and Bantoum villages who distinguished between children born and children living, and only 83.7 percent of Bamiléké children in the Western Province survive beyond age five in the statistically more reliable sample of the World Fertility Survey [1983:78]).[8] These figures indicate that there are substantial risks to children's survival in Bangangté. Bangangté mothers fear for their children's survival, however, based on what they see around them and on their own sorrow. The death of a child is a spectacular and tragic event in Bangangté and serves as a warning to every Bangangté women of the vulnerability of her offspring to fate and disease. Fertility is fragile.

In the past, it was in the interest of the mfen and those who benefited from his strength that Bangangté have a large, fertile population. Wealth and power depended upon gaining the allegiance of large numbers of people. The king's wealth in people gave him a large pool of men to be warriors, of women to be exchanged for alliances and wealth, and of agricultural producers to provide redistributable surpluses. One of the simplest ways of increasing one's followership was by having fertile dependent kin who created numerous descendants. In contemporary Bangangté, the number of those counted in the census as inhabitants of Bangangté kingdom determines Bangangté's ranking as a *"chefferie du premier degré"* (chieftancy of the first degree) and thus both its prestige and the salary of the mfen.

Actors viewing Bangangté society from outside the system of divine kingship beliefs also saw population as an indicator of the health of society. Colonial civil servants and plantation owners were interested in a rapidly reproducing population in the Grassfields to insure a labor pool for public works projects and commercial agriculture in the more developed southern Cameroon (DeLancey 1978; Kuczynski 1939:100; Rapport annuel 1935:115, 1937:97; Reichskolonialamt 1914:xiv, 78). As early as the German colonial period, foreign merchants were concerned about the maintenance of the Grassfields population to assure them of consumers for their imported products (Rudin 1938:346). During the early decades of the colonial period, missionaries also hoped for a rapidly reproducing population among their converts. They wanted to increase the absolute numbers and the proportion of Bangangté citizens whose souls they could save, and they attributed the apparent decline in Bangangté fertility to the breakdown of morals and the spread of venereal disease.[9]

In contemporary Bangangté, the Cameroonian state is pro-natalist for reasons having nothing to do with divine kingship beliefs. A growing population is deemed necessary for development and to maintain the rural agricultural work force. Family planning facilities and contraceptive drugs and devices are nearly nonexistent outside of Yaoundé and Douala, and were not legalized until 1991 (following the fieldwork on which this ethnography is based). Government family planning programs and maternity benefits aim at encouraging maternal and child health through properly spaced births, not at limiting births (Essama, personal communication, January 1986). Neither the pro-natalist maternity benefits for civil servants in the 1980s nor health-promoting family planning facilities reach the ordinary rural Bangangté woman. She continues to hope for numerous offspring for the psychological, social, and economic benefits that children provide her, and to relate her reproductive success to the state of the mfen and the institution of divine kingship.

Food, Poverty, and Women's Voices

The imagery of food and cooking is central to Bangangté women's understandings of procreation. Disturbances in cooking and eating are prominent in Bangangté images of the causes of infertility. Women express concerns about poverty in the language of food, complaining of the hunger of poverty. The image of hunger is persistent, despite the fact that most rural residents can grow sufficient food to feed themselves. Food and poverty are important elements of the ways that rural Bangangté women voice their concerns about infertility and their visions of the relation of population to cultural identity.

Food figures prominently in the symbolic elaboration of Bangangté notions of kingship, fortune, and procreation. The mfen of Bangangté is the feeder of his people, directly through convening feasts and handing out beans and palm oil at his installation ceremonies, and indirectly through granting rights of land use and mystically insuring agricultural fertility. He also figuratively "eats" his people by demanding tribute from them, and in the past through his power over their life and death. Such imagery is common in other societies with divine kingship, where processes of acquiring power are typically expressed in metaphors of eating wealth, including humans, like food (Feeley-Harnik 1985:277). These concepts linking kingship and food reiterate Bangangté images of the procreative kitchen and express the king's power over the immediate necessities of life.

Bangangté women's talk about food is also linked to their experience of downward social mobility, a process of the feminization of poverty experienced throughout rural Africa (S. F. Moore 1994). Women's poverty threatens their ability to maintain social ties and bear and raise the next generation of Bangangté citizens. Food is central for Bangangté women in maintaining ties with their cowives, neighbors, and kin and in creating that feeling of oneness (*nchu' ntu*) that Bangangté seek. In Bangangté it is impossible to think of people living together without sharing food. Commensality is both a symbolic expression of solidarity and the venue of socializing that contributes to solidarity. *Ju,* eating cooked vegetable sauces, is an act of social commensality, drawing people together around a woman's cooking hearth. Its violent mirror image in *fed,* the tearing at food and flesh associated with the antisocial eating of witches and vampires, indicates the importance of feeding and eating in Bangangté social life.

Throughout the world, food symbolizes a variety of social relations (Douglas 1966; Leach 1964; Lévi-Strauss 1963, 1966, 1967; Meigs 1984; Mintz 1985, 1996; Tambiah 1969; Weiss 1996). Forms of commensality may be models of social organization that participants present to themselves, as in Iteso beer parties (Karp 1980). Who eats what with whom and how has long been recognized as a marker of identity and group boundaries (Feeley-Harnik 1981). Bangangté identify certain foods as "very Bangangté" or "very Bamiléké." Bangangté even associate one of these foods, the viscous sauce nkwi, as promoting recovery from the trauma of childbirth. Nkwi figured into much commentary about what foods I should and could eat with what amount of gusto; these comments and observations were one way that Bangangté women tried to define a stranger and the level of familiarity and trust they could give her.

The theft of food disturbs women's ability to maintain their households and social ties. The theft of reproductive chances, through disease, domestic conflict, and witchcraft, contributes to rural women's status loss. The violent imagery of plundered kitchens, cannibalistic witchcraft, and theft that permeates Bangangté women's accounts of infertility and child loss arises from the context of rural female poverty. Growing, selling, and exchanging food is essential for women's survival in an increasingly cash-oriented environment. Food is both a social and a material resource for poor, rural Bangangté women.

Infertility increases Bangangté women's risk of poverty and thus their fears of hunger, of not being able to provide for themselves and for others. Infertility can weaken a husband's interest in and support of a woman or lead to divorce, and it takes away a sense of adult accomplishment and social and economic security in old age. Bangangté women fear the consequences of infertility. They also worry about their place in the future if Bangangté lifeways are not reproduced. The weakness of the mfen causes them to fear economic consequences of his effect on human and agricultural fertility. Their incomes decline as the fertility of the land and the number of children (the potential labor power) decline. With no royal control, the social soup spoils, and threats from witchcraft increase. Women thus link poverty and their concern about food to their anxieties regarding reproductive health and social reproduction. The views Bangangté women hold about procreation, food, poverty, and kingship are necessary to understand the place of kingship and the gender-specific consequences of its transformation in the 1990s.

Much of the data for this book is based on women's talk, and Bangangté women talk a lot about food and procreation. My analysis has suggested that rural Bangangté women's preoccupation with culinary imagery, procreation, and the theft of food and babies is their way of talking about their view of authentic Bangangté culture, the past, and feelings of present vulnerability. Relieving women's suffering regarding their fears of failed procreation requires a change in the context in which their anxieties emerge. Do their voices and laments contribute to this change?

Fear and *threat* are central terms in the description and analysis of Bangangté women's experience. Rowlands and Warnier suggest that the asocial use of occult powers and the fear of these powers are forms of popular political action and resistance to the increasing hegemony of the Cameroonian state (1988).[10] In this framework, fear of witchcraft and of infertility is part of the "hidden transcripts" of resistance (Scott 1990), and talking about it is "doing things with words" (Austin 1962). I agree with Rowlands and Warnier that ordinary Bangangté men's and women's suspicion that the new elite only reach their positions by practicing witchcraft serves to limit rural allegiance to the national state and its local representatives. Rural women who fear direct witchcraft attacks on their reproductive health, however, accuse their equally downwardly mobile cowives and neighbors rather than the new elite. Their beliefs are more suggestive of suffering and competition for scarce material, social, and spiritual resources than of resistance to domination (be it domination by men, by the state, or by capital).

But Bangangté women are "doing something with words" when they complain about infertility and threats to their reproductive health. Identifying rural Bangangté women's expressions of reproductive threats merely as displaced fears, covering real problems in a mantle of metaphor, creates a dichotomy between the material and the ideal that impedes our understanding of Bangangté women's lives. Most importantly, it is not adequate to Bangangté understandings of social life. In terms of Bangangté concepts regarding the interconnections among health and polity in their divine kingship, fears of infertility and failed reproduction in all their breadth are a very Bangangté way to initiate discussion on themes of real fears. For example, any Bangangté, properly socialized, understands expressions about the small number of children in the royal compound, that "the royal compound has stopped" (*nchwed tin,* i.e., it is sterile), as coded messages about the state of the Bangangté polity. Any Bangangté husband understands that when his wife serves him a meal without palm oil, she is complaining about his negligence of his material and sexual duties toward his wife and the maintenance of her household. These symbolic statements are much more than tiny "rituals of rebellion" (Gluckman 1963) relieving the pressure of social conflicts and allowing the structures and ideologies of male dominance to endure. Women use metaphor and symbol tactically in everyday verbal interactions, negotiating relations of gender, kinship, and power (Gal 1991) with regard to procreation, population management, and the social reproduction of a distinctive cultural identity.

Ethnographic examples abound of women's "muted" and often subversive discourses being embedded in formal speech genres (proverbs, songs, poetry, and folklore) (e.g., Abu-Lughod 1986; Karp 1987; Raheja and Gold 1994). The metaphoric expressions in the idiom of infertility that structures much of Bangangté women's commentary on social life are embedded not in formal speech genres but in everyday conversations and interactions. Mutedness depends on the listener. Rural Bangangté women's voices are "muted" (Ardener 1972) in certain contexts. They have little or no power within the Cameroonian state and the world economy to effect change that would secure their self-esteem and physical and economic well-being. Bangangté women need a voice where it makes a difference. Perhaps, by complaining discreetly but insistently, via culturally recognized metaphors, they can at least temporarily reverse the decline of the Bangangté kingship. Their nostalgic view of a past "when they were many" is understandable in a present that offers few opportunities to rural Bangangté women.

Women's complaints about the apparently physical matters of fertility and infertility connect ideas about the body, the mind, and the state of society. Examining Bangangté women's fears of infertility has revealed for us some of the enduring insights of medical anthropology, but has also taken us beyond the realm of medical concerns. The symbolism of procreation, fertility, infertility, and royal social reproduction has emerged from the particular history and political, economic, and cultural context of the Cameroonian Grassfields kingdom of Bangangté. It is put to use by various actors, all with their particular interests, within this very same context. We cannot understand world population problems and responses to population policy without understanding this socially meaningful communication—often expressed through metaphor—and its contexts. Bangangté women are doing what they can with words, expressing their anxieties about threats to their wombs and threats to cultural continuity, urging all who will listen to restore health and order to their world.

Kings of Bangangté

The dynasty of the fifteen *mfennga,* or kings of Bangangté, extends from the legendary past of the founder, Ngami, to the late 1990s.

No.	King	Period of Reign
1.	Ngami	
2.	Tshamngo	
3.	Nenaton	
4.	Mbiatat	
5.	Ngassam I	
6.	Nya I	died during initiation period at La'kwa
7.	Nzike I	
8.	Nya II	
9.	Ngassam II	1885–1891
10.	Yomi	1891–1895
11.	Tchatchoua	1895–1910
12.	Nzike II Salomon	1910–1943
13.	Pokam Njiké Robert	1943–1974
14.	Njiké Pokam François	1974–1987
15.	Nji Monluh Seidou Pokam	1987–present

Notes

Introduction

1. I use *manage* in the sense of "therapy management," a concept developed by John Janzen and defined as the process in which "medical clients . . . diagnose illness, select therapies, and evaluate treatments" (1978a:xviii).

2. In regional demographic surveys conducted from 1960 through 1965, "Bamiléké country" showed a total fertility rate of 6.3 (children born to the average woman in her lifetime, assuming age-specific fertility rates remain constant), in contrast to a range from 3.8 to 5.6 for the south Benoue to western Cameroon regions. Findings of the 1978 World Fertility Survey show an average completed fertility of 6.4 for the Western Province (including both Bamiléké and Bamoum peoples), in contrast to 4.9 for Cameroon as a whole. Marital fertility over the past twelve months at the time of the World Fertility Survey of 1978 was 8.3 for the Western Province (6.9 for Cameroon). Marital fertility at the time of the Cameroon General Census of 1987, one year after the fieldwork for this study, was 8.8 (8.1 urban, 9.0 rural) for the Western Province (7.0 for Cameroon) (Wakam 1994:350, 352, 353). At the time of the 1991 Demographic and Health Survey, the national total fertility rate was 5.8 (Balépa, Fotso, and Barèrre 1992a:32). A comparison with previous regional data is difficult, as the DHS report lumps together data from the West and Littoral provinces (although West and Northwest have more cultural similarities). The total fertility rate for the West and Littoral provinces in 1991 was 5.96, higher than the national rate, but only the third highest from four regional groupings (Balépa, Fotso, and Barèrre 1992a:31). The difference between the total fertility rate and descendence indicates a fertility transition may be occurring in the Western and Littoral provinces (Balépa, Fotso, and Barèrre 1992a:33).

3. There are many linguistically closely related terms for what has variously been translated as king, paramount chief, chief, and subchief in the Cameroonian Grassfields. *Mfen* is the Bangangté term, and *fo* is the term common to the Bamiléké kingdoms near the provincial capital of Bafoussam. *Fon,* the term best known in the anthropological literature, is the term for kings (or paramount chiefs) in the Western (English-speaking) Grassfields. I translate *mfen* as "king" to retain the sense of royalty that pervades this important office within a system of divine kingship.

Chapter One

1. Since I conducted this fieldwork in 1986, Claude Njiké-Bergeret has become a celebrity. She is "La Reine Blanche" (the white queen), the subject of a 1995 French television documentary in the series *Envoyé Spécial*. Her autobiography, *Ma Passion Africaine* (My African passion) was published in 1997. For this reason and with her permission, I use Claude's real name in this book, although I use pseudonyms for the other wives of the king.

2. See Voorhoeve (1964) for a discussion of Bamiléké praise names, and Pradelles de Latour (1986) for an analysis of their kinship significance in Bangwa chiefdom.

3. Building a wife's kitchen-hut is an important part of marriage for nonroyals and thus almost always precedes the wife's first pregnancy. See chapter 3.

4. Translated as "Illness: Belly. Plugged [fallopian] tubes. Unstopping fecundity."

5. This meets with Weber's definition of social status (1968).

6. Comparison with the Nso' of the western Grassfields, a kingdom sharing many aspects of political and kinship structure, vocabulary, and witchcraft beliefs with Bangangté, throws light on the relative importance of incest as a source of misfortune in varying circumstances. In her study of Nso' incest, Kaberry points out that the seriousness of sexual offenses varied with the status of those involved (1969:176). As in Bangangté, not the sexual offense itself but the mistrust and dissension incest causes (that can lead, for example, to witchcraft) are stressed by Nso'. Kaberry cites two forms of incest in Nso' that are relevant to Paulette's case. First, when a lineage head and his daughter have intercourse, his marriage with the daughter's mother is dissolved. This is considered the man's offense. In Bangangté, however, the lineage head was the mfen, enormously more powerful than, and not able to be accused by, his most recent wife. Second, when a couple marries and later discovers they are kin, the act only becomes incest once the relationship is known. The marriage is dissolved and the woman cannot remarry. If the marriage continues, as it had for Paulette and the mfen at the time of Paulette's complaints, the wife and her children are no longer under protection of the woman's ancestors and likely to die. Such an explanation, however, was never raised by Paulette or her healer, probably due (1) to the high status and relative invulnerability of the mfen, and (2) to the easy availability of other explanations stemming from stereotypes of contentious and dangerous relations among cowives.

7. This does not mean that Paulette or women like her would equate childlessness with independence. There is an increasing number of unmarried mothers in Cameroon, reflected in press reports of the 1970s and 1980s. Some of these unwed mothers are independent urban women, some live in their fathers' compounds in rural areas. The women I knew and talked to were largely either unmarried and childless, or married (with or without children).

8. In the past, distinctions of types of healers within the current category "indigenous" may have been made more finely by nonexperts. Today the differ-

ence between "custom" and "white, Western, imported, of the city" is so important as to overshadow other distinctions in a folk typology. See den Ouden's discussion of the paired concepts "black" and "white" among two other Bamiléké groups (1987:3).

9. According to the wives who stayed in the royal compound, mfen Njiké Pokam had married 17 women in addition to the wives he inherited. At the time of his death in February 1987, 13 of these 17 had run away. While her marginality may have been extreme, Paulette's flight appears more the norm than the exception for royal wives during this reign.

Chapter Two

1. By using the terms *Bangangté* and *Bamiléké* I do not mean to reify a timeless ethnicity. I use these labels rather as a shorthand to represent people's understandings and social construction of the categories Bangangté or Bamiléké. See also Webster 1991:269n4.

2. The complete legend of the founding of the Bangangté dynasty is reported in Nkwenga (1965:95–97). The founder of the Bangangté chiefship, Ngami, was a hunter who left his natal village near Banka with his twin brother, Kammi. Kammi found a home in the village of Bangang-Fokam, where he became chief. Ngami continued to Bangangté, where he resided in Tela' ("center of the village") with Njanzwe, one of four local chiefs. Ngami distributed the meat from his hunt so generously that Njanzwe gave him land. With Njanzwe's permission Ngami formed an association of hunters called Manjo (later a mutual aid and military association of youths). He was able to force nearly all the young men of the four chiefdoms of Bangangté to join Manjo and take an oath of allegiance to him. After creating this base of support, Ngami then tricked Njanzwe with praising words and wine, claiming that the titles distinguishing between nobles and chiefs were reversed in Bangangté. To correct this "mistake" Njanzwe traded titles with Ngami. He then sat Ngami on a banana trunk to, as he thought, install him as a noble. However, Njanzwe unwittingly made Ngami chief and demoted himself to the nobility. Thus, through hunting skill and trickery a stranger was able to install himself as chief of the central Bangangté villages Tela' and Ntaleme.

3. For example, Tardits cites the following figures: African production of coffee in tons, Bangangté: 1939, 0; 1947, 2 tons arabica (Tardits 1960:76); number of coffee plants, Bangangté: 1947, 37,044; 1956, 284,428 arabica, 1,515,950 robusta (Tardits 1960:77); size of coffee plantations, 1942: Bangangté: 34 plantations of less than one hectare, 1 of 1 to 2 ha, 1 of more than 2 ha (Tardits 1960:79).

4. These include Bangang-Fokam, Bangwa, Bamena, Batchingou, Balengou, Bahouc, Bakong, Bangoulap, Bazou, Bagnou, and Bandounga.

5. Three conflicting sources exist for Bangangté population figures. Boog 1986 is an officially stamped population estimate for Ndé Division, signed by the prefect, Jean-Calvin Boog, on January 2, 1986, and based on 1984 estimates by the Service Provincial Statistique de l'Ouest. It shows the following figures.

Administrative Unit	Surface Area	1976 (Census)	Population 1984 Estimates		
			Urban	Rural	Total
Bangangté Subdiv.	923 km²	48,002	12,832	45,519	58,351
Bazou Subdivision	243 km²	15,232	7,450	11,066	18,516
Tonga Subdivision	349 km²	9,410	9,139	2,301	11,440
Ndé Division	1,515 km²	72,644	29,421	58,886	88,307

The figures drawn from the 1976 census do not coincide with those of the published 1976 census, which divides the population by administrative unit, by urban/rural areas, and by sex, as follows:

	Population, Both Sexes		
	Urban	Rural	Total
Bangangté Subdivision	9,854	35,055	44,909
Bazou Subdivision	5,721	8,522	14,243
Tonga Subdivision	7,018	1,772	8,790
Ndé Division	22,593	45,349	67,942
	Population, Masculine		
Bangangté Subdivision	4,799	15,129	19,928
Ndé Division	10,615	19,555	30,170
	Population, Feminine		
Bangangté Subdivision	5,055	19,926	24,981
Ndé Division	11,978	25,794	37,772

(*Source:* République Unie du Cameroun, Ministère de l'Economie et du Plan, Direction de la Statistique et de la Comptabilité Nationale. Recensement Général de la Population et de l'Habitat d'Avril 1976, Volume 1, Tome 3:169)

The third source is Dongmo's population and area chart of Bamiléké kingdoms, drawn from the 1976 census, grouping kingdoms together by population density. Bangangté and Bandounga kingdoms, with population densities of 23 and 24 inhabitants/km² respectively, are grouped together with a total population of 23,428. Unfortunately the surface area was left blank in this case, and one gets different figures (992 and 1042) when calculating the difference by row or column (Dongmo 1981:84). In addition to the questionable reliability of both sources (and of the census), administrative units and kingdoms are not equivalent, making comparison of their areas and population figures difficult. The census contains no data on populations owing allegiance to the Bangangté kingdom but living elsewhere, probably because ethnic identity is a sensitive issue in this diverse country.

6. Anthropologists studying Bamiléké kinship disagree whether it is a patrilin-

eal or dual descent system, and most emphasize agnatic relations. M.-L. and C.-H. Pradelles de Latour (1985, 1994n, respectively) describe the neighboring Bangwa as a patrilineal people. Tardits (1960) calls the Bamiléké bilinear, but discusses only agnatic descent. Hurault (1962) describes the Bamiléké kinship system "as if it were double descent," but warns that Bamiléké lineages, particularly the patri-lineage, are not "true" lineages. His discussion of descent nonetheless emphasizes the "more evident" patrilineal ties. Den Ouden (1987:6) describes kinship among the Bamiléké of Tsa and Ngang chiefdoms in Bamboutos district as "a limited patrilineal descent system." Brain (1972) is the only scholar of the Bamiléké to emphasize maternal ties in his treatment of *atsen'ndia* uterine kin groups among the Bangwa-Fontem of Cameroon's Northwest Province.

7. Bangangté belief in ancestral wrath may become a self-fulfilling prophecy as well as an interpretation of past events. A Bangangté person, cognizant of some wrongdoing or neglect of ancestral skulls, may become so distraught as to make some sort of misfortune inevitable. A missionary physician suggested that fear resulting from beliefs in ancestral wrath and witchcraft may explain some cases of sterility where no organic cause can be found. Distress at her incestuous and unap-proved marriage may have contributed to Paulette's misfortunes, discussed in chapter 1.

8. In a sample of 38 women from Bantoum, Batela' and Ntamleme, excluding the wives of the mfen, brideprice was paid to the father or father's heir for the mar-riages of 16 women, another 16 were married under the *ta nkap* regime (of which the rights in six women were "cashed in" as brideprice was paid to the mother, mother's father, chief, or other marriage ward, and 10 women were married with no brideprice exchange). Of the remaining six informants, one knew that bride-price was paid but did not know to whom, three did not know anything about the financial arrangements surrounding their marriages, and two were single.

9. Robert Brain (1972:53–59) is the only scholar of the Bamiléké to analyze the importance of uterine relationships. He discusses the *atsen'ndia* among the Bangwa of Fontem, in the Northwest Province of Cameroon. He calls it the "solidary group par excellence" (1972:53). The Bangwa *atsen'ndia,* whose relations receive some jural recognition with regard to partial inheritance of property and bridewealth rights, appears to be more institutionalized than the *pam nto'* group in Bangangté kinship.

10. Witchcraft substance, *ntok,* enabling one to be a *ngafettok* ("person who eats ntok," also called *ndum*), a vampire or person who transforms him/herself and eats others, is inherited through uterine lines. *Ntok* is located in the intestines, and those who "share" the same intestines or "come from" the same belly will also share the presence or absence of this trait.

11. They also speak of "the mother who has raised me," referring to foster moth-ers who may have cared for them as youths. The moral obligation one has toward one's mother is extended to these childhood caregivers. When royal wives com-plained about the mfen, they sometimes cited his neglect of his foster mother, the eldest royal wife still living in the compound. "Even though his own mother is no longer living, he still gives his old nurse nothing."

12. Of 33 children within the royal compound, 11 lived in the house of their own mother, four lived in houses of their mothers' cowives (two of these four had been abandoned when their mothers had fled the royal compound), three children were grandchildren or great-nieces staying with an elderly royal wife, two were nieces or cousins of their foster mothers, one was the child of his foster mother's friend, and two were niece and nephew of the mfen who lived in the palace but ate with different royal wives. Of the elderly royal wives, five lived with no children, and two had foster wards. Only one elderly wife with living children still lived in the royal compound.

13. My sample of 38 Bangangté women from Bantoum, Batela', and Ntamleme indicates the proportion of polygynous vs. monogamous households in Bangangté today. Two of the 38 women were single, and one widow gave no data on her marriage. Of the remaining 35, 22 were or had been in polygynous marriages, 13 in monogamous marriages; four of these women were divorced, one was in her second marriage, and seven were widowed. Of the 35 households for which I have data, the total average number of wives per household was 2.17. Within the 22 polygynous households, the average number of wives per household was 2.864, ranging from two wives ($n = 11$) to six wives ($n = 1$).

14. This high-dry-sterile vs. low-moist-fertile distinction is common throughout the Bamiléké territory. It has been discussed for the neighboring Bangwa by Marie-Lorraine Pradelles de Latour, who links it also to language usage of young men. Pidgin, used by young Bangwa men to flirt with women, is called "dry speech," speech that allows one to lie, hide, dissemble (1985:366).

15. The royal compound is an exception. Graves of the chiefs are kept secret, to prevent a usurper from stealing a royal skull, thus taking spiritual legitimacy away from the rightful heir. Unlike most heirs, the mfen does not sacrifice to his ancestors directly, but has royal servants and *minnyi* do these rites for him. Graves of royal wives are found directly in front of their houses, just as with commoners. Royal wives receive no ostentatious tombs, however, only an upside-down beer or Coca-cola bottle to mark the grave.

16. That is, they do not plant maize, beans, or peanuts between the rows of coffee.

17. Distance to fields may also be increased by resettlement plans, such as in Bantoum I, where villages were grouped together along the roadside during the civil war in the 1950s and 1960s. Both men and women of Bantoum now walk up to eight kilometers to get to their fields near the original villages.

18. Bantoum I, which in 1967 had 986 inhabitants, counting its four quarters, has the following voluntary associations:

> a rotating credit association for each of its four "quarters" (Bitchoua I, Bitchoua II, Noumntse, and Bantoum I were "regrouped" during the civil war in 1960), of which all but one are mixed sex, the fourth quarter having a separate association for men and women
> a mutual aid society and rotating credit association for wives of civil servants
> three dance groups, two of which meet on days of the seven-day week (*ndanji*

and *lali*) and one of which meets on a day of the eight-day week (*ngú,* the termite dance)

four village committees, with widely varying attendance (a women's community development group, a health committee, a village development committee, and a committee organizing labor for a water project)

a credit union committee, started by German volunteers in the late 1970s

a Catholic and a Protestant chapel

a mutual aid society of women who work their fields together on Wednesdays and Thursdays

19. *Ndap* stems from the verb *ne lapte,* to thank, in Medumba, the Bangangté language. Pradelles de Latour (1986:115) cites the same etymology for the neighboring Bangwa of Ndé District. When discussing *ndap* in French, Bangangté will use the terms *nom de remerciement* and *éloge.* Voorhoeve uses *éloge* in his linguistic study of these honorifics (1964).

20. A woman with the *ndap* So'nju is the daughter of the mfen of Bangangté. Her daughter's *ndap me* (matrilineal *ndap*) is Ncânko. Ncânko's daughter's *ndap* is So'nju. Any woman with the *ndap* Ncânko, when singing her praises, would call this granddaughter "my mother," including her real mother.

21. Here I am not judging the Bangangté mfen, past or present, but am citing expressions many Bangangté citizens made in 1986, criticizing their terminally ill mfen who was caught between demands of traditionalism and modernization.

22. Of the king's wives who stayed in the royal compound, two had three children, three had two children, two wives of childbearing age and six of seven elderly wives had no children.

23. A number of authors investigating divine kingship in Africa discuss this issue of the creation of strangeness. Hocart (1936) and Fortes (1968) discuss the transformation of persons into the embodiment of the idea of kingly office. Richards describes how Bemba kings embody royal traditions in themselves, their relations with kin and subjects, and their rituals to maintain a charter of divine kingship in the absence of writing (1939, 1969). Beidelman (1966), interpreting Kuper's early Swazi data (1947), most specifically addresses the creation of a "stranger" king via the annual *ncwala* ritual; the king must both participate in and transcend the complexities of social life. Sacrifice, cannibalism, and incest are common images in installation rites that make the king "strange" in a fearful way. At the same time, the king often symbolically and literally feeds his people, through giving handfuls of beans and oil as in Bangangté installation rites, through giving feasts, or through sacred hearth and kitchen ceremonies in Bemba royal installation (Richards 1939:48–50).

24. Notué and Perrois (1984) have written a thorough study of Bamiléké secret societies. They use the example of Bandjoun, a chiefdom that has retained more traditional functions, and royal pomp fit for tourists, than nearly any other Bamiléké chiefdom.

25. Such happened in the outlying village of Maham in early 1983.

26. See Feeley-Harnik (1985:285) on divine kingship, especially in Africa, and the king's two bodies.

27. The thesis that the success of traditional courts may be encouraged by fear of incursion by the state in colonial and postcolonial settings has been nicely presented in an essay entitled "Dispute resolution in the shadow of the Leviathan" (Spittler 1980, my translation of title).

Chapter Three

Chapter 3 is revised from "Cooking Inside: Kinship and Gender in Bangangté Idioms of Marriage and Procreation." *American Ethnologist* 22, no. 3 (1995): 483–501. Reprinted by permission of the American Anthropological Association.

1. *Country Sunday* is the Pidgin term used throughout the Western Grassfields, and understood by most in the Eastern Grassfields, to which Bangangté belongs. Observance of country Sundays is an act of expressing fealty to a particular sovereign as ritual leader and to his ancestors (see Goheen 1992:389). In Bangangté, country Sunday is called *li' ngá* and commemorates the death of Nyâmi, the founding hunter king. Within the traditional eight-day week, there are actually three days on which work with the hoe is prohibited to women, *li' ngá, ntanbu'* (commemorating the death of Pokam, the king's father), and *ntala'* (market day). Royal wives are prohibited from hoe cultivation on an additional two days.

2. Rotating credit associations among Bangangté in urban areas are sometimes, but rarely, of mixed sex. In Bantoum, a women's rotating credit association had one male member, a literate man with the function of secretary.

3. French is an exception, since it is a "school" language. Because fewer girls than boys attended school in past generations, few women over 35 spoke French fluently in the mid-1980s.

4. A number of women stated the following interpretations of dream symbols as common knowledge *among women:* killing a snake is bad; a snake approaching means the dreamer will soon get children; a red river indicates imminent sickness; and a black river is a good, healthy sign.

5. *Carrier* is defined by Berger, Berger, and Kellner as "an institutional process or a group that has produced or transmitted a particular element of consciousness" (1973:98). They borrow the concept from Weber.

6. These associations of sex, the woman's hearth, and blood with women's roles and procreation are widespread in central, eastern, and southern Africa. For example, sex, blood, and fire are an important symbolic cluster in Richards's classic study of the Bemba girls' initiation rite, Chisungu (1956:30–36).

7. Bangangté informants did not explicate the meaning of salt in this context. Perhaps it refers to the possibility that a woman who has conceived before marriage may have had sexual relations with more than one man. Married men contribute salt to their wives' kitchen larders.

8. Within the royal compound, sexual relations are referred to as "work" when the royal wives speak in French: "Elle travaille à la chefferie." In Bangangté language, one says "*a be'a ntun nchwed*" (she is in the below of the palace compound) or "*a num ntsue a ntun nchwed*" (she lives in the below of the palace compound). When one says "*a nen fa' ntun nchwed*" (she has gone to work in the below of the

palace compound), it means she has gone to help her cowife whose turn it is to do the domestic duties of wife-of-the-day. This assumes she will come back to her own house in one of the women's quarters at night.

9. The "measuring" of procreation is expressed with the same verb denoting measuring cooking ingredients, distinct from the verb for measuring length or distance.

10. No Bangangté could specify what that amount is.

11. God the potter is both above all and nourishes the earth. Nsi is close to the ancestors, who are in the earth and through the earth have a relationship with divinity. The earth from which the first people were made was low, fresh, cool, and humid (Goldschmidt 1986:210), all qualities describing fertile land and the fecund, complicated areas of royal compounds.

12. In other Bangangté contexts, and throughout the Bamiléké region, water is also associated with fertility, such as in the distinction between moist and fertile vs. dry and barren land. Water is used in therapy to strengthen or fortify as well as to wash or purify sufferers.

13. For comparative material on Gambian women's concepts of the health and aging effects of pregnancy, see Bledsoe 1997.

14. As early as 1937, there were few professional midwives in Bangangté (Egerton 1938:236). I describe the health-care alternatives available at different historical periods to Bangangté women in chapter 5 and in another publication (Feldman-Savelsberg 1990).

15. Girls' seclusion at puberty, *nja,* was practiced until at least the mid-1940s. This ritual enclosure involved much of the cooking, eating, and fattening symbolism of procreation. When education for girls began to expand some 30 years ago, schooling took the place of nja for those families who could spare their daughter's labor and spend resources preparing her for adult life. Now some elderly explicitly refer to schooling as *nja.* They perceive girls sitting in school doing no physical labor, eating up household resources, and preparing themselves for marriage. After healer Tondji of Banekane's wife finished her account of nja saying "the children do not do it anymore," Tondji commented, "The school comes. So the children had to learn this new law (*kan*)." Another explicit ritual enclosure is still experienced by two queens, who spend nine weeks enclosed with the new king, emerging for the coronation in a public ceremony rife with the imagery of birth, cooking, and wealth.

16. Nzikam Djomo describes mothers' rites to leave seclusion and to resume agricultural work in Babouantou (1977:98–104). It is likely that such rites once existed for Bangangté, but they are either no longer remembered or for some reason were hidden from the researcher. Rites similar to those Nzikam Djomo describes for mothers exist in Bangangté for widows of the mfen, and are stretched over a seven year period that ends with the reopening of the sacred field of mafam to cultivation.

17. Among the Bamiléké, being of the "same blood" as one's mother and her uterine kin is self understood and highly valued. By contrast, among the strongly patrilineal Bambara and Mandinka of urban Mali, children are thought to inherit

only their father's "blood." The process of breastfeeding, rather than breastmilk as a product, forms the kinship link between children and their mothers in urban Mali (Dettwyler 1988:179).

18. If the couple also has a civil or church wedding, this takes place from one week to several years after the traditional ceremony. Timing seems dependent upon how much urgency the couple feels in having a civil or church wedding as well as upon the financial resources they need to spend on celebrations.

Chapter Four

Chapter 4 has been revised from an earlier article. Reprinted from "Plundered Kitchens, Empty Wombs: Fear of Infertility in the Cameroonian Grassfields." *Social Science and Medicine* 39, no. 4 (1994): 463–74. Copyright 1994, with permission from Elsevier Science.

1. This civil war is variously called the "UPC Rebellion" and the "Bamiléké Rebellion." It started as a trade union movement, and developed into a guerrilla war conducted by an outlawed political party calling for independence and reunification of British and French Cameroon. As independence neared, and following independence, it became simultaneously a struggle against the new French-supported president, Ahmadou Ahidjo, a struggle of disinherited and urban underemployed Bamiléké against chiefs and nobles they deemed exploitative, and an excuse for local land disputes to be settled through violence. See chapter 2 of this book, as well as Joseph (1977) and Bayart (1979) for further discussion of the "troubles."

2. In his study of public autopsy among the Bamiléké of Dschang, Miaffo cites death with a swollen belly as one form of "bad death," caused by impurity and necessitating special precautions during burial to protect the living (1977:95). "Swollen-belly disease" is likewise a shameful and polluting death among the Kom of the western Grassfields (Shanklin 1988:13).

3. This scheme follows, and cuts across, Foster and Anderson's classification of medical systems according to "personalistic" and "naturalistic" causality concepts (Foster 1976). A personalistic medical system attributes the cause of illness to the use of suprasensory forces directed toward the afflicted individual by the action of a malevolent agent, be it human, nonhuman, or supernatural. A naturalistic medical system explains the cause of illness through natural elements that provoke an equilibrium loss within the body of the individual.

4. Two teams of practitioners and researchers on health care in Africa have pointed out how therapy, even in biomedical institutions, is often used as a diagnostic tool in Africa. Wim Thijs, a general practitioner at Bangwa Protestant Hospital 15 kilometers from Bangangté, reports that due to lacking funds and equipment many diagnostic tests are skipped in his practice. Only when the patient does not respond favorably to the most likely therapy is a new diagnosis and treatment put forth. Feierman, in collaboration with his wife, a physician, indicates that both traditional and biomedical therapies are employed in northeastern Tanzania to make a final diagnosis according to what works. The longer the patient remains sick, the more therapies are tried and the wider the social net is cast to draw people into the therapy management group (1981).

5. These rites are performed at sacred places, most often a small grove of trees creating a moist and dark sanctuary, or a single large tree. Specific streams, where enemies were turned away in legendary battles or where royal widows undergo rites of innocence, are also considered sacred places. It is believed that sacred trees and groves are sites where one can most easily approach or be close to Nsi. For Bangangté, their moistness is evidence of divine fertility or creative force. Minnyis (see note 7) will sometimes indicate which sacred spots are the most propitious to perform rites to appease Nsi. Locally produced clay bowls, a grinding stone, and a felled tree trunk are usually present at sacred sites to facilitate the sacrifice of palm oil, ground melon seeds, mushrooms, or poultry (*ngap nsi,* chicken of god). See map of royal compound (fig. 9, chap. 2) for locations of sacred sites.

6. Hurault discusses the relations of ancestor worship, breath/spirit of the ancestors, and one's personal god for the closely related Bamiléké of Bandjoun (1962:115). His description of these connections is more detailed than data I have gathered from Bangangté informants, who rarely talk about personal gods (*nsiam* in Bangangté, *mbem* in Bandjoun). "Breath" (*zwiak* in Bangangté, *jüenye* in Bandjoun) is considered intermediate between the human being and the divine. A link is forged between the *jüenye* of the ancestors and the *mbem,* one's personal god, in that only other gods and one's own ancestors can disturb one's mbem. When faced with adversity or illness, one says in Bandjoun "*Mbem a poq,*" "My mbem has become hostile to me." The healing of a person depends upon the good wishes of his or her mbem. Hurault cites informants in Batie and Bandjoun as stating "He will recover, if his mbem so wishes," and "*mbem e fien e,*" "His mbem has sold him" when a situation appears hopeless.

7. *Minnyi*s are visionaries possessed by divine power to see causes of misfortune and to cure a varying range of illnesses. All minnyis go through a trying time of initial possession and apprenticeship/initiation. The closest gloss for minnyi in the anthropological literature is spirit medium.

8. The other Bangangté word for medicine is *fu,* literally leaf or herb. *Fu* refers to remedies made of leaves, roots, barks, and kaolin, which may or may not be infused with the mystical powers of kà. "Simple" remedies are always considered fu, not kà. This distinction between two kinds of medicine, applied loosely by nonspecialist Bangangté, appears widespread in the Cameroonian Grassfields. The Wiya (Wimbum ethnic group) of Ndu distinguish between *mshep* (medicines) and *nshep* (medicine); the plural refers to public and harmless (i.e., curative) medicines, and the singular to the secret and dangerous realm of magic, associated with traditional title and office holders and the moral legitimacy of political hierarchy (Bühler and Probst 1988).

9. In Batie and Bandjoun, if a pregnant woman dies both she and her children are suspected of being *ndum.* The husband of this woman is also shunned, as it is believed he carries *tfie,* a serious "stain," which is sexually transmitted and will kill the man's consorts when they become pregnant (Hurault 1962:122). Bangangté hold similar ideas regarding pollution following the death of a pregnant woman, but do not relate it to ntok.

10. *Ntok* is similar to "witchcraft of the night" in the Western Grassfields king-

dom of Nso (Kaberry 1969:179). Witches of the night bring misfortune to agnates and individuals whose office or power they covet, and do so invisibly, secretively, under cover of the night.

11. This invisible world is often visualized as a distant mountain, sometimes identified as Mount Kupé in the south of Cameroon. Hence the other common name for *famla'* in the Mungo valley and in the Western (English-speaking) Grassfields is *kupé* (Notué and Perrois 1984:104; Bühler and Probst 1988:13). Warnier (1985) suggests that belief in *famla'* may have its origin in precolonial slave trade.

12. At least two concrete cases allegedly involving *famla'* are reported in the literature. Hurault cites a case of "ritual murder" for personal gain in Batie in 1955 (1962:121). I have reported on "the case of Etienne and the witches' *tontine*" in an earlier presentation (Feldman 1984:26–27). *Famla'* is a common topic of conversation throughout southern and western Cameroon, especially in taxi parks. Other ethnic groups fear the Bamiléké for their involvement in *famla'*, and deem this ability to sacrifice one's kin not surprising for a people who touch and even honor human remains.

13. See also Bledsoe 1997 on reproductive capacity.

14. Bangangté worry that the contraceptive pill also contributes to the breakdown of marital morality. They fear that contraceptive pills "ruin one's insides." This imported contraceptive device is little understood and not easily available in Bangangté. Its threat is in causing permanent infertility rather than temporary contraception. Renne's studies of IUDs and abortion in Nigeria reveals a similar mistrust of biomedical contraceptive methods (1994).

15. My Bangangté informants did not talk about the relationship of postpartum care to the new mother's continuing reproductive capacity. But statements of elderly women bemoaning what they perceive as increasingly narrow child spacing indicate that Bangangté may conceive of a need to recover from the strains of pregnancy and childbirth to maintain the ability to carry a pregnancy to a healthy outcome, similar to Bledsoe's findings among Gambian women (1997).

16. The data in this section are based on interviews and a written questionnaire given to staff at Bangangté Divisional Hospital, Bangwa Protestant Hospital, Centre de Santé Developpé de Bantoum, Fetom P.M.I. (Protection Maternelle et Infantile, an outreach clinic of Bangwa Hospital in one quarter of Bangangté town), and Ad Lucem Dispensaire (a Catholic health center on the northeast edge of Bangangté town). Fifty-three questionnaires from staff at every level of every department in the five institutions were returned.

17. Fernandez, based on fieldwork among the Fang of Gabon, suggests a very different reason for recently observed promiscuity in central African societies. The observation and experience of increasing sterility in a society plagued with sexually transmitted diseases may lead men and women to seek proof of their potency or fertility wherever they can. In addition, premarital sex and motherhood, formerly severely sanctioned, may now be necessary for young women to prove their ability to have children to potential husbands (Fernandez 1982).

18. These trends are similar to findings from the 1991 Demographic and Health

Survey of Cameroon, which found 40.2 percent of women aged 15–50 in the Western and Littoral Provinces to be in polygynous unions, compared to 38.6 percent in the national sample. In both regional and national samples, the percentage of women in polygynous unions decreases with decreasing age (e.g., 67 percent of women aged 45–49 vs. 24.9 percent of women aged 15–19 in polygynous unions in the Western and Littoral Provinces [Balépa, Fotso, and Barrère 1992a: 69]).

Chapter Five

1. Although the coastal peoples of Cameroon had had direct contact with European traders for centuries, the Bangangté and other Grassfields peoples experienced their first direct contact with Europeans only during the second decade of German colonial rule, that is, after 1895. Grassfields peoples previously had obtained numerous trade items of European origin, including beads and guns, through Duala middlemen.

2. The most detailed reports are from observers working among peoples closest to the important centers of German population: Plehn (1894:89–98) on Duala and Bakweri medicine, Zenker (1895:66–67) on Jaunde (Ewondo) medicine. The Duala and Bakweri live, respectively, around the port city of Douala and the cooler upland city of Buea, near the coast. The Ewondo live in the area surrounding Yaoundé, a city in the central rain forest that became the administrative capital in the final years of German colonization.

3. This valley is the site where mfen Njiké's wives had their largest farms in the mid-1980s and where several of his widows still resided in 1997.

4. Specifically Bamiléké labor, as distinguished from other Grassfields laborers, is documented in reports of railway construction and the creation of German cocoa, coffee, and rubber plantations in 1910 (Tardits 1960:87).

5. A series of medical surveys from a later period, conducted by British mandate forces in 1949 and cited by DeLancey (1978:160), exemplify the different disease rates in the Grassfields and plantation areas, and thus the grave medical problems faced by Bamiléké labor migrants. Only 5.53 percent of 8,264 surveyed inhabitants of Bafut (Western Grassfields) had malaria, as compared to 39.16 percent of 8,008 surveyed inhabitants of the plantation area. In the Grassfields, 9.08 percent of those surveyed suffered from filarial infections (e.g., elephantiasis, onchercerciasis) as compared to 50.64 percent of those surveyed in the plantation lowlands.

6. Most but not all government reports complain about decreasing population in the Grassfields. During his 1914 trip to Bana district, which included Bangangté, Zimmermann observed impressively dense population and the development of urban centers (1916:24).

7. Unfortunately, the Woermann archives have been destroyed. No mention of the offering of a cash prize, its date, or of studies submitted in the competition for this prize exist in the State Archives of Hamburg.

8. Tardits's sources are no longer to be found in French or Cameroonian archives. Relly's account of labor recruitment practices and the state of health of

Bamiléké labor recruits is found in "Rapport de tournée effectuée par M. H. Relly dans la chefferie de Baham, 16 au 25 octobre" (Tardits 1960:124).

9. Reports of the military medical services to France and of the French administration of Cameroon to the League of Nations are full of statistics on the activities of these mobile medical teams (e.g., on the assignment of physicians and their teams to specific ethnic areas: Beaudiment, Cavalade, and Maze 1930; on activities in the Bamiléké area: Vaisseau 1951:27, 32; Vaucel 1939:238, 332).

10. In that year, 1,125 Bamiléké women delivered their babies in government centers. The unfavorable political climate probably refers to agitation by Bamiléké veterans returning from World War II and involved in organizing the UPC trade union.

11. This history of public health institutions in Bangangté is based on the testimony of Tooua Raymond, elderly pharmacist of Bangangté Hospital and nearly lifelong resident of Bangangté. The 1936 annual report of the government health services mentions that the Bangangté dispensary building was in bad physical shape. At that time the Région de Noun had three physicians and 45 other public health employees, and boasted two hospitals (in Dschang and Foumban), one mother–child clinic (in Dschang), and four dispensaries in Bamiléké towns including Bangangté (Lefèvre 1936:23, 32, 33).

12. This remains true today. Debarge cites the following figures: 43 percent adult female, 25 percent adult male, 20 percent children between 2 and 15, and 12 percent infant patients (1934:66).

13. As Feierman (1986:140–41) points out, "In reality, western technology is not the only source of medical innovation. . . . Local non-Islamic medical traditions also alter themselves; they do not await the stimulus of contact with western technology. When household structures and disease patterns change, healers are forced to adapt or to be perceived as irrelevant. Local African practitioners are the creators of medical knowledge, not merely recipients of a medical tradition."

14. For an exemplary case study of the emergence of a new health-care institution that creatively combines elements of divergent medical systems see Mullings's discussion of spiritualist healing in urban Ghana (1984).

15. Some traditional practitioners refer to themselves as *ngafu* or *ngazenu,* rejecting implications of the ambivalent powers of owning kà. They are usually referred to as *ngakà,* with all its implications of social and asocial potential, by their clients.

16. This is the only instance in which Bangangté talk about spirit possession. *Zwiak,* breath, is sometimes referred to in the singular as "spirit," meaning the spirit of an individual. Neither minnyis nor others are possessed by their own or another's zwiak.

17. None of the participants in the following case explained the meaning of washing in raffia wine at the time of the rite. However, all referred to the event as a rite of reconciliation. In other contexts, sharing raffia wine is a way to express trust and unity among friends and even among parties with divergent interests (such as the parents of bride and groom at a wedding ceremony). "Cooked" raffia wine has acquired the special properties of a *cadi;* Bangangté believe it works like a poison ordeal, sparing those who keep the oath they have made upon it and

harming those who break the oath or swear in bad faith. All metaphoric uses of *nâ*, to cook, in Bangangté imply mysterious transformation of materials. Raffia wine is "cooked" by the *bandansi*, initiated members of a royal organization charged with overseeing the morality of the kingdom.

18. Hours (1985) describes the waiting corridors and benches of the two public biomedical institutions he studied in Douala as highly reminiscent of the waiting areas of police stations.

19. After the consultation, or when Nana was out of the room, several of Nana's patients described their long itineraries with "charlatan" or "fraudulent" healers to me, expressing their hope that they had finally found a "true" healer.

Chapter Six

1. The same expression, *to cry* or *pleurer,* is used both in Pidgin English and in French, to denote public mourning following the death of a close relative. Bangangté use both Pidgin and French expressions in everyday talk. They also use the Bangangté term, *vue. Vue* is an inclusive term for many forms of mourning and celebrating the dead, distinguished in practice by all Bangangté.

2. In 1997 I observed an even more bitter discourse of decline in the context of the politicization of ethnicity. Lively debate ensued in a bush taxi traveling from Yaoundé to Bangangté. Some said the mfen was "improving things at the palace," restoring the physical glory of the compound. Others countered that he was "far from the people" because of his support of the party in power (RDPC) while most Bangangté (indeed most Bamiléké and Western Grassfielders) supported the Social Democratic Front and suffered for their vocal opposition to the government. King Nji Monluh himself denied support for any one political party.

3. Even gender definitions are not fixed, depending upon varying sets of relationships and performances (Butler 1990; Weston 1993).

4. Rosaldo likewise critiques the anthropological study of death and grief for focusing on mortuary ritual, rather than on the wider range of experiences, emotions, and positions persons hold in relation to a death (1989:14–15).

5. *Bwopa'* is not referred to in German archival records, but Bangangté say it was built by the Germans at the end of Tchatchoua's and the beginning of Njiké II's reigns. Egerton refers to it as a "fearful . . . [and] . . . ambitious building, two storeys high, with a sort of loggia in front of it," and in bad repair so that "the only time I made the ascent, His Majesty was most solicitous about my safety" (1938:69). The "loggia" is a brick arcade typical of German colonial architecture in Cameroon. Egerton also mentions the current palace, begun during Egerton's visit in 1937 and for which the Chef de Subdivision, Monsieur Cazal, "acted as architect and clerk of the works" (1938:70). Bangangté describe Cazal as a particularly hard taskmaster who used forced labor for road building. They claim that this house was not completed in its present shape until the reign of mfen Pokam (1943–74), when the latter removed some interior walls to enlarge the salon. Nkwenga (1965:102–3) writes that upon Pokam's accession to the throne, only the foundations of the house designed by Cazal were completed. Pokam abandoned the con-

struction project to make a coffee plantation in the Noun valley. He completed construction of the present palace in 1955.

6. Articles 228 and 251 of the Cameroonian penal code of 1967 outlaw healers and antisorcery specialists (Rowlands and Warnier 1988:127). For an account of the ambiguous position of witchcraft in the Cameroonian courts, see Geschiere with Fisiy (1994).

7. For similar beliefs in a South American context, see Taussig (1980b).

8. The 1991 DHS shows a mortality rate of 109.3 per 1,000 for children under five in the Western and Littoral Provinces (lumped together as one region), compared to a national average of 126.3 per 1,000 (Balépa, Fotso, and Barrère 1992a:135; 1992b:18).

9. These missionaries did not recognize in writing their own contribution to the breakdown of morals, believing that Bangangté regulations of sexual and marital relations should be replaced by European Christian ones (Journal des Missions Evangéliques 1929:241).

10. Balshem makes a similar point in a very different context, identifying the rhetoric about cancer and "fate" among working-class residents of Philadelphia as a form of action, resistance to the individualization of guilt in hegemonic health education efforts (1991).

Glossary

Note: The prefix "ne" has been deleted from all infinitives

bagde'	(bagdə')	spoiled
bandansi		people of the house of god; members of a palace association charged with regulating and protecting the morals of the chiefdom
ba'tu	(bɑ' tu)	entry gate to royal compound, literally, houses of the head
bweh	(bwɛ)	camwood powder
bwo	(bwɔ)	good, healthy, beautiful (also mebwo)
bwopa'	(bwɔpa')	the good house; two-storey house built in German colonial era for the mfen
che' mfen	(cə' mfən)	royal retainer, literally, mfen's hat
chongwa	(coŋwa)	oversalted
dokta	(doktɑ)	doctor, nurse (from "Wes Cos" Pidgin)
du'nsi'	(dʉ' nsi')	sacrifice site
fa'		to work
famasi		pharmacy (from "Wes Cos" Pidgin)
famla'		witches' rotating credit association, with sacrifice of kin; term used throughout Bamiléké area; see nzo
famncwɛd		site of the first royal compound in Bangangté
fed	(fɛd)	to eat, using the teeth to cut or tear apart
fenkang	(fənkaŋ)	tree of peace; plant of the grass family used as sign of peace
fi		cool, fresh
fite	(fitə)	to cool
fon		generally recognized Grassfields term for paramount chief, widely used in the Anglophone (western Grassfields) area
fu		medicine ("simple"), herb, leaf

ju	(jʉ)	to eat, referring to sauces of ground, soft vegetable foods; socially positive commensuality
kà		medicine ("complicated"), magic, magical power
kan		law, norms
kebwo'	(kəbwɔ)	"complicated" (refers to persons and places), possessing mysterious powers and, for persons, being able to manipulate the weight of one's voice; all Bamiléké say "compliqué" in French
ko'		curse
kum		meeting, association
ku'nga		secret regulatory society; mfen's masked police force
la'	(lɑ')	compound, village
la'kam	(lɑ'kam)	residence of new mfen during interval between initiation and the birth of a daughter and a son
la'kwa	(lɑ'kwa)	mfen's initiation house
lem	(ləm)	blood
lem kebwo	(ləm kəbwɔ)	bad blood, making a woman sterile; believed incurable
li kebwo	(li kəbwɔ)	misfortune, literally, bad forehead
ma	(mɑ)	in a downhill direction
mabengoup	(mabəŋgup)	first queen, title of royal wife
mafam		sacred land cultivated by royal women, site of battle with Bamoum
mafen	(mâfən)	sacred forest and "complicated" part of royal compound
makokwa		title of third wife of mfen
mamfen	(mamfən)	queen mother
ma' ngut nze'	(mɑ' ŋgʉt nze')	ancestors, literally melon vines
manjo		male youth age-grade association
masou		association of royal and influential women
mbe	(mbə)	sacrifice sites, sacred forests or small groves
mbu nchwed	(mbu ncwɛd)	double avenue leading from gate to palace in royal compound, literally, foot of the royal compound
Medumba	(mədʉmba)	Bangangté language, part of the Mbam-Nkam group of Bantu languages, sometimes called semi-Bantu
mekat	(məkat)	white man

men fi	(mɛn fi)	newborn, literally, fresh person
mfen	(mfən)	paramount chief
mfi'		to measure (as in ingredients, volume)
mfi' mentun	(mfi' mentʉn)	to measure a person, that is, to procreate
minnyi	(mɪnnyi)	spirit medium
mongwe		moon, month
na		to cook
nânda	(nândɑ)	marriage, to cook inside
ncheb	(nceb)	fetish
nchwed,	(ncwɛd),	
mân nchwed	(mân ncwɛd)	royal compound
nchu' ntu	(ncʉ' ntʉ)	one heart, unity
nda	(ndɑ)	house
ndâ nja	(ndâ njɑ)	seclusion or circumcision house
ndâ nsi	(ndâ nsi)	the house of god
ndâ nzo	(ndɑ nzɔ)	the house of mystery, that is, famla'
ndap		praise name
ndjip pennjwi		midwife, literally, the eldest woman
ndonn	(ndɔnn)	custom, difficultés du coutume
ndum	(ndʉm)	vampire, person who has ntok, also ngafettok
nen	(nɛn)	to go
ne yen mongwe	(nə yɛn moŋgwe)	menstruation, literally, to see the moon
nga		person of . . . (indicator of profession or state)
ngafu		herbalist healer
ngakà		healer, magician
nga la	(ŋga lɑ')	compound head
nga ngome	(ŋga ŋgamə)	diviner, manipulator of the spider oracle
nga ngokwet	(ŋga ŋgokwɛt)	patient
nganzenu	(ŋganzɛnu)	sage, person who sees, healer
nganzo	(ŋganzɔ)	member of famla', witch
ngap nsi		chicken of god, that is, sacrificed poultry
ngo	(ŋgɔ)	country, chiefdom
ngokwet	(ŋgokwɛt)	illness
ngwala'	(ŋgwɑlɑ')	mfen's representative, highly ranked retainer
niam la'	(niam lɑ')	the mfen's kitchen, literally, behind the compound
nja	(njɑ)	puberty rite: seclusion and fattening of girls; circumcision of boys

njwi		woman
njwi mfen	(njwi mfən)	royal wife, wife of the mfen
nkam		noble
nkam be'e	(nkam bə'ə)	council of nine highest nobles, advisers to the mfen
nkam tan la'		quarter chief
nkwi		viscous sauce considered the quintessential Bamiléké food
Nsi		God
ntan	(ntɑn)	market
ntok	(ntɔk)	anthropophagic witchcraft, requiring substance in belly (also called ntok)
ntse kebwo	(ntsə kəbwɔ)	bad water, making a woman sterile; believed curable
ntu kebwo	(ntʉ kəbwɔ)	bad heart, that is, potential for witchcraft
ntun nda	(ntʉn ndɑ)	lineage, literally, foundation of the house
nu'u		to mix
nza'	(nzɑ')	decorative scarification
nzo	(nzɔ)	mystery; witches' rotating credit association; same as famla'
nzwikam		second queen, title of royal wife
nzwimânto		panther, animal double of the mfen
paa'		madness
pagla'		part of the village, referring to the two women's quarters of the royal compound
pam	(pɑm)	belly
pam nto'	(pam ntɔ')	uterine relations, literally, sack of intestines
pan pan	(pɑn pɑn)	simple or natural illness (no supernatural causation)
pa' tu		skull house
pen	(pən)	porridge (foofoo)
sheb	(shəb)	to catch, seize, as ancestors seize descendants to make them ill
sop		title of nobility
ta		father
tak		fresh ground maize with greens and palm oil, used as sacrifice to "feed" ancestors
tâmfen	(tâmfən)	title of nobility, literally, father of mfen
ta nkap		marriage form with marriage lords who have right to brideprice or off-

		spring of another's daughter; literally, father of money/brideprice
tela	(tɛlɑ')	center of the village or compound, refers also to women's quarter of the royal compound
tontine [Fr.]		rotating credit association
tsiyang		title of fourth wife of mfen
tu		head, skull (often used to refer to ancestors)
ven	(vɛn)	to carve or cut for nza' scarification
vu	(vʉè)	mourning, death celebration
yen	(yɛn)	to see
zi		an ordeal (cadi) to prove guilt or innocence
ziag		animal double, totem
zimewu	(zɪməwʉ)	the mfen's "madame," a favorite wife who accompanies him on official occasions
zwiak	(zwiɑk)	breath, locus of the spirit and symbol of life

References

Abu-Lughod, L.
  1986 Veiled Sentiments: Honor and Poetry in a Bedouin Society. Berkeley: University of California Press.
  1993 Writing Women's Worlds: Bedouin Stories. Berkeley: University of California Press.
Ardener, E.
  1962 Divorce and Fertility: An African Study. London: Oxford University Press.
  1970 Witchcraft, economics, and the continuity of belief. In M. Douglas, ed., Witchcraft Confessions and Accusations, 141–60. London: Tavistock.
  1972 Belief and the problem of women. In J. S. La Fontaine, ed., The Interpretation of Ritual. London: Tavistock. (Reprinted in S. Ardener, ed. [1975], Perceiving Women, 1–17. New York: Wiley.)
Arens, W.
  1980 Taxonomy versus dynamics revisited: The interpretation of misfortune in a polyethnic community. In I. Karp and C. Bird, eds., Explorations in African Systems of Thought. Bloomington: Indiana University Press, 165–80.
Arens, W., and I. Karp
  1989 Introduction. In W. Arens and I. Karp, eds., Creativity of Power: Cosmology and Action in African Societies, xi–xxix. Washington: Smithsonian Institution Press.
Armstrong, E.
  1983 Political Anatomy of the Body: Medical Knowledge in Britain in the Twentieth Century. Cambridge: Cambridge University Press.
Austin, J. L.
  1962 How to Do Things with Words. New York: Oxford University Press.
Balépa, M., M. Fotso, and B. Barrère
  1992a Enquête Démographique et de Santé Cameroun 1991. Yaoundé: Direction Nationale du Deuxième Recensement Général de la Population et de l'Habitat. Columbia, MD: Macro International.
  1992b Cameroon Demographic and Health Survey 1991: Summary Report. Yaoundé: National Department of the Second General Population and Housing Census. Columbia, MD: Macro International.

Balshem, M.
1991 Cancer, control, and causality: Talking about cancer in a working-class community. *American Ethnologist* 18 (1): 152–72.

Bannerman, R. H.
1982 Traditional medicine in modern health care. *World Health Forum* 3 (1): 8–26.

Barbier, J. C., G. Courade, and P. Gubry
1978 L'Exode rural au Cameroun. Yaoundé: ONAREST, ISH.

Basel Mission
n.d. Ärztliche Mission in Kamerun. Unpublished MS in Basel Mission Archives, Basel, Switzerland.

Bayart, J.-F.
1979 L'Etat au Cameroun. Paris: Presses de la Fondation Nationale des Sciences Politiques.
1993 The State in Africa: The Politics of the Belly. London: Longman.

Beaudiment, Cavalade, and Maze
1930 Rapport sur la Prospection du Foyer Endemo-Epidemique de Trypanosomiase de Bafia. (Archives Techniques-Marseille, Box 1, Rapports Annuels SDN 1928–31.)

Becker, G.
1994 Metaphors in disrupted lives. *Medical Anthropology Quarterly* 8 (4): 383–410.

Beidelman, T. O.
1966 Swazi royal ritual. *Africa* 36:373–405.
1986 Moral Imagination in Kaguru Modes of Thought. Bloomington: Indiana University Press.

Beneria, L., and G. Sen
1981 Accumulation, reproduction, and women's role in economic development: Boserup revisited. *Signs* 7 (2): 279–98.

Berger, P., B. Berger, and H. Kellner
1973 The Homeless Mind: Modernization and Consciousness. New York: Random House.

Biya, P.
1987 Communal Liberalism. London: Macmillan.

Blank, D.
1985 The modern elite and traditional titles in Babungo. Paper presented at the Conference of the Grassfields Working Group, Bamenda, December.

Bledsoe, C.
1997 Reproduction and Aging in the Rural Gambia: African Empirical Challenges for the Culture of Western Science. Unpublished MS.

Bleek, W.
1976 Witchcraft, gossip and death: A social drama. *Man* (N.S.) 11:526–41.

Boddy, J.
1989 Wombs and Alien Spirits: Women, Men and the Zar Cult in Northern Sudan. Madison: University of Wisconsin Press.

Boog, J.-C.
1986 Département du Ndé, Population (1984 Estimation Service Provinciel Statistique Ouest). Bangangté, January 2, 1986.
Boserup, E.
1970 Woman's Role in Economic Development. London: George Allen and Unwin.
Boston Women's Health Book Collective
1984 The New Our Bodies, Ourselves. New York: Simon and Schuster.
Boswell, D. M.
1969 Personal crises and the mobilization of the social network. In J. C. Mitchell, ed., Social Networks in Urban Situations, 245–96. Manchester: Manchester University Press.
Bourdieu, P.
1977 Outline of a Theory of Practice. Cambridge: Cambridge University Press.
Brain, R.
1972 Bangwa Kinship and Marriage. Cambridge: Cambridge University Press.
Browner, C. H.
1986 The politics of reproduction in a Mexican village. *Signs* 11 (4): 710–24.
Browner, C. H., and S. T. Perdue
1988 Women's secrets: Bases for reproductive and social autonomy in a Mexican community. *American Ethnologist* 15 (1): 84–97.
Bühler, B., and P. Probst
1988 Medicine as a political category: The case of the Wiya-Wimbum of the Cameroon Grassfields. Paper presented at the conference "Ethnomedical Systems in Sub-Saharan Africa," African Studies Centre, Leiden University, The Netherlands, June.
Butler, J.
1990 Gender Trouble. New York: Routledge.
Caldwell, J. C., and P. Caldwell.
1987 The cultural context of high fertility in sub-Saharan Africa. *Population and Development Review* 13 (3): 409–38.
Calhoun, C.
1994 Social theory and the politics of identity. In C. Calhoun, ed., Social Theory and the Politics of Identity, 9–36. Oxford: Blackwell.
Cartron, Médecin Commandant
1934 Étude démographique comparée des pays Bamiléké et Bamoum (Cameroun). *Annales de Médecine et des Pharmacies Coloniales* 37:350–63.
Chavunduka, G. L., and M. Last
1986 African medical professions today. In M. Last and G. L. Chavunduka, eds., The Professionalization of African Medicine, 259–69. Manchester: Manchester University Press in association with the International African Institute.
Collier, J. F., and S. J. Yanagisako
1987 Gender and Kinship: Essays Toward a Unified Analysis. Stanford: Stanford University Press.

Comaroff, J.
1980 Healing and the cultural order: The case of the Barolong boo Ratshidi of southern Africa. *American Ethnologist* 7 (4): 637–57.
1981 Healing and cultural transformation: The Tswana of southern Africa. *Social Science and Medicine* 15B:367–78.
1982 Medicine: Symbol and ideology. In P. Wright and A. Treacher, eds., The Problem of Medical Knowledge, 49–68. Edinburgh: Edinburgh University Press.
1985 Body of Power, Spirit of Resistance: The Culture and History of a South African People. Chicago: University of Chicago Press.
1993 The diseased heart of Africa: Medicine, colonialism, and the black body. In S. Lindenbaum and M. Lock, eds., Knowledge, Power and Practice: The Anthropology of Medicine and Everyday Life, 305–29. Berkeley: University of California Press.
Conrau, G.
1898 Einige Beiträge über die Völker zwischen Mpundu und Bali. Wissenschaftliche Beihefte zum Deutschen Kolonialblatte: Mittheilungen von Forschungsreiseneden und Gelehrten aus den Deutschen Schutzgebieten 11 (3): 194–204.
1899 Im Lande der Bangwa. Wissenschaftliche Beihefte zum Deutschen Kolonialblatte . . . 12 (4): 201–9.
Cordell, D., and J. Gregory
1994 African Population and Capitalism: Historical Perspectives. Madison: University of Wisconsin Press.
Csordas, T., and A. Kleinmann
1996 Therapeutic process. In Medical Anthropology: Contemporary Theory and Method, 3–20. Westport, CT: Praeger.
Debarge, J.
1934 La Mission Médicale au Cameroun. Paris: Société des Missions Evangéliques.
De Boeck, F.
1995 Lorsque la faim court le pays: La faim et l'alimentation parmi les Luunda du Zaire. In R. Devisch, F. De Boeck, and D. Jonckers, eds., Alimentations, Traditions et Développements en Afrique Intertropicale, 85–116. Paris: Harmattan.
De Heusch, L.
1980 Heat, physiology and cosmogony: Rites de passage among the Thonga. In Explorations in African Systems of Thought, eds. I. Karp and C. Bird. Bloomington: Indiana University Press.
1982 The Drunken King, or the Origin of the State. Bloomington: Indiana University Press.
DeLancey, M. W.
1978 Health and disease on the plantations of Cameroon, 1884–1939. In G. W. Hartwig and K. D. Patterson, eds., Disease in African History, 153–79. Durham, NC: Duke University Press.

Delaney, C.
1986 The meaning of paternity and the virgin birth debate. *Man* (N.S.) 21:494–513.
1987 Seeds of honor, fields of shame. In D. Gilmore, ed., Honor and Shame and the Unity of the Mediterranean. American Anthropological Association Special Volume no. 22, 35–48. Washington, DC: American Anthropological Association.
1991 The Seed and the Soil: Gender and Cosmology in Turkish Village Society. Berkeley: University of California Press.
den Ouden, J. H. B.
1980 Incorporation and changes in the composite household. The effects of coffee introduction and food crop commercialization in two Bamiléké chiefdoms, Cameroon. In C. Presvelou and S. Spijkers-Zwart, eds., The Household, Women and Agricultural Development, 41–67. Wageningen: H. Veenman and Zonen, B.V.
1987 In search of personal mobility: Changing interpersonal relations in two Bamiléké chiefdoms, Cameroon. *Africa* 57 (1): 3–27.
de Rosny, E.
1981 Les Yeux de Ma Chèvre: Sur les Pas des Maîtres de la Nuit en Pays Douala (Cameroun). Paris: Plon.
Dettwyler, K. A.
1988 More than nutrition: Breastfeeding in urban Mali. *Medical Anthropology Quarterly* (N.S.) 2 (2): 172–83.
Devisch, R.
1985 Se Recréer Femme: Manipulation Sémantique d'une Situation d'Infécondité chez les Yaka du Zaire. Berlin: Dietrich Reimer.
1993 Weaving the Threads of Life: The Khita Gyn-eco-logical Healing Cult among the Yaka. Chicago: University of Chicago Press.
Diduk, S.
1989 Women's agricultural production and political action in the Cameroon Grassfields. *Africa* 59 (3): 338–55.
Dieckmann, N., and H. Joldersma
1982 Cultivating the Fields and Plaiting Mats: The Changes in the Situation of Women in a Bamiléké Chiefdom, Cameroon. Wageningen: Agricultural University.
Diehn, O.
1956 Kaufmannschaft und Deutsche Eingeborenenpolitik in Togo und Kamerun von der Jahrhundertwende bis zum Ausbruch des Weltkrieges. Unpublished doctoral dissertation, Universität Hamburg. Found in Staatsarchiv Bremen.
Dongmo, J.-L.
1981 Le Dynamisme Bamiléké (Cameroun). Vol. 1, La Maîtrise de l'espace agraire. Yaoundé: Université de Yaoundé.
Douglas, M.
1966 Purity and Danger: An Analysis of the Concepts of Pollution and Taboo. London: Routledge and Kegan Paul.

1970 Introduction. In M. Douglas, ed., Witchcraft Confessions and Accusations, xiii–xxxviii. London: Tavistock.

Doyal, L.
1979 The Political Economy of Health. Boston: South End Press.

Durkheim, E., and M. Mauss
1903 (1976) Primitive Classification. Trans. and introduction by R. Needham. Chicago: University of Chicago Press.

Ebin, V.
1982 Interpretations of infertility: The Aowin people of south-west Ghana. In C. P. MacCormack, ed., Ethnography of Fertility and Birth, 141–59. London: Academic.

Egerton, C.
1938 African Majesty: A Record of Refuge at the Court of the King of Bangangté in the French Cameroons. London: George Routledge and Sons.

Elias, N.
1939 (1982) The Civilizing Process: Vol. 2, Power and Civility. English translation of Über den Prozess der Zivilisation. New York: Random House.

Evans-Pritchard, E. E.
1937 Witchcraft, Oracles and Magic among the Azande (abridged edition, 1976). Oxford: Oxford University Press.
1940 The Nuer. Oxford: Clarendon Press.

Farinaud, Médecin Colonel
1944 Rapport Annuel, Année 1944. Yaoundé: Cameroun Français, Service de Santé.
1945 Rapport Annuel, Année 1945. Yaoundé: Cameroun Français, Service de Santé.

Farmer, P.
1988 Bad blood, spoiled milk: Bodily fluids as moral barometers in rural Haiti. *American Ethnologist* 15 (1): 62–83.

Feeley-Harnik, G.
1981 The Lord's Table: Eucharist and Passover in Early Christianity. Philadelphia: University of Pennsylvania Press.
1985 Issues in divine kingship. Annual Review of Anthropology 14:273–313.
1991 A Green Estate: Restoring Independence in Madagascar. Washington, DC: Smithsonian Institution Press.
1995 Plants and people, children or wealth? Shifting grounds of "choice" in Madagascar. *PoLAR* (Political and Legal Anthropology Review) 18:45–64.

Feierman, S.
1981 Therapy as a system-in-action in northeastern Tanzania. *Social Science and Medicine* 15B:353–60.
1985 Struggles for control. *African Studies Review* 28:73–147.
1986 Reply to Imperato. *African Studies Review* 29 (2): 140–41.

Feierman, S., and J. Janzen, eds.
1992 The Social Basis of Health and Healing in Africa. Berkeley: University of California Press.

Feldman, P.
1984 Social change and the interpretation of misfortune: Recent Bamiléké witchcraft afflictions. Paper presented to The Atlantic History, Culture and Society Seminar, Johns Hopkins University, February 28, 1984.
1985 Bamiléké women and misfortune. Unpublished MS.

Feldman-Savelsberg, P.
1990 "Then we were many": Bangangté Women's Conceptions of Health, Fertility and Social Change in a Bamiléké Chiefdom, Cameroon. Ph.D. dissertation, Department of Anthropology, Johns Hopkins University. Ann Arbor, MI: University Microfilms International.
1994 Plundered kitchens, empty wombs: Fear of infertility in the Cameroonian Grassfields. *Social Science and Medicine* 39 (4): 463–74.
1995 Cooking inside: Kinship and gender in Bangangté idioms of marriage and procreation. *American Ethnologist* 22 (3): 483–501.
1997 Stolen babies and personal mobility: Gender, fertility, and social inequality in Bangangté. Unpublished MS.

Fernandez, J.
1965 Symbolic consensus in a Fang reformative cult. *American Anthropologist* 67 (4): 902–29.
1982 Bwiti. Princeton: Princeton University Press.
1986 Persuasions and Performances: The Play of Tropes in Culture. Bloomington: Indiana University Press.

Fisher, L.
1984 Colonial Madness: Mental Health in the Barbadian Social Order. New Brunswick, NJ: Rutgers University Press.

Fisiy, C., and P. Geschiere
1991 Sorcery, witchcraft and accumulation: regional variations in south and west Cameroon. *Critique of Anthropology* 11 (3): 251–78.

Fjellman, S. M., and M. Goheen
1984 A prince by any other name? Identity and politics in highland Cameroon. *American Ethnologist* 11 (3): 473–86.

Fortes, M.
1968 On installation ceremonies. Proceedings of the Royal Anthropological Institute 1967:5–20.

Foster, G. M.
1976 Disease etiologies in non-western medical systems. *American Anthropologist* 78:773–82.

Foster, G. M., and B. G. Anderson
1978 Medical Anthropology. New York: Wiley.

Foucault, M.
1973 Birth of the Clinic. New York: Pantheon.

Frank, O., and G. McNicoll
1987 An Interpretation of Fertility and Population Policy in Kenya, Center for Policy Studies Working Papers, 131. New York: Population Council.

Frankenberg, R., ed.

1988   Gramsci, Marxism, and Phenomenology: Essays for the Development of Critical Medical Anthropology. Special issue, *Medical Anthropology Quarterly* (N.S.) 2 (4): 323–464.

Frazer, J. G.

1922   The Golden Bough (abridged ed.). London: Macmillan.

Frisch, R. E.

1975   Critical weight, a critical body composition, menarche, and the maintenance of menstrual cycles. In E. S. Watts, F. E. Johnson, and G. W. Lasker, eds., Biosocial Interrelations in Population Adaptation, 319–52 (cited in MacCormack 1982:7). The Hague: Mouton.

1978   Population, food intake and fertility. *Science* 119:22 (cited in MacCormack 1982:7).

Gal, S.

1991   Between speech and silence: The problematics of research on language and gender. In M. Di Lionardo, ed., Gender at the Crossroads of Knowledge: Feminist Anthropology in the Postmodern Era, 175–203. Berkeley: University of California Press.

Geary, C. M.

1986   On Legal Change in Cameroon: Women, Marriage, and Bridewealth. Working Papers in African Studies, 113. Boston: African Studies Center, Boston University.

Geschiere, P.

1980   Child-witches against the authority of their elders: Anthropology and history in the analysis of witchcraft beliefs of the Maka (southeast Cameroon). In R. Schefold, J. W. Schoorl and J. Tennekes, eds., Man, Meaning and History: Essays in Honour of H.G. Schulte Nordholt, 268–99. The Hague: Martinus Nijhoff.

1982   Village Communities and the State. London: Routledge and Kegan Paul.

Geschiere, P., with C. Fisiy

1994   Domesticating personal violence: Witchcraft, courts and confessions in Cameroon. *Africa* 64 (3): 323–41.

Ghomsi, E.

1971   La naissance des chefferies Bamiléké et les relations entre divers groupements avant la conquête allemande. *Revue Camerounaise d'Histoire* 1:94–121.

Giddens, A.

1976   New Rules of Sociological Method: A Positive Critique of Interpretative Sociologies. New York: Basic Books.

Gillies, E.

1976   Introduction. In E. E. Evans-Pritchard, Witchcraft, Oracles and Magic, vii–xxxiii. Oxford: Oxford University Press.

Gluckman, M.

1950   Kinship and Marriage among the Lozi of Northern Rhodesia and the Zulu of Natal. In A. R. Radcliffe-Brown and Daryll Forde, eds., African Systems of Kinship and Marriage. London: Oxford University Press.

1954　Rituals of Rebellion in South-East Africa. Frazer Lecture, 1952. Manchester: Manchester University Press.

1955　The utility of the equilibrium model in the study of social change. *American Anthropologist* 70:219–35.

1963　Rituals of rebellion in South East Africa. In Order and Rebellion in Tribal Africa: Collected Essays. New York: Free Press.

Goheen, M.

1992　Chiefs, sub-chiefs and local control: Negotiations over land, struggles over meaning. *Africa* 62 (3): 389–412.

1996　Men Own the Fields, Women Own the Crops: Gender and Power in the Cameroon Grassfields. Madison: University of Wisconsin Press.

Goldschmidt, D.

1986　Le Corps chez les Bamiléké de Bandjoun (Cameroun). Thèse présentée pour le Doctorat en Médecine, Diplôme d'État, Université Louis Pasteur, Faculté de Médecine de Strasbourg.

Goody, J.

1958　(Ed.) The Developmental Cycle in Domestic Groups. Cambridge: Cambridge University Press.

1976　Farming, labour and sex. Chapter 4 in Production and Reproduction: A Comparative Study of the Domestic Domain, 31–40. Cambridge: Cambridge University Press.

Gottlieb, A.

1992　Under the Kapok Tree: Identity and Difference in Beng Thought. Chicago: University of Chicago Press.

Greenhalgh, S.

1990　Toward a political economy of fertility: Anthropological contributions. *Population and Development Review* 16 (1): 85–106.

1994　Controlling births and bodies in village China. *American Ethnologist* 21 (1): 3–30.

1995　Anthropology theorizes reproduction: Integrating practice, political economic, and feminist perspectives. In S. Greenhalgh, ed., Situating Fertility: Anthropology and Demographic Inquiry, 3–28. Cambridge: Cambridge University Press.

Guenther, M. G.

1976　From hunters to squatters. In R. Lee and I. DeVore, eds., Kalahari Hunter-Gatherers, 120–34. Cambridge: Harvard University Press.

Guyer, J. I.

1981　Household and community in African studies. *African Studies Review* (2/3): 87–137.

1987　Feeding African Cities: Studies in Regional Social History. Bloomington: Indiana University Press in association with International African Institute.

Hahn, R. A., and A. D. Gaines, eds.

1985　Physicians of Western Medicine. Dordrecht: Reidel.

Hammel, E.

1990　A theory of culture for demography. *Population and Development Review* 16 (5): 455–85.

Handwerker, L.
1995 The hen that can't lay an egg. (*Bu Xia Dan de Mu Ji*): Conceptions of Female Infertility in Modern China. In J. Terry and J. Urla, eds., Deviant Bodies: Critical Perspectives on Difference in Science and Popular Culture, 358–86. Bloomington: Indiana University Press.

Handwerker, W. P.
1990 Politics and reproduction: A window on social change. In W. P. Handwerker, ed., Births and Power: Social Change and the Politics of Reproduction, 1–38. Boulder: Westview.

Hannerz, U.
1987 The World in Creolization. *Africa* 57 (4): 546–59.

Haraway, D.
1988 Situated knowledges: The science question in feminism and the privilege of partial perspective. *Feminist Studies* 14:575–99.

Harris, M., and E. B. Ross
1987 Death, Sex, and Fertility: Population Regulation in Pre-industrial and Developing Societies. New York: Columbia University Press.

Hartwig, G.
1972 Long distance trade and the evolution of sorcery among the Kerebe. *International Journal of African Historical Studies* 4:505–25.

Harwood, A.
1988 Editorial introduction: A discussion about "discourse." *Medical Anthropology Quarterly* (N.S.) 2 (2): 99–101.

Heald, S.
1982 The making of men: The relevance of vernacular psychology to the interpretation of a Gisu ritual. *Africa* 52 (1): 15–36.

Héritier, F.
1984 Stérilité, aridité, sécheresse: Quelques invariants de la pensée symbolique. In M. Augé and C. Herzlich, eds., Le Sens du Mal: Anthropologie, Histoire, Sociologie de la Maladie, 123–54. Paris: Editions des Archives Contemporaines.

Hocart, A. M.
1936 (1970) Kings and Councillors: An Essay in the Comparative Anatomy of Human Society. Chicago: University of Chicago Press.

Hoch-Smith, J., and A. Spring
1978 Introduction. In J. Hoch-Smith and A. Spring, eds., Women in Ritual and Symbolic Roles, 1–23. New York: Plenum.

Hours, B.
1985 L'État Sorcier: Santé Publique et Société au Cameroun. Paris: Harmattan.

Hunt, N.
1993 Negotiated Colonialism: Domesticity, Hygiene, and Birth Work in the Belgian Congo. Madison: University of Wisconsin Press.

Huntington, R.
1988 Gender and Social Structure in Madagascar. Bloomington: Indiana University Press.

Hurault, J.
1962   La Structure Sociale des Bamiléké. Paris: Mouton.
Hutter, Lieutenant
1892   Cermonien beim Schliessen von Blutfreundschaft bei den Graslandstäm-
men im Kamerun-Hinterland. Wissenschaftliche Beihefte zum
Deutschen Kolonialblatte: Mittheilungen von Forschungsreisenden und
Gelehrten aus den Deutschen Schutzgebieten 5 (4): 176–84.
Inhorn, M.
1994a   Quest for Conception: Gender, Infertility, and Egyptian Medical Traditions. Philadelphia: University of Pennsylvania Press.
1994b   Interpreting infertility: Medical anthropological perspectives. Social
Science and Medicine 39 (4): 459–61.
1996   Infertility and Patriarchy: The Cultural Politics of Gender and Family
Life in Egypt. Philadelphia: University of Pennsylvania Press.
Janzen, J.
1978a   The Quest for Therapy: Medical Pluralism in Lower Zaire. Berkeley:
University of California Press.
1978b   The comparative study of medical systems as changing social systems.
Social Science and Medicine 12:121–29.
1982   Lemba, 1650–1930: A Drum of Affliction in Africa and the New World.
New York: Garland.
1987   Therapy management: Concept, reality, process. Medical Anthropology
Quarterly (N.S.) 1:68–84.
Jordan, B.
1993   Birth in Four Cultures: A Crosscultural Investigation of Childbirth in
Yucatan, Holland, Sweden and the United States. Montreal: Eden.
Joseph, R. A.
1977   Radical Nationalism in Cameroun: Social Origins of the UPC (Union
des Populations du Cameroun) Rebellion. Oxford: Clarendon.
Journal des Missions Evangéliques
1929   Rapport annuel. Journal des Missions Evangéliques, 104.
Kaberry, P. M.
1952   Women of the Grassfields: A Study of the Economic Position of Women
in Bamenda, British Cameroons. London: Her Majesty's Stationery
Office.
1962   Retainers and royal households in the Grassfields of Cameroon. Cahiers
d'études Africaines 3:282–98.
1969   Witchcraft of the sun: Incest in Nso. In M. Douglas and P. M. Kaberry,
eds., Man in Africa, 175–95. London: Tavistock.
Karp, I.
1980   Beer drinking and social experience in an African society: An essay in
formal sociology. In I. Karp and C. S. Bird, eds., Explorations in African
Systems of Thought, 83–119. Bloomington: Indiana University Press.
1987   Laughter at marriage: Subversion in Performance. In D. Parkin and D.
Nyamwaya, eds., Transformations of African Marriage, 137–54. Manchester: Manchester University Press for the International African Institute.

1989 Power and capacity in rituals of possession. In W. Arens and I. Karp, eds., Creativity of Power: Cosmology and Action in African Societies, 91–109. Washington: Smithsonian Institution Press.

Kertzer, D. I.
1993 Sacrificed for Honor: Italian Infant Abandonment and the Politics of Reproductive Control. Boston: Beacon Press.
1995 Political-economic and cultural explanations of demographic behavior. In S. Greenhalgh, ed., Situating Fertility: Anthropology and Demographic Inquiry, 29–52. Cambridge: Cambridge University Press.

Kiernan, J. P.
1982 The "Problem of Evil" in the context of ancestral intervention in the affairs of the living in Africa. Man (N.S.) 17:287–301.

Kleinman, A.
1980 Patients and Healers in the Context of Culture. Berkeley: University of California Press.

Koenig, D. B.
1977 Sex, Work and Social Class in Cameroon. Unpublished Ph.D. dissertation, Northwestern University.

Kollehlon, K. T.
1984 Women's work role and fertility in Liberia. Africa 54 (4): 31–45.

Kreager, P.
1997 Population and identity. In D. Kertzer and T. Fricke, eds., Anthropological Demography: Toward a New Synthesis, 139–74. Chicago: University of Chicago Press.

Kuczynski, R.R.
1939 The Cameroons and Togoland: A Demographic Study. London: Oxford University Press.

Kuper, H.
1944 A ritual of kingship among the Swazi. Africa 14:230–56.
1947 An African Aristocracy: Rank among the Swazi. London: Oxford University Press.
1963 The Swazi: An African Kingdom. New York: Holt, Rinehart, Winston.
1972 A royal ritual in a changing historical context. Cahiers d'etudes Africaines 12:593–615.
1978 Sobhuza: Ngwenyama and King of Swaziland. London: Duckworth.
1986 The Swazi: A South African Kingdom (2d ed.). New York: Holt, Rinehart, Winston.

Lakoff, G., and M. Johnson
1980 Metaphors We Live By. Chicago: Chicago University Press.

Last, M., and G. L. Chavunduka, eds.
1986 The Professionalisation of African Medicine. Manchester: Manchester University Press.

Layne, L. L.
1990 Motherhood lost: Cultural dimensions of miscarriage and stillbirth in America. Women and Health 16 (3/4): 69–98.

1992   Of fetuses and angels: Fragmentation and integration in narratives of pregnancy loss. *Knowledge and Society: The Anthropology of Science and Technology* 9:29–58.

Leach, E.
1964   Anthropological aspects of language: Animal categories and verbal abuse. In E.H. Lenneberg, ed., New Directions in the Study of Language, 23–62. Cambridge, MA: MIT Press.

Lee, R.
1984   The Dobe !Kung. Ed. G. Spindler and L. Spindler. Toronto: Holt, Rinehart and Winston.

Lefèvre, Médecin Colonel
1936   Rapport Annuel, Année 1936. Yaoundé: Service de Santé, Territoires du Cameroun.

LeVine, V.
1964   The Cameroons from Mandate to Independence. Berkeley: University of California Press.

LeVine, V., and R. P. Nye
1974   Historical Dictionary of Cameroon. Metuchen, NJ: Scarecrow Press.

Lévi-Strauss, C.
1963   (1949) The effectiveness of symbols. Chapter 10 in Structural Anthropology. New York: Basic Books.
1966   The Savage Mind. Chicago: University of Chicago Press.
1967   The Raw and the Cooked: Introduction to a Science of Mythology, vol. 1. New York: Harper and Row.

Lewis, I. M.
1966   Spirit Possession and Deprivation Cults. *Man: Journal of the Royal Anthropological Institute* 1:306–29.

Lindenbaum, S.
1979   Kuru Sorcery: Disease and Danger in the New Guinea Highlands. Palo Alto: Mayfield.
1987   The mystification of female labors. In J. F. Collier and S. J. Yanagisako, eds., Gender and Kinship: Essays Toward a Unified Analysis, 221–43. Stanford: Stanford University Press.

Long, N.
1968   Social Change and the Individual: A Study of the Social and Religious Responses to Innovation in a Zambian Rural Community. Manchester: Manchester University Press.

MacCormack, C. P.
1977   Biological events and cultural control. *Signs* 3 (1): 93–100.
1982   Biological, cultural and social adaptation in human fertility and birth: A synthesis. In C. P. MacCormack, ed., Ethnography of Fertility and Birth, 1–24. London: Academic.

Malinowski, B.
1929   The Sexual Life of Savages in North-Western Melanesia: An Ethnographic Account of Courtship, Marriage, and Family Life among the

Natives of the Trobriand Islands, British New Guinea. London: George Routledge and Sons.

Martin, E.

1987 The Woman in the Body: A Cultural Analysis of Reproduction. Boston: Beacon Press.

1991 The egg and the sperm. *Signs* 16 (3): 485–501.

Marwick, M. G.

1952 The social context of Cêwa witch beliefs. *Africa* 22 (2): 120–35; 22 (3): 215–33.

1965 Sorcery in Its Social Setting. Manchester: Manchester University Press.

Mason, K. O., and A. M. Taj

1987 Differences between women's and men's reproductive goals in developing countries. *Population and Development Review* 13 (4): 611–38.

Mauss, M.

1938 (1979) A category of the human mind: The notion of Person, the notion of 'Self.' In M. Mauss, ed., Sociology and Psychology: Essays. Trans. Ben Brewster, 57–94. London: Routledge and Kegan Paul.

Mayer, P.

1954 Witches. Inaugural Lecture, Rhodes University, Grahamstown.

Meigs, A.

1984 Food, Sex, and Pollution: A New Guinea Religion. New Brunswick, NJ: Rutgers University Press.

Meillassoux, C.

1981 (1975) Maidens, Meal and Money: Capitalism and the Domestic Community. Cambridge: Cambridge University Press.

Miaffo, D.

1977 Rôle Social de l'Autopsie Publique Traditionelle chez les Bamiléké. Mémoire pour D.E.S., Department of Sociology, University of Yaoundé.

Middleton, J.

1960 Lugbara Religion: Ritual and Authority among an East African People. London: Oxford University Press.

Mintz, S.

1985 Sweetness and Power: The Place of Sugar in Modern History. New York: Viking.

1996 Tasting Food, Tasting Freedom: Excursions into Eating, Culture, and the Past. Boston: Beacon Press.

Mitchell, J. C.

1956 The Yao Village. Manchester: Manchester University Press.

1965 The meaning in misfortune for urban Africans. In M. Fortes and G. Dieterlen, eds., African Systems of Thought. London: Oxford University Press.

Modell, J.

1989 Last chance babies: Interpretations of parenthood in an in vitro fertilization program. *Medical Anthropology Quarterly* (N.S.) 3 (2): 124–38.

Moore, H.
1994 A Passion for Difference: Essays in Anthropology and Gender. Bloomington: Indiana University Press.

Moore, S. F.
1994 Anthropology and Africa: Changing Perspectives on a Changing Scene. Charlottesville: University Press of Virginia.

Mullings, L.
1976 Women and economic change in Africa. In N. Hafkin and E. Bay, eds., Women in Africa, 239–64. Stanford: Stanford University Press.

1984 Therapy, Ideology and Social Change: Mental Healing in Urban Ghana. Berkeley: University of California Press.

Muna, W. F. T.
1981 How I encountered the sophisticated traditional healer. *Journal of the American Medical Association* 246 (22): 2618–19.

Myerhoff, B.
1978 Bobbes and zeydes: Old and new roles for elderly Jews. In J. Hoch-Smith and A. Spring, eds., Women in Ritual and Symbolic Roles, 207–41. New York: Plenum.

Ndachi Tagne, D.
1986 La Reine Captive. Paris: Harmattan.

Ndonko, F. T.
1986 Une étude sociologique de la chance comme représentation chez les Bamiléké. Unpublished MS.

1987a La force de la Tradition: Un Chef Bamiléké Explique. An interview with *Mfen* Nji Monluh Seidou Pokam, April 1987, Bangangté. Excerpts published under the title "Le futur chef Bangangté, Pokam Seidou Nji Monluh, entre en période d'initiation au 'La'kwa'," Cameroon Tribune 3865:19, May 8, 1987.

1987b Representations Culturelles de l'Epilepsie chez les Bamiléké: Le Cas de Maham. Yaoundé: Mémoire de Maîtrise en Anthropologie, Department of Sociology, University of Yaoundé.

Ngomsi, E.
1986 Peoples of the Western Province, Lecture presented at American Cultural Center, Yaoundé, March 6.

Ngongo, L.
1982 Histoire des Forces Religieuses au Cameroun. Paris: Karthala.

Ngubane, H.
1981 Aspects of clinical practice and traditional organization of indigenous healers in South Africa. *Social Science and Medicine* 15B:361–65.

Njiké-Bergeret, C.
1997 Ma Passion Africaine. Paris: Éditions C.L. Lattès.

Njinga, J.
1938 Réponse à l'Enquête No. I-C sur l'Alimentation des Indigènes. Bangangté, July 10, 1938 (from the archives of Claude Tardits).

Nkwenga, J.
1965 Histoire de la chefferie de Bangangté. *Abbia* 9/10:91–129.

Nkwi, P. N.
1987 Traditional Diplomacy: A Study of Inter-chiefdom Relations in the Western Grassfields, Northwest Province of Cameroon. Yaoundé: University of Yaoundé.

Nkwi, P. N., and F. T. Ndonko
1988 The perception of epilepsy: The Maham of the Nde Division West Province of Cameroon. Paper presented at the conference "Ethnomedical Systems in Sub-Saharan Africa," African Studies Centre, Leiden University, The Netherlands, June.

Nkwi, P. N., and F. Nyamnjoh
1997 Cameroon regional balance policy and national integration: Food for an uncertain future. In P. N. Nkwi and F. B. Nyamnjoh, eds., Regional Balance and National Integration in Cameroon, 8–16. Leiden: African Studies Centre and Yaoundé: ICASSRT.

Nkwi, P. N., and A. Socpa
1997 Ethnicity and Party Politics in Cameroon: The Politics of Divide and Rule. In P. N. Nkwi and F. B. Nyamnjoh, eds., Regional Balance and National Integration in Cameroon, 138–49. Leiden: African Studies Centre and Yaoundé: ICASSRT.

Nkwi, P. N., and J.-P. Warnier
1982 Elements for a History of the Western Grassfields. Yaoundé: Department of Sociology, University of Yaoundé.

Northern, T.
1984 The Art of Cameroon. Washington, DC: Smithsonian Institution.

Notué, J. P., and L. Perrois
1984 Contribution à l'Étude des Sociétés Secrètes chez les Bamiléké (Ouest Cameroun). Yaoundé: ISH and ORSTOM.

Nzikam, Djomo, E.
1977 Les Rites Relatifs à la Naissance chez les Fe'e Fe'e de Babouantou (Pùàntù). Yaoundé: Mémoire pour D.E.S., Department of Sociology, University of Yaoundé.

Ohadike, D. C.
1981 The influenza pandemic of 1918–19 and the spread of cassava cultivation on the Lower Niger: A study in historical linkages. *Journal of African History* 22:379–91.

Ongoum, L.-M.
1985 Poèmes de femmes bamiléké. In J. C. Barbier, ed., Femmes du Cameroun: Mères Pacifiques, Femmes Rebelles, 283–97. Paris: Karthala.

Ott, S.
1979 Aristotle among the Basques: The "cheese analogy" of conception. *Man* (N.S.) 14 (4): 699–711.

Packard, R.
1980 Social change and the history of misfortune among the Bashu of Eastern Zaire. In I. Karp and C. Bird, eds., Explorations in African Systems of Thought, 237–67. Bloomington: Indiana University Press.

Parkin, D. J.
1968   Medicines and men of influence. *Man* (N.S.) 3:424–39.
Parsons, T.
1951   The Social System. New York: Free Press.
Patterson, K. D.
1981   Health in Colonial Ghana: Disease, Medicine, and Socio-Economic Change, 1900–1955. Waltham, MA: Crossroads.
1983   The influenza epidemic of 1918–19 in the Gold Coast. *Journal of African History* 24 (4): 485–502.
Plehn, F.
1894   Über einige auf Krankheit und Tod bezügliche Vorstellungen und Gebräuche der Dualaneger. Wissenschaftliche Beihefte zum Deutschen Kolonialblatte . . . 7 (2): 89–99.
Powers, M. N.
1980   Menstruation and reproduction: An Oglala case. *Signs* 6 (1): 54–65.
Pradelles de Latour, C.-H.
1986   Le Champ de Langage dans une Chefferie Bamiléké du Cameroun. Thèse du Doctorat d'État, Paris: École des Hautes Études en Sciences Sociales.
1994   Marriage Payments, Debt and Fatherhood among the Bangoua: A Lacanian Analysis of a Kinship System. *Africa* 64 (1): 21–33.
Pradelles de Latour, M.-L.
1985   Paroles d'hommes, images de femmes. In J. C. Barbier, ed., Femmes du Cameroun: Mères Pacifiques, Femmes Rebelles, 357–68. Paris: Karthala.
Press, I.
1980   Problems in the definition and classification of medical systems. *Social Science and Medicine* 14B (1): 45–57.
Preuss, Dr.
1891a   Bericht des Dr. Preuss über die Reise von Kamerun den Mungo stromaufwärts nach Mundame. Wissenschaftliche Beihefte zum Deutschen Kolonialblatte: Mittheilungen von Forschungsreisenden und Gelehrten aus den Deutschen Schutzgebieten 4 (1): 28–38.
1891b   Bericht des Dr. Preuss über Buea. Wissenschaftliche Beihefte zum Deutschen Kolonialblatte . . . 4 (3): 128–53.
Price, N.
1996   The changing value of children among the Kikuyu of Central Province, Kenya. *Africa* 66 (3): 411–36.
Quinn, N.
1977   Anthropological studies on women's status. *Annual Review of Anthropology* 6:181–225.
Raheja, G.
1995   The limits of partriliny: Kinship, gender and women's speech practices in rural North India. In M. J. Maynes et al., eds., Gender, Kinship, Power: A Comparative and Interdisciplinary History, 149–46. New York: Routledge.

Raheja, G., and A. Gold
1994   Listen to the Heron's Words: Reimagining Gender and Kinship in North India. Berkeley: University of California Press.

Rapp, R.
1988   Chromosomes and communication: The discourse of genetic counseling. *Medical Anthropology Quarterly* (N.S.) 2 (2): 158–71.
1993   Accounting for amniocentesis. In S. Lindenbaum and M. Lock, eds., Knowledge, Power and Practice: The Anthropology of Medicine and Everyday Life, 55–76. Berkeley: University of California Press.

Rapp, R., and F. Ginsburg
1991   The politics of reproduction. *Annual Review of Anthropology* 20:311–43.
1995   (Eds.) Conceiving the New World Order: The Global Politics of Reproduction. Berkeley: University of California Press.

Rapport annuel . . . à l'Assemblé Générale
1935   Rapport annuel adressé par le Gouvernement français au Conseil de la Société des Nations sur l'administration sous mandat du territoire du Cameroun pour l'année 1935. Paris: Imprimerie Générale Lahure.
1937   Rapport annuel . . . au Conseil de la Société des Nations . . . pour l'année 1937. Paris: Imprimerie Générale Lahure.
1951   Rapport Annuel du Gouvernement Français à l'Assemblé Générale des Nations Unies sur l'Administration du Cameroun placé sous la Tutelle de la France. Paris: Gouvernement Français.

Rasmussen, S. J.
1989   Accounting for belief: Causation, misfortune, and evil in Tuareg systems of thought. *Man: Journal of the Royal Anthropological Institute* 24:124–44.
1995   Spirit Possession and Personhood among the Kel Ewey Tuareg. Cambridge: Cambridge University Press.

Reichskolonialamt
1911   Die Deutschen Schutzgebiete in Afrika und der Südsee 1909/1910. Amtliche Jahresberichte. Berlin: Ernst Siegfried Mittler und Sohn, Königliche Hofbuchhandlung.
1912   Die Deutschen Schutzgebiete in Afrika und der Südsee 1910/1911. Amtliche Jahresberichte. Berlin: Ernst Siegfried Mittler und Sohn, Königliche Hofbuchhandlung.
1913   Die Deutschen Schutzgebiete in Afrika und der Südsee 1911/1912. Amtliche Jahresberichte. Berlin: Ernst Siegfried Mittler und Sohn, Königliche Hofbuchhandlung.
1914   Die Deutschen Schutzgebiete in Afrika und der Südsee 1912/1913. Amtliche Jahresberichte. Berlin: Ernst Siegfried Mittler und Sohn, Königliche Hofbuchhandlung.

Rémy, G.
1982   Études epidemiologiques et approches géographiques des maladies en Afrique tropical: Mélanges pour un dialogue. *Cahiers d'Études Africaines* 22 (1–2): 85–86.

Renne, E.
1994   Fashions in fertility control: Local and institutional interpretations of IUDs. Paper presented at Situating Fertility: Global Visions and Local Values, SSRC Workshop. John Hopkins University, February.

République Unie du Cameroun. Ministère de l'Economie et du Plan, Direction de la Statistique et de la Comptabilité Nationale
1976   Recensement Général de la Population et de l'Habitat d'Avril 1976, vol. 1, tome 3.

Retel-Laurentin, A.
1974   Infécondité en Afrique Noire: Maladies et conséquences sociales. Paris: Masson et Cie.

Reynolds, P.
1986   The training of traditional healers in Mashonaland. In M. Last and G. L. Chavunduka, eds., The Professionalisation of African Medicine, 165–88. Manchester: Manchester University Press.

Richards, A. I.
1939   Land, Labour and Diet in Northern Rhodesia: An Economic Study of the Bemba Tribe. London: Oxford University Press.
1956   Chisungu: A Girl's Initiation Ceremony among the Bemba of Zambia. London: Tavistock.
1961   African kings and their royal relatives. *Journal of the Royal Anthropological Institute* 91:135–50.
1969   Keeping the king divine. Proceedings of the Royal Anthropological Institute 1968:23–25.

Rolland, P.
1951   Quelques aspects sociologiques de la vie des Bamiléké de la Subdivision de Bagangté [*sic*]. Typescript from the archives of Claude Tardits, dated October 31, 1951.

Rosaldo, R.
1989   Culture and Truth: The Remaking of Social Analysis. Boston: Beacon Press.

Rowlands, M.
1996   The consumption of an African modernity. In M. J. Arnoldi, C. M. Geary, and K. L. Hardin, eds., African Material Culture, 188–213. Bloomington: Indiana University Press.

Rowlands, M., and J.-P. Warnier
1988   Sorcery, power and the modern state in Cameroon. *Man* (N.S.) 23 (1): 118–32.

Rudin, H.
1938   Germans in the Cameroons, 1884–1914. New Haven: Yale University Press.

Sanday, P. R.
1973   Toward a theory of the status of women. *American Anthropologist* 75:1682–1700.

Sandelowski, M.
   1991   Telling stories: Narrative approaches in qualitative research. *Image: Journal of Nursing Scholarship* 23:161–66.
   1993   With Child in Mind: Studies of the Personal Encounter with Infertility. Philadelphia: University of Pennsylvania Press.
Sapir, J. D.
   1977   The fabricated child. In J. D. Sapir and J. C. Crocker, eds., The Social Use of Metaphor: Essays on the Anthropology of Rhetoric Press, 193–223. Philadelphia: University of Pennsylvania.
Sapir, J. D., and J. C. Crocker
   1977   Introduction. In J. D. Sapir and J. C. Crocker, eds., The Social Use of Metaphor: Essays on the Anthropology of Rhetoric. Philadelphia: University of Pennsylvania Press.
Sargent, C. F.
   1982   The Cultural Context of Therapeutic Choice: Obstetrical Care Decisions Among the Bariba of Benin. Boston: D. Reidel.
   1988   Born to die: Witchcraft and infanticide in Bariba culture. *Ethnology* 27 (1): 79–95.
   1989   Maternity, Medicine, and Power: Reproductive Decisions in Urban Benin. Berkeley: University of California Press.
Sargent, C. F., and R. E. Davis-Floyd
   1997   Childbirth and Authoritative Knowledge: Cross-Cultural Perspectives. Berkeley: University of California Press.
Sarraut, A.
   1923   La mise en valeur des colonies françaises. Paris: Payot.
Scheper-Hughes, N.
   1992   Death Without Weeping: The Violence of Everyday Life in Brazil. Berkeley: University of California Press.
Scheper-Hughes, N., and M. Lock
   1987   The mindful body: A prolegomenon to future work in medical anthropology. *Medical Anthropology Quarterly* (N.S.) 1 (1): 6–41.
Schmidt, A.
   1955a   The water of life. *African Studies* 14 (1): 23–28.
   1955b   Die rote Lendenschnur: Als Frau im Grasland Kameruns. Berlin: Dietrich Reimer.
Scott, J.
   1990   Domination and the Arts of Resistance: Hidden Transcripts. New Haven: Yale University Press.
Sewell, W. H.
   1992   A theory of structure: Duality, agency, and transformation. *American Journal of Sociology* 98 (1): 1–29.
Shanklin, E.
   1988   Even witches have friends: Witchcraft in a matrilineal society. Paper presented at the conference "Ethnomedical Systems in Sub-Saharan Africa," African Studies Centre, Leiden University, The Netherlands, June 1988.

Shaw, R.
1985   Gender and the structuring of reality in Temne divination: An interactive study. *Africa* 55 (3): 286–303.
Simmel, G.
1964   Conflict: The Web of Group-Affiliations. New York: Free Press.
Singer, M., L. Davison, and G. Gerdes
1988   Culture, critical theory, and reproductive illness behavior in Haiti. *Medical Anthropology Quarterly* (N.S.) 2 (4): 370–85.
Skultans, V.
1976   Empathy and healing: Aspects of spiritualist ritual. In J. B. Loudon, ed., Social Anthropology and Medicine, 190–222. London: Academic.
Société des Missions Evangéliques de Paris
1960   Rapport Annuel de la Société des Missions Evangéliques chez les peuples non chrétiens. Paris: SMEP.
Soen, D., and P. de Comarmon
1969–70   The secret societies and age groups of the Bamiléké and their potential adaptability to cooperative organization. *Wiener Völkerkundliche Mitteilungen* 11–12:71–88.
Sontag, S.
1978   Illness as Metaphor. New York: Farrar, Straus and Giroux.
Sop Nkamgang, M.
1976   La Femme dans la Pensée Nègre (cited in Miaffo 1977:111). Yaoundé.
Spittler, G.
1980   Streitregelung im Schatten des Leviathan: Eine Darstellung und Kritik rechtsethnologischer Untersuchungen. Zeitschrift für Rechtssoziologie, 4–32.
Spring, A.
1978   Epidemiology of spirit possession among the Luvale of Zambia. In J. Hoch-Smith and A. Spring, eds., Women in Ritual and Symbolic Roles, 165–90. New York: Plenum.
Stacey, J.
1988   Can There Be a Feminist Ethnography? *Women's Studies International Forum* 11:21–27.
Stack, C. B.
1974   All Our Kin: Strategies for Survival in a Black Community. New York: Harper and Row.
Strathern, M.
1984   Domesticity and the denigration of women. In D. O'Brien and S. W. Tiffany, eds., Rethinking Women's Roles: Perspectives from the Pacific, 13–31. Berkeley: University of California Press.
1992   Reproducing the Future: Anthropology, Kinship, and the New Reproductive Technologies. New York: Routledge.
Tambiah, S.
1969   Animals are good to think and good to prohibit. *Ethnology* 7:423–59.

Tardits, C.
1960 Contribution à l'Étude des Populations Bamiléké de l'Ouest Cameroun. Paris: Editions Berger-Levrault.
1981 (Ed.) Contribution de la Recherche Ethnologique à l'Histoire des Civilisations du Cameroun. Paris: Éditions du Centre National de la Recherche Scientifique.
1985 Aimer, danser, manger. In J. C. Barbier, ed., Les Femmes au Cameroun, 119–31. Paris: Harmattan.
Taussig, M.
1980a Reification and the consciousness of the patient. *Social Science and Medicine* 14B:3–13.
1980b The baptism of money and the secret of capital. Chapter 7 in The Devil and Commodity Fetishism in South America, 126–39. Chapel Hill: University of North Carolina Press.
Thomas, J. M. C.
1963 Les Ngbaka de la Lobaye: Le Dépeuplement Rural chez une Population Forestière de la République Centrafricaine. Paris: Mouton.
Thomas, K.
1970 The relevance of social anthropology to the study of English witchcraft. In M. Douglas, ed., Witchcraft Confessions and Accusations, 47–79. London: Tavistock.
1971 Religion and the Decline of Magic. London: Weidenfeld and Nicolson.
Thompson, E. P.
1972 Anthropology and the discipline of historical context. *Midland History* 1 (3): 41–55.
Turner, B. S.
1981 For Weber: Essays on the Sociology of Fate. Boston: Routledge and Kegan Paul.
Turner, V. W.
1954 Schism and Continuity in an African Society. Manchester: Manchester University Press.
1967 The Forest of Symbols: Aspects of Ndembu Ritual. Ithaca: Cornell University Press.
1968 (1981) The Drums of Affliction. Oxford: Oxford University Press.
Tyler, S.
1987 The Unspeakable: Discourse, Dialogue, and Rhetoric in the Postmodern World. Madison: University of Wisconsin Press.
Unschuld, P. U.
1979 Medical Ethics in Imperial China: A Study in Historical Anthropology. Berkeley: University of California Press.
USAID Office of Nutrition
1978 United Republic of Cameroon. National Nutrition Survey. Final Report. Washington, DC: U.S. Agency for International Development.
Vaisseau, Médecin-Colonel
1948 Rapport Annuel, Année 1948. Yaoundé: Cameroun Français, Service de la Santé Publique.

1951   Rapport Annuel, Année 1951. Yaoundé: Cameroun Français, Service de la Santé Publique.

van der Geest, S.
1988   The Production of Popular Medical Knowledge: Marketplace Conversations in Cameroon. Paper presented at "Anthropologies of Medicine: A Colloquium on West European and North American Perspectives," Hamburg, December 4–8.

van Velsen, J.
1967   The extended case method and situational analysis. In A. L. Epstein, ed., The Craft of Social Anthropology, 129–49. London: Tavistock.

Vaucel, Médecin Lieutenant-Colonel
1939   Rapport Annuel, Année 1939. Yaoundé: Service de Santé, Territoire du Cameroun.

Vaughan, M.
1983   Idioms of madness: Zomba Lunatic Asylum, Nyasaland, in the colonial period. *Journal of Southern African Studies* 9 (2): 218–38.
1991   Curing Their Ills: Colonial Power and African Illness. Stanford: Stanford University Press.

Voorhoeve, J.
1964   Notes sur les noms d'éloges Bamiléké. *Cahier d'Études Africaines* 15 (4): 452–55.
1976   Contes Bamiléké. Tervuren: Musée Royale de l'Afrique Centrale.

Wakam, J.
1994   De la Pertinence des Théories "Economistes" de Fécondité dans le Contexte Socio-Culturel Camerounais et Négro-Africain. Yaoundé: IFORD (Institut de Formation et de Recherche Démographiques).

Ware, H.
1977   Women's work and fertility in Africa. In S. Kupinsky, ed., The Fertility of Working Women, 1–34. New York: Praeger.

Warnier, J.-P.
1985   Échanges, Développement et Hiérarchies dans le Bamenda Pré-Colonial (Cameroun). Stuttgart: Franz Steiner Verlag Wiesbaden.

Watkins, S. C.
1987   The fertility transition: Europe and the third world compared. *Sociological Forum* 2 (4): 645–73.

Weber, M.
1963   (1922) The Sociology of Religion. Boston: Beacon Press.
1968   Economy and Society. Berkeley: University of California Press.

Webster, D.
1991   Abafazi Bathonga Bafihlakala. *African Studies* 50 (1–2): 243–71.

Weiss, B.
1996   The Making and Unmaking of the Haya Lived World: Consumption, Commoditization, and Everyday Practice. Durham, NC: Duke University Press.

Weston, K.
1993   Do clothes make the woman? Gender, performance theory, and lesbian eroticism. *Genders,* no. 17: 1–21.

Whyte, S. R.
1982 Men, women and misfortune in Bunyole. *Man* (N.S.) 16 (3): 350–66.
Wilson, M. H.
1957 Rituals of Kinship among the Nyakyusa. London: Oxford University Press.
1959 Divine Kings and the "Breath of Men." The Frazer Lecture for 1959. Cambridge: Cambridge University Press.
Wissenschaftliche Beihefte
1894 Über das Gebiet zwischen Mundame und Baliburg. *Wissenschaftliche Beihefte zum Deutschen Kolonialblatte* . . . 7 (2): 99–104.
Wolff, N. H.
1979 Concepts of causation and treatment in the Yoruba medical system: The special case of barrenness. In Z. A. Ademuwagun et al., eds., African Therapeutic Systems, 125–31. Waltham, MA: Crossroads.
World Bank
1984 World Development Report. New York: Oxford University Press.
World Fertility Survey
1983 Enquête Nationale sur la Fécondité du Cameroun, 1978. Rapport Principal, Vol. 1. Yaoundé: MINEP.
Wright, P., and A. Treacher, eds.
1982 The Problem of Medical Knowledge. Edinburgh: Edinburgh University Press.
Young, A.
1982 The anthropologies of illness and sickness. *Annual Review of Anthropology* 11:257–85.
Zenker, G.
1895 Jaunde. *Wissenschaftliche Beihefte zum Deutschen Kolonialblatte* . . . 8 (1): 36–69.
Ziemann, H.
1904 Zur Bevölkerungs- und Viehfrage in Kamerun. Ergebnisse einer Expedition in die gesunden Hochländer am und nördlich vom Manengubagebirge. *Wissenschaftliche Beihefte zum Deutschen Kolonialblatte* . . . 17 (3): 136–74.
Zimmermann, E.
1916 Wirtschaftliches und politisches aus Nordkamerun zwischen Logone und Benue; Wirtschaftliche Lage in unseren Kolonien. Verhandlung des Vorstandes und der Mitgliederversammlung des Kolonial-Wirtschaftlichen Komittees e.V.: Wirtschaftlicher Ausschuss der Deutschen Kolonialgesellschaft 1:11–48.

Index

Action Médicale Indigène (AMI), 148
Adultery, 80–81, 94–95, 115–16, 128;
   infidelity, 94, 115, 117–18
Agnatic kinship, 51, 169, 170, 207n. 6
Ahidjo, President Ahmadou, 47, 187,
   212n. 1
Ancestors (*ma'ngut nze'*), 49, 51–52,
   80, 106–8, 213n. 6; misfortune and,
   3, 112; skull worship, 51, 106, 107,
   122, 123, 131; wrath of, 70, 94, 103,
   109, 207n. 7
André, 41
Ardener, Edwin, 186
Associations, voluntary, 66, 208n. 18;
   male youth (*manjo*), 60, 205n. 2;
   rotating credit (*tontines*), 10, 40, 60,
   61, 76; witches', 109, 113, 185, 186,
   214nn. 11–12
Authority, 31–32, 62–63

Bafoussam, 148
Bakongo, 138
Bamiléké, 43–45, 46, 185
Bamoum kingdoms, 146
Bamum palace, 24
Bandjoun, 88
Bangangté, 1, 17; historical context of,
   43, 45–48, 205n. 2; social change for,
   41–42, 194
Bangangté Divisional Hospital, 157,
   172
Bangwa, 148
Bangwa Protestant Hospital, 157,
   212n. 4

Bariba, of Benin, 165
Beidelman, T. O., 182, 209n. 23
Beliefs and therapeutic choice, 165–67
Bemba, 63, 209n. 23
Bergeret, Charles, and Yvette Bergeret,
   150
Biomedical institutions, 126–27, 151,
   155, 156–59; and childbirth, 88,
   163–64. *See also specific institutions*
Biomedical practitioners, 157, 166,
   172
Biomedical treatment, 144, 155. *See
   also* Health care
Biya, President Paul, 47, 187
Bledsoe, C., 3, 7
Blood, 85, 211n. 17
Body parts, characteristics of, 110–11
Boswell, D. M., 171
Brain, Robert, 207n. 9
Breastmilk, quality of, 89
Breath/spirit (*zwiak*), 107, 213n. 6
Brideprice, 130, 207n. 8
Bridewealth, 53–54, 56, 90, 115

Caldwell, J. C., and P. Caldwell, 3
Cameroon, Republic of, 42, 43, 46–47,
   196
Cameroonian church (EEC), 150
Cameroon People's Democratic Move-
   ment, 47
Cartron, Médecin Commandant, 147
Cash crops, 45, 75, 147
Cash economy, 124–25
Che'elou, 19, 22, 23–24, 175–77

Childbirth, 87–90, 119, 155, 163–64, 195

Childlessness, 33, 78, 100, 125, 204n. 7; and social status, 30, 33, 130. *See also* Infertility

Children: education of, 69, 76, 122, 211n. 15; fosterage of, 23–24, 57, 207n. 11; as infants, 88–90, 149–50; king's, 19, 208n. 12; and kinship, 55–56, 89, 92; mortality of, 120–21, 149–50, 195–96; socialization of, 42, 48, 122–23, 191–92; threats to survival of, 106, 119–23

Christianity, 140, 148, 149. *See also* Missionaries, medical

Civil servants, 185, 189

Civil war, 46, 67, 112, 212

Cocoa production, 45, 58, 75, 147

Coffee production, 45, 58, 59, 75, 147, 205n. 3

Colonization, European, 43, 115–16, 196; French practices, 45, 46, 144–48; German, and indigenous medicine, 45, 140–44; and kingship, 183–84

Commensality, 48–49, 96, 123–24, 197–98

Compound (*la'*), 57–59, 61–62, 69

Conception, 85–86, 116, 130–31

Conrau, G., 140–41, 143

Contraceptives, 3, 194, 196, 214n. 14

Cooking inside, marriage as (*na nda*), 4, 11, 71, 74, 78, 90–91, 95–97

Cooking metaphors. *See* Culinary imagery

Corinne (royal wife), 24–25

Council of nine (*nkam be'e*), 21, 63, 66

Country Sunday (*li'ngá*), 75, 210n. 1

Credit associations, rotating. *See* Associations, voluntary

Culinary imagery, 88, 179; for adultery, 115, 116; for gestation, 86, 87, 117–18, 119–20; for infertility, 99–100; kitchen metaphors, 4, 95–97, 113–14, 166; for procreation, 73, 90–92, 95–97, 113, 191; and sex, 71, 84

Cultural creolization, 158

Cultural identity, 5, 177–78, 179, 197. *See also* Identity

Custom (*ndonn*), 32, 102–3, 105, 111, 130, 163, 193

"Daughters," young wives as, 22–26

Death, 106–7, 175, 213n. 9; of children, 120–21, 149–50, 195–96; in colonial era, 140, 141, 142; of the king, 119, 131, 190

Debarge, Josette, 148–49, 158

Delaney, C., 4–5, 180

Demographic and Health Survey (1991), 120

Demography and fertility, 2–3, 4. *See also* Population

Descent, 50–51. *See also* Matrilineage; Patrilineage

Development, 81, 186, 189, 194

Diagnosis, 154, 155, 212n. 4; healer's, 27, 28, 161, 166; resistance to revealing, 157, 158

Dieckmann, N., 76

Disease, 102, 140, 141–44, 145–46, 215n. 5. *See also* Illness; Sexually transmitted disease

Divination, 36, 151, 159, 174

Divine kingship. *See* Kingship, divine

Divorce, 125, 130

Djomo, Nzikam, 211n. 16

Domestic violence, 20

Drugs, manufactured, 155

Dysentery, 141, 142

Economic crisis (1990s), 7, 47, 124, 185, 190

Education, 77, 130; of children, 69, 76, 122, 211n. 15

Egerton, C., 24, 115–16, 121, 163–64, 217n. 5

Eglise Evangélique de Cameroun (EEC), 150

Egyptian women, 138, 170, 181
Elites, 7, 20, 188–89, 193, 199; nobles, 60, 63, 66, 113, 205n. 2; and social order, 38, 184, 185, 186
Emotions, 105, 107, 116; women and, 80, 111, 129, 132
Envy, 22, 118, 132
Epilepsy, 93, 110, 115, 121
Ethnicity, 47, 185, 193–94
Evangelization, 148, 149–50
Exogamy, 91. *See also* Marriage

Family, rejection by, 21
Family enterprise, healing as, 159–60, 162
Family planning programs, 196
Farinaud, Médecin Colonel, 146
Farmer, P., 89
Fate, personal, 5–6, 7, 112
Father-by-money marriage, 53–54, 55, 56, 207n. 8
Feierman, S., 133, 170, 212n. 4, 216n. 13
Felix (indigenous healer), 156, 158–59; royal wife consultation, 26–27, 28, 29, 32, 34
Fernandez, J., 214n. 17
Fertility, 2–3, 128–29, 193; in colonial period, 142, 143, 146; and commensality, 123–24; rates, 203n. 2; royal, 61, 182; and social relations, 97–98, 156; and venereal disease, 196; water and, 211n. 12
Fetishes, 109–10, 116–17, 140
Fetus, 86–87, 88, 113–14, 117–18
Food: for ancestors, 51; colonial investigation of, 141–42; and fertility, 12, 123–24; ideological focus on, 181; *ju* (vegetable sauce), 124, 197; *nkwi* (sauce), 88–89, 198; and procreation, 33–34, 125, 197–98; and sex, 71; and social networks, 42, 59, 134; women's role in, 45, 75–76, 81, 83
Fosterage of children, 23–24, 57, 207n. 11

France, colonial policies of, 45, 46, 144–48
Frank, O., 3
Frazer, J. G., 7, 8

Gambia, 3, 7
Gender, 179; differences, 8; division of labor by, 75–76, 97; and identity, 180–81; images, 78–84; and procreation, 4–5, 11–12; relations, 183, 190, 191; segregation by, 58, 70, 73–74, 76, 78; and social status, 38
German colonization, 45, 140–44
Gestation, 86–87, 117–18, 119–20. *See also* Pregnancy
Ghost Town (Villes Mortes) movement, 47
God: *nsi,* 85–86, 102, 105, 211n. 11; personal (*mbem*), 213n. 6
Golden Bough (Frazer), 7, 8
Goldschmidt, D., 88
Gossip, 34, 60, 78–79
Greenhalgh, Susan, 2

Haitian women, 89, 181
Hannerz, U., 158
Healers, indigenous. *See* Indigenous healers (*ngakà*)
Health care: access to, 132–33; beliefs about, 165–67; costs and fees for, 170–71; French military, 144–48; and gender segregation, 76–77; German colonial, 140–44; history of, 137; indigenous, 143, 150, 158–59; for infertility, 34–35; innovation in, 216n. 13; medical missionaries, 140, 148–50; and the state, 69; support networks for, 125, 130, 167–69, 170, 173–74; and therapy management, 133, 164–65, 167, 169–70. *See also* Medicine; Therapy
Health care institutions, 151–52, 171, 172, 173. *See also* Biomedical institutions

Health-care practitioners. *See* Biomedical practioners; Indigenous healers (*ngakà*)
Hearth sharing, 55
Herbal medicine (*fu*), 155, 159, 160, 161, 173, 213n. 8
Hierarchy, 30, 31, 70, 127, 157–58. *See also* Social status
Household (*nda*), 57
Hua of New Guinea, 181
Hurault, J., 67, 213n. 6

Ideal society, 113, 179, 190
Identity, 8, 41–42, 59, 184; cultural, 5, 177–78, 179, 197; and ethnicity, 194; politics of, 13–14; and procreation, 11, 30, 73, 180–81; and social connection, 31, 49, 193–94
Illness, 133, 155, 162; causes of, 101–4, 105, 107–8. *See also* Disease; Reproductive illness
Incest, 11, 21, 114–15, 204n. 6; prevention of, 93, 94
Indigenous healers (*ngakà*), 149, 151–53, 158–60; discretion of, 163; fees for, 171; patient interaction with, 172; and reproductive disorders, 29–30, 155–56, 161, 166; and royal family, 26–27, 165; witch distinction, 108–9, 110
Indigenous health care, 143, 150, 158–59
Indigenous medicine, 140, 141, 173. *See also* Herbal medicine (*fu*)
Infant mortality, 149, 195–96
Infertility: anxiety about, 2, 126; and colonial medicine, 140; culinary symbolism for, 99–100; as idiom, 178; indigenous medicine and, 27, 129, 159, 160–61; as legal case, 153–54; and marital strife, 160–61; and medical pluralism, 135, 137; and poverty, 125–26, 173–74, 198; and social relations, 3, 5–7, 180; treat-

ment of, 13, 34–35, 155; and women's vulnerability, 101. *See also* Reproductive illness
Infidelity, 94, 115, 117–18. *See also* Adultery
Inhorn, M., 126, 138, 170, 181
Innovation, medical, 216n. 13
Iteso of Kenya, 36

Jamot, Eugène, 145–46
Janzen, J., 102, 138
Jealousy, 22, 33, 79, 95, 117, 192–93
Jeanne, 28, 93, 169–70, 172
Joldersma, H., 76
Josette (first queen), 17, 24, 26, 118–19, 192
"Journée de Mari," 81
Judge, king as, 62
Jural responsibility, 169–70
Justine, 192–93

Kaberry, P. M., 204n. 6
Karp, I., 36
King (*mfen*), 7–9, 17, 115–16; authority of, 61–63; behavior of, 20, 106, 195; decline of, 13, 47–48, 70, 198; double nature of, 67–68; illness of, 20, 119, 131, 190; political autonomy of, 183–84; and royal wives, 16, 22, 33, 63, 66; strangeness of, 63, 209n. 23; vitality of, 182; wealth of, 196
Kingdom, 60–61, 68–69, 106
Kingship, divine, 141, 197, 209n. 23; and colonization, 183–84; decline of, 37, 178–79, 182, 187, 190–91; and population, 194–95; power of wives in, 7–9
King's wives. *See* Royal wives
Kinship ties, 4, 96–97, 207n. 6; agnatic, 51, 169, 170, 207n. 6; by blood, 211n. 17; of children, 55–56, 89, 92; descent, 50–51; loosening of, 162; strife in, 69–70; and urbanization, 18. *See also* Ancestors (*ma'ngut nze'*); Marriage; Matrilin-

eage; Patrilineage; Uterine group (*pam nto'*)
Kitchen metaphors, 4, 95–97, 113–14, 166. *See also* Culinary imagery
Kleinman, A., 165
Kom, kingdom of, 112
Kongo therapeutics, 102
Kuczynski, R. R., 146
Kujamaat-Diola folktale, 181
Kuru Sorcery (Lindenbaum), 126

Labor: colonial recruitment of, 139, 140, 141–43, 144, 145, 147; gendered division of, 75–76, 97; wage, 48, 70, 75, 76, 124, 133; of women, 75–76, 128–29, 190
Labor migration, 18, 48, 70, 122, 215n. 5; and women, 6, 46, 124, 133
Land, 58–59, 147; disputes, 67, 133–34, 188–89
Lassauvagerie, Médecin-Lieutenant, 148
Latrines, locking of, 117, 125
Law (*kan*), 50, 103, 106
Legal case, infertility as, 153–54
Leprosy, 145, 146
Lindenbaum, S., 126
Lineage. *See* Descent; Matrilineage; Patrilineage
Louise (second queen), 16–17

Madness, 107–8
Magic (*ka*), 108, 109
Marriage, 52—54, 93; adultery/infidelity in, 80–81, 94–95, 115–16, 117–18, 128; as cooking inside (*na nda*), 4, 11, 71, 74, 78, 90, 91, 95–97; father-by-money, 53–54, 55, 56, 207n. 8; fertility rates for, 203n. 2; infertility and strife in, 160–61; and lineage, 73–74, 90, 91–92, 96, 97; nonarranged, 114–15; royal, 15, 20–21, 24–26, 94, 114–15. *See also* Polygyny
Martin, E., 4

Matrilineage, 50, 54; and marriage, 73–74, 92, 96, 97. *See also* Uterine group (*pam nto'*)
McNicoll, G., 3
Medical pluralism, 1, 135, 150–53
Medicine, 108, 151; creolized, 158–59; herbal, 155, 159, 160, 161, 173, 213n. 8; indigenous, 140, 141, 173; missionary, 140, 142–43, 148–50, 165–66, 196
Medicine-kitchen, 159–60, 162
Meigs, A., 181
Melon vines, ancestors as, 49, 51
Men: and adultery, 94–95; gender image of, 82–83; image of women by, 79, 80; institutional experience of, 77; labor of, 46, 75, 76, 124, 133; opportunities for, 185; responsibility of, 58–59; as witches, 109
Metaphor, women's use of, 181–82, 199–200
Mfen. See King
Mfen Meshinke' of Bantoum, 135, 136, 143, 155, 166
Miaffo, D., 79
Midwifery, traditional, 88, 144, 163–64
Migration. *See* Labor migration
Ministry of Agriculture, 81
Misfortune: adultery, 95; ancestral wrath, 51–52, 106–7; breaches of norms, 106; causes of, 101–12; fetishes, 109–10; god, 105; infertility, 101; witchcraft, 108–9, 112
Missionaries, medical, 140, 142–43, 148–50, 165–66, 196
Miteu, 160–61
Mobility, personal, 8, 29–30, 31, 125. *See also* Social status
Mother-daughter cowife institution, 22–26
Motherhood, 30, 32, 33, 89, 121–22, 214n. 15
Müller, 45
Mullings, L., 171

Names, praise (*ndap*), 21, 49, 60, 91, 209nn. 19–20
Nana (indigenous healer), 155, 159–60, 161
Ndachi Tagne, D., 24, 74
Ndonko, F. T., 110
Neighborhood (quarter), 59–60
New Guinea, 181
Ngami, (king), 205n. 2
Njanzwe, 205n. 2
Njiké-Bergeret, Claude, 17, 22, 83, 204n. 1; as foster mother, 26, 28, 35
Njiké Pokam François (king), 17, 19–21, 68, 93; decline of, 187–88; and land dispute, 188–89
Njiké II Salomon (king, 1912–43), 115, 143
Nji Monluh Seidou Pokam (king), 47, 68, 217n. 2
Nobles, 60, 63, 66, 113, 205n. 2. *See also* Elites
Noun valley, 146–47
Nso' incest, 204n. 6
Nutrition, 128
Nyombab, 121

Occult power, 185–86, 187, 199. *See also* Sorcery; Supernatural power (*kà*); Vampires (*ndum*); Witchcraft
One heart (*nchu' ntu'*), 48, 189–90
Ouden, Den, 70
Ovulation, 128

Palace, 61–62, 217n. 5. *See also* Royal compound (*nchwed*)
Palace association (*bandansi*), 153, 154, 156
Palm oil, 59, 85, 90, 91
Parsons, T., 35
Paternity, 119
Patients: beliefs of, 166; costs for, 171; isolation of, 149–50; practitioner relationship, 156, 157–58
Patrilineage, 50, 191, 207n. 6; and

marriage, 73, 74, 90, 91–92, 96, 97; and pregnancy, 87
Paulette (royal wife), 18–19, 28, 37; "belly" problems of, 26–27; healer's diagnosis of, 34–36, 159, 166; marriage of, 15, 20–21, 24–26, 94, 114–15; perception of affliction, 32–34; personal mobility of, 29–30, 31; reproductive complaints of, 10–11, 15; social status of, 31–32, 39
Personal god (*mbem*), 213n. 6
Placenta, burial of, 89
Political autonomy, king's, 183–84
Political struggles, 187
Polygyny, 46, 58, 208n. 13, 215n. 18; of royal court, 9, 31–32; and sexually transmitted disease, 127, 128; support network of, 133, 168–69
Population, 43, 194, 196, 206; colonial decline, 142, 146–47
Possession, 35–36, 107–8, 153
Poverty: and infertility, 125–26, 173–74, 198; of women, 6–7, 124–25, 181, 197
Praise name (*ndap*). *See* Names, praise
Pregnancy, 86–87, 117–18, 130–31, 166, 213n. 9; false, 118–19, 192
Preuss, Dr., 140
Procreation, 95–97; culinary imagery for, 73, 90–92, 95–97, 113, 191; and food, 33–34, 125, 197–98; and identity, 11, 30; and kingship, 183; and social issues, 11, 178, 180–82; symbolism of, 3–5; threats to, 2, 113–14; women's role in, 85
Promiscuity, 82, 127, 128, 214n. 17
Prostitution, 25, 127
Protection rites, 156
Protestant missions, 148. *See also* Missionaries, medical
Puberty seclusion (*nja*), 89, 211n. 15

Quarter chiefs, 67, 134
Quarter (neighborhood) system, 59–60, 67

Queen mothers (*mamfen*), 16–17, 63, 66. *See also* Royal wives

Reconciliation rites, 153–54, 216n. 17
Reine Captive, La (Tagne), 74
Relly, M. H., 145
Reproduction and social status, 10, 129–34
Reproductive illness, 54; and biomedical practitioners, 127–28, 154–55; and cultural identity, 177–78, 179; and gestation, 117; and health-care institutions, 137; indigenous medicine and, 155–56, 159, 160; jural responsibility for, 169–70; and royal wives, 29, 37; and social change, 38, 39, 180; and social relations, 48; support network for, 168; therapy for, 29–30, 138, 162–63; threats of, 1–2; and witchcraft, 199. *See also* Infertility; Sexually transmitted disease
Resources, material, 170–71
Richards, A. I., 63, 209n. 23
Rituals, 89, 156, 211nn. 15–16; for reconciliation, 153–54, 216n. 17
Rosaldo, R., 179
Rotating credit associations. *See* Associations, voluntary
Rowlands, M., 199
Royal compound (*nchwed*), 16, 61–62, 105, 208n. 12; decline of, 175, 177; map of, 64–65
Royal family, 6, 34, 165; decline of, 36–37, 131, 178–79, 194–95
Royal retainers (*che' mfen*), 66
Royal wives, 6, 9–10, 19, 79; declining power of, 20, 178–79; first queen, 17, 21, 22, 26, 177; as queen mothers, 16–17, 63, 66; ranking of, 21–26; social status of, 25, 30–33, 37–38, 39. *See also names of specific royal wives*
Royal women's association (*masou*), 37

Sacred forest (*mâfen*), 62, 153, 160, 213n. 5

Sacred land (*mafam*), 188–89
Sanke (royal wife), 23–24
Sapir, J. D., 181
Sargent, C. F., 165
Seclusion rites, 89, 211nn. 15–16
Secrecy, in fertility treatment, 26, 163, 167
Secret societies (*kum*), 66
Seed and the Soil, The (Delaney), 4–5
Semen, 85, 86
Service de Santé de la France Outre-Mer, 145
Service d'Hygiène Mobile et de Prophylaxie (SHMP), 146, 147–48
Sex and cooking, 71, 84
Sex, extramarital, 80, 82, 87, 94–95. *See also* Adultery; Infidelity
Sexual intercourse, 86, 87, 89, 92
Sexually transmitted disease, 147, 149, 173, 196, 214n. 17; in colonial period, 140, 142, 143; and polygyny, 127, 128
Sexual mores, 116
Shanklin, E., 112
Shaw, R., 36
SHMP. *See* Service d'Hygiène Mobile et de Prophylaxie
Sick role, 35
Sierra Leone, 36
Skull worship, ancestral, 51, 106, 107, 122, 123, 131
Slave trade, 45
Sleeping sickness (trypanosomiasis), 145–46
Social change, 3, 9, 38, 39, 180, 182
Social distance in healing institutions, 156
Social isolation, 34, 35
Socialization of children, 42, 48, 122–23, 191–92
Social relations: and fertility, 5–7, 48, 138–39, 156, 174; and food, 48–49, 198; and health care beliefs, 166–67; and illness, 162; and kingship, 140–41; and marriage, 95–97

Social reproduction, 42, 101, 192; and identity, 193–94; and procreation imagery, 11, 178, 181; royal, 2, 179
Social status, 56, 184, 192; and health care, 156; and reproductive health, 10, 129–34, 181; of royal wives, 25, 30–33, 37–38, 39. *See also* hierarchy
Social structure and demographics, 4
Société des Missions Evangéliques de Paris, 148
Society, ideal, 113, 179, 190
Sorcery, 28, 95, 109, 140, 193
Spirit/breath (*zwiak*), 107, 213n. 6
Spirit medium (*minnyi*), 107–8, 151, 152–53, 213nn. 5, 7
State, 77, 81; power and kingship, 68–69, 187; and social order, 185, 186
Sterility, 117, 127–28
Strangeness, king's, 63, 209n. 23
Strike, general, 47
Strumpell (German colonial official), 45
Supernatural power (*kà*), 108, 132, 185–86, 187, 213n. 8; king's, 8, 63
Support networks, 134; for health care, 125, 130, 167–69, 170, 173–74; therapy management groups, 133, 164–65, 167, 169–70
Surgery, 149, 155

Taiwan, 165
Tanzania, 170, 212n. 4
Tardits, C., 24
Temne society of Sierra Leone, 36
Theft, 7, 117–18, 125, 126, 198
Therapy: and cause of illness, 103; choice, 13, 165–67; as diagnostic tool, 212n. 4; and German colonialism, 140–44; Kongo, 102; management groups, 133, 164–65, 167, 169–70; for reproductive disorders, 29–30, 138, 162–63; and social relations, 138–39
Thijs, Wim, 212n. 4

Tontines. *See* Associations, voluntary
Trading networks, 45
Transportation costs, 171
Treatment, biomedical, 144, 155
Turkey, 4, 180–81

Union des Populations Camerounaise (UPC), 46
Unity, rhetoric of, 194
Urban/rural movement, 18
Uterine group (*pam nto'*), 49–50, 54–56, 97, 207n. 9; and marriage, 73–74; and reproductive illness, 110, 169, 170

Vaccinations, 144, 146, 147
Vampires (*ndum*), 110, 118, 125, 192, 207n. 10; eating of, 109, 124, 197
Vaughan, M., 148
Village, 59–60
Vitality, kingdom's, 178, 179, 182
Vulnerability, women's, 8–9, 101, 190–92, 199

Wage labor, 48, 70, 75, 76, 124, 133
Warnier, J. P., 199
Washing ritual, 156
Water, 91, 166, 211n. 12
Wealth, 110, 184, 196
Wife-beating, 20
Witchcraft, 7, 108–12, 185–86, 213n. 10; accusations of, 59–60, 67; and ancestral wrath, 52; anthropophagic, 109, 124, 126, 197, 207n. 10; control of, 191; and illness, 102, 103, 105; and infertility, 9, 99–100, 199; jealousy and, 79, 95, 192–93; and land disputes, 134; and polygyny, 32; and social relations, 12, 132; sorcery, 28, 95, 109, 140, 193; vulnerability to, 46
Witches' association (*famla'*), 109, 113, 185, 186, 214nn. 11–12
Wolff, N. H., 108
Woman in the Body, The (Martin), 4
Women: and adultery, 80–81, 94–95;

education of, 77, 130, 211n. 15; Egyptian, 138, 170, 181; and emotional stress, 80, 111, 129; fears of, 12–13, 131; fertility of, 3, 7, 14, 128–29, 182; food production by, 45, 75–76, 81, 83, 134; gender image of, 78–80; health of, 102, 144; ideal, 95; identity of, 97; information for, 59–60, 78–79; and labor migration, 46, 133; labor of, 75–76, 128–29, 190; menopausal, 83; metaphors in lives of, 181–82, 199–200; occult power of, 36, 109, 185; poverty of, 6–7, 124–25, 181, 197; roles of, 85, 179–80; status of, 38–39, 129–34, 184; support networks for, 81–82, 167–69; therapeutic choices of, 164–65; view of men by, 82; voices of, 193, 200; vulnerability of, 8–9, 101, 190–92, 199. *See also* Motherhood; Royal wives; Uterine group (*pam nto'*)

World Fertility Survey (1978), 120, 195, 203n. 2

Youth association (*manjo*), 60, 205n. 2

Zande witchcraft, 52
Ziemann, H., 140

DATE DUE